# Rapid Review of ECG

Tapas Kumar Koley

# Rapid Review of ECG

## Self-Assessment Questions, Case Studies and Clinical Correlation

Springer

Tapas Kumar Koley
Department of Medicine
Kasturba Hospital
Darya Ganj, Delhi, India

ISBN 978-981-99-9115-0 ISBN 978-981-99-9116-7 (eBook)
https://doi.org/10.1007/978-981-99-9116-7



This Springer imprint is published by the registered company Springer Nature Singapore Pte Ltd.
The registered company address is: 152 Beach Road, #21-01/04 Gateway East, Singapore 189721, Singapore

# Preface

Welcome to the exciting world of electrocardiography (ECG), an invaluable tool in the realm of cardiovascular medicine. ECG plays a vital role in patient care. This book has been meticulously crafted to provide you with a comprehensive understanding of ECG interpretation, while also offering opportunities for self-assessment, practical case studies, and meaningful clinical correlations.

In the fast-paced environment of healthcare, the ability to swiftly interpret an ECG is a skill that can make a significant difference in patient outcomes. As healthcare professionals, we are constantly faced with the challenge of identifying and diagnosing cardiac abnormalities in a timely manner. This book aims to equip you with the knowledge and confidence needed to interpret ECGs rapidly and effectively.

To facilitate your learning, the book has been divided into seven parts. There are a total of twenty nine chapters, and we have included self-assessment questions throughout the book. These questions serve as checkpoints, allowing you to gauge your understanding of the material covered and reinforce key concepts. The answers and explanations provided will help solidify your knowledge and address any areas that may require further attention.

In addition to self-assessment questions, this book offers a range of case studies that present real-life scenarios encountered in clinical practice. Each case study provides an ECG, accompanied by relevant clinical information. By analyzing these cases, you will have the opportunity to apply your knowledge to practical situations, honing your skills in interpreting ECGs in a clinical context. The comprehensive explanations and discussions following each case will further enhance your understanding and highlight the importance of ECG interpretation in patient care.

Understanding the clinical relevance of ECG findings is crucial for accurate diagnosis and management. Therefore, throughout this book, we emphasize the correlation between ECG findings and various cardiac conditions. By exploring the connections between ECG abnormalities and underlying pathophysiology, you will develop a holistic approach to interpreting ECGs and appreciate the clinical significance of each finding.

We recognize that mastering ECG interpretation is not a solitary pursuit but rather an ongoing process. As you progress through this book, we encourage you to engage in active learning, seeking opportunities to practice your skills and seek guidance from experienced clinicians. Remember, proficiency in ECG interpretation comes with practice and exposure to diverse clinical scenarios.

We hope that this book serves as a valuable resource in your journey to becoming a proficient ECG interpreter. Our aim is to provide you with the knowledge, self-assessment tools, case studies, and clinical correlations necessary to enhance your expertise in this essential skill. We wish you success in your endeavours and hope that the knowledge gained from this book translates into improved patient care.

New Delhi, India Tapas Kumar Koley

# Acknowledgments

Writing this ECG book has been a challenging yet rewarding journey, and I am profoundly grateful to all those who have contributed their time, expertise, and support to make this project a reality. Without their dedication and encouragement, this endeavour would not have been possible.

Thank you to the esteemed professors and experts in cardiology for sharing their knowledge, to my colleagues and collaborators for their support, and to the patients and participants for their valuable contributions. Special thanks to the reviewers, editors, and publishing team for their efforts. I am also thankful to my family, friends, and all the readers for their encouragement. Your support has been instrumental in making this book possible and advancing the understanding of electrocardiography.

To everyone who has been part of this project in one way or another, I offer my sincerest thanks. Your contributions have shaped this book and will undoubtedly impact the understanding and practice of ECG interpretation for years to come.

With utmost appreciation,

Tapas Kumar Koley

# Contents

# About the Author

**Tapas Kumar Koley, MBBS, MD Medicine** graduated from Burdwan Medical College and completed his postgraduation at the Postgraduate Institute of Medical Sciences, Rohtak, India. He has several articles and international book publications and has delivered numerous presentations at conferences and CMEs. He has been an ECG tutor for All About Staffing, an affiliate of Hospital Corporation of America. He is the resource person for the National Institute of Health and Family Welfare, India, to train doctors on medical negligence. He is working as Senior Specialist Physician at Kasturba Hospital, Delhi.

# Abbreviations

| | |
|---|---|
| APC | Atrial premature complex |
| ASD | Atrial septal defect |
| AV | Atrioventricular |
| BBB | Bundle branch block |
| BPM | Beats per minute |
| CAH | Combined atrial hypertrophy |
| CVH | Combined ventricular hypertrophy |
| ECG | Electrocardiograph (UK) |
| EKG | Electrokardiograph (USA) |
| LA | Left atrium |
| LAD | Left axis deviation |
| LAH | Left atrial hypertrophy |
| LBBB | Left bundle branch block |
| LGL | Lown Ganong-Levine |
| LV | Left ventricle |
| LVH | Left ventricular hypertrophy |
| PAT | Paroxysmal atrial tachycardia |
| PCI | Percutaneous coronary intervention |
| PDA | Patent ductus arteriosus |
| PSVT | Paroxysmal supraventricular tachycardia |
| Q-Tc | Corrected Q-T interval |
| RA | Right atrium |
| RAD | Right axis deviation |
| RAH | Right atrial hypertrophy |
| RBBB | Right bundle branch block |
| RV | Right ventricle |
| RVH | Right ventricular hypertrophy |
| SA | Sinoatrial |
| SSS | Sick sinus syndrome |

| | |
|---|---|
| SVT | Supraventricular tachycardia |
| VF | Ventricular fibrillation |
| VSD | Ventricular septal defect |
| VT | Ventricular tachycardia |
| WPW | Wolff-Parkinson-White |

# Part I
# Basic Principles

# Chapter 1
# Cardiac Electrophysiology

**Learning Objectives**

After studying this chapter, the reader will learn about:

- Historical perspective
- Electrophysiology
- Origin of intracellular potential
- Action potential
- Generation of ECG
- Conduction of electrical impulse

Electrocardiogram (abbreviated as ECG or EKG in some countries) is the graphical recording of the change in potentials of the electrical field produced by the heart. The word ECG is derived from the German language. In German, it is elektro-kardiographie. As English is more dominant in today's world, the acronym ECG is more widely used today. It is recorded by means of metal electrodes connected by cables to an ECG machine. The recorded electrical activity is depicted as a series of graph-like tracings, or waves in a paper or digitally displayed in a screen. The shapes and frequencies of these tracings reveal cardiac abnormalities.

Today ECG is one of the most important tools to study the cardiac anatomy and physiology. It helps in diagnosis of various cardiac abnormalities including myocardial infarction and ischaemia, cardiac arrhythmias, conduction defects, myocardial hypertrophy and congenital heart diseases. The fact that ECG is only a laboratory test should always be borne in mind. Normal ECG may be observed in patients with heart disease and normal healthy persons may have a nonspecific change in ECG.

## Tips and Tricks of ECG

- The ECG should be read and analysed only after examination of the patient and should be interpreted based on the clinical findings.


T. K. Koley, *Rapid Review of ECG*,
https://doi.org/10.1007/978-981-99-9116-7_1

## 1.1 Historical Perspective

In May 1887, Augustus D Waller published the first single lead ECG with a capillary electrometer. He, however, failed to realize the clinical importance and significance of his discovery. Willem Einthoven, considered the father of electrocardiography, worked in The Netherlands for years, first with an electrometer and later with a string galvanometer to generate clinically relevant ECG in the early 1900s. He coined the term *elektrokardiogramm* in German and subsequently labelled the waveforms as P, Q, R, S, T and U. He described numerous abnormalities in this field and created the bipolar lead system.

The early years of studies in ECG were dominated by Einthoven and Sir Thomas Lewis, who are credited with bringing the ECG from the laboratory to the bedside of the patient. After several years of such efforts, the ECG gained importance in clinical practice and was accepted as a useful tool in cardiac evaluation. In 1924, Einthoven was awarded the Nobel Prize for his invaluable contribution to the field. Initially, the ECG machines were huge and required the help of several persons to operate them. Subsequent developments over several decades have resulted in the current computerized versions of the ECG machine. More than a century has elapsed after the first recording of ECG, yet the standard 12-lead ECG is still an essential part of complete cardiac evaluation.

## 1.2 Electrophysiology

The human heart lies behind the sternum in the mediastinal cavity (Fig. 1.1). Together with the blood vessels and blood, it constitutes the body's circulatory system. The top of the heart known as the base is located at the level of the second

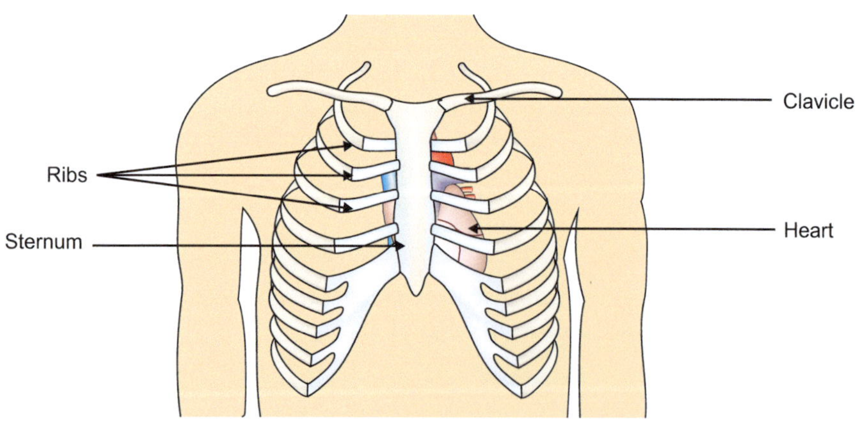


**Fig. 1.1** Position of human heart in the mediastinal cavity

intercostal space, while the bottom of the heart, called the apex, is tilted to the left side of the body and rests on the diaphragm. It is well protected inside the rib cage. The heart is made up of four chambers: right atrium, left atrium, right ventricle and left ventricle. Interatrial septum separates the two atria and the two ventricles are separated by interventricular septum (Fig. 1.2). From electrophysiological angle, the heart is made up of only two chambers. The two atria form one chamber and the other chamber is formed by the two ventricles. The two atria may be considered as a single electrophysiological unit because they are activated by a single process of activation; similarly, the two ventricles may also be considered a single electrophysiological unit, as they are also activated by a single activation process. Electrophysiologically, the left ventricle together with the interventricular septum is the most important structure. The thickness of left ventricle is almost thrice that of the right ventricle, which makes the right ventricle less significant haemodynamically, electrophysiologically and electrocardiologically.

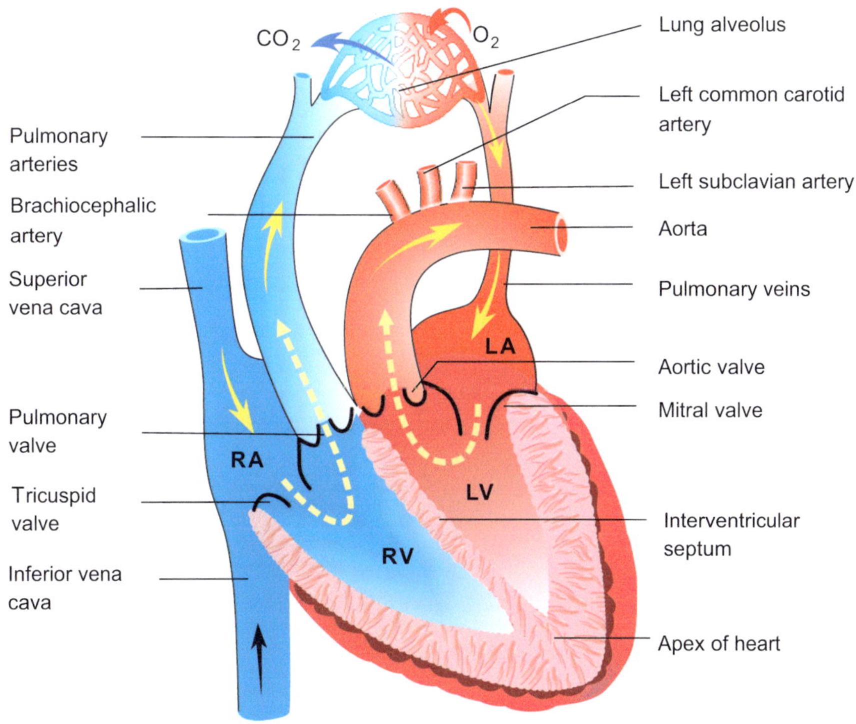


**Fig. 1.2** Anatomy of human heart

### *1.2.1 Generation of Intracellular Potential*

To understand the origin and conduction of electrical impulse, it is important to know the four primary properties of cardiac myocytes. These are:

- Automaticity: It is the ability of the cells to generate electrical impulse spontaneously. This property is specific for pacemaker cells, for example, cells of SA node.
- Excitability: It is the ability of cardiac myocytes to respond to an electric impulse, which results from shifting of ions across the cell membrane.
- Conductivity: It is the ability of cardiac myocytes to receive and further transmit electric impulse to other cells.
- Contractility: It is the ability to shorten and cause muscle contraction.

Out of these four properties, only contractility is the mechanical function of the heart, and the other three are electrical functions of the heart.

#### 1.2.1.1 Sodium Potassium Pump

Sodium potassium pump (Fig. 1.3) maintains a potential difference of −90 mV across the cardiac cell membrane. This is known as resting membrane potential and the main factor responsible for this is the gradient of potassium ions ($K^+$) across the cell membrane. The extracellular $K^+$ ion concentration is about 5 mEq/L, and the

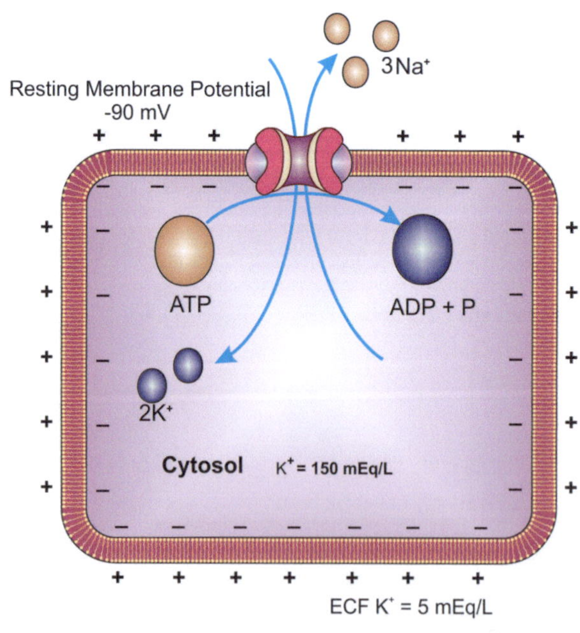


**Fig. 1.3** Sodium potassium pump

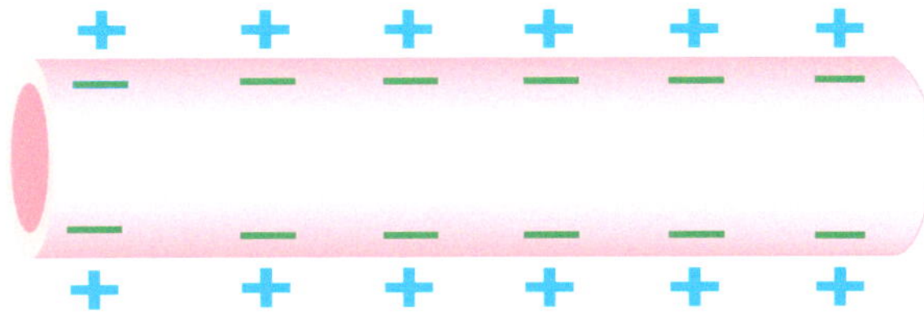


**Fig. 1.4** Myocardial cell (cardiac myocyte). At resting state, the inside of cell is negatively charged and the outside is positively charged

intracellular concentration is 150 mEq/L. This 30:1 $K^+$ gradient is responsible for generation of resting membrane potential. Due to concentration gradient across the cardiac cell membrane and high permeability of potassium ions, outward diffusion of the positively charged potassium creates a negative electrical potential inside the cell relative to the outside. Thus, the outside of the cell is positively charged and the inside is negatively charged (Fig. 1.4). The distribution of sodium ions ($Na^+$) is exactly opposite of $K^+$ ions. Sodium and calcium ions contribute very less to resting membrane potential as the resting cardiac cell membrane permeability for these ions is very low.

#### 1.2.1.2 Action Potential

The electrical activity of the heart depends upon the generation of action potential by the cardiac cell due to an electrical stimulus. Action potential refers to changes in membrane potential over time (Fig. 1.5). It has five phases: phase 0, 1, 2, 3 and 4. The phase 0 starts at the onset of depolarization of a cardiac myocyte (Fig. 1.6) and during this phase there is an abrupt increase in the permeability of the sodium ions. They enter into the cell (calcium ions also enter to a lesser degree) and cause a sharp rise in the potential to positivity (about +20 mV). As a result, the inside of the cell becomes positive and the outside of the cell negative. This is called the depolarization of the cell.

After depolarization, there is a gradual return to resting membrane potential. In phase 1, there is a rapid return of potential to about 0 mV. This is due to a sudden stoppage of sodium channels. In phase 2, there is a plateau. This is due to slow entry of calcium ions into the cell. In phase 3, there is a slow return to resting membrane potential. This is due to extrusion of potassium ions from the cell. As a result again the inside of the cell becomes negative and the outside becomes positive. The cell gradually returns to −90 mV (phase 4). The aim of repolarization is to bring back the cell to the resting state so that depolarization can occur again. The movement of ions is facilitated by sodium-potassium pump.

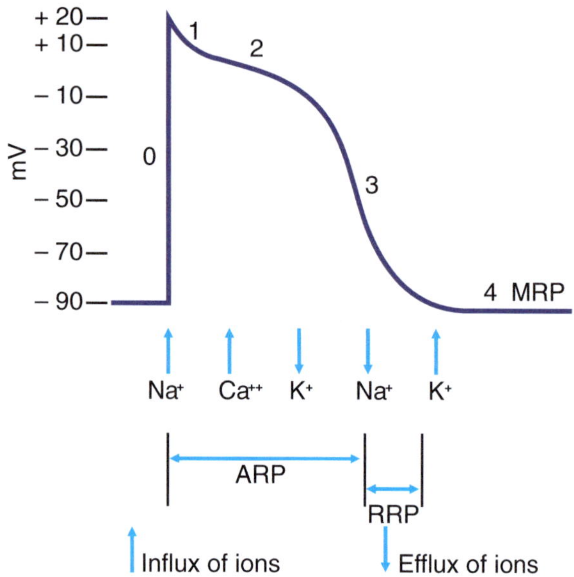


**Fig. 1.5** Action potential. *MRP* membrane resting potential, *0* depolarization, *1, 2, 3* phases of repolarization, *ARP* absolute refractory period, *RRP* relative refractory period

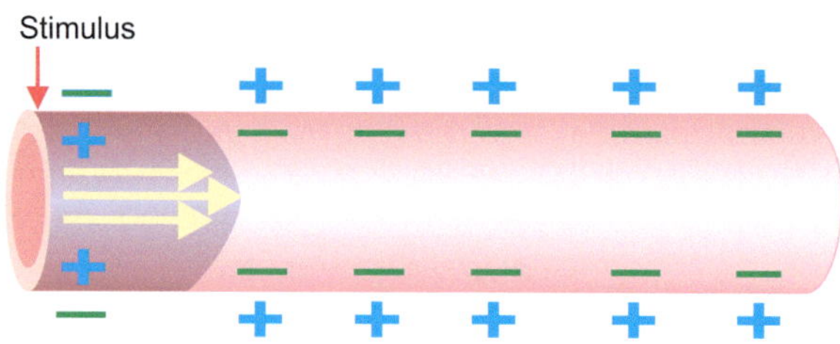


**Fig. 1.6** Depolarization of cardiac myocyte after stimulus

#### 1.2.1.3 Refractoriness of Myocardium

During the phases 0, 1, 2 and 3 of the action potential no stimulus however strong will propagate another action potential. This is known as absolute refractory period. After this there is a period during which a strong stimulus can produce a response. This is the relative refractory period. After this there is a period of supernormal excitability during which a weaker stimulus can evoke a response. This coincides with the terminal part of phase 3 and beginning of phase 4.

**Tips and Tricks**

- Depolarization and repolarization are electrical events and they are not same as systole and diastole.

- Depolarization just precedes systole and repolarization just precedes diastole.

#### 1.2.1.4 Difference of Sinoatrial (SA) Node from Other Parts of Myocardium

The action potential of SA node is different from other parts of the myocardium. The pacemaker cells of SA node do not require an electrical stimulus to generate action potential, unlike other cardiac myocytes. The specialized function associated with the pacemaker cells is their spontaneous depolarization with no true resting potential. When spontaneous depolarization reaches the threshold voltage, it triggers a rapid depolarization followed by repolarization.

1. The resting membrane potential is low, about −60 to −70 mV.
2. A prepotential is present in phase 4. There is a gradual rise in resting membrane potential that is responsible for the automaticity of SA node.
3. Depolarization is slower.
4. The peak of action potential is rounded and repolarization is a slow curve, where the phases 1, 2 and 3 cannot be defined separately.

### *1.2.2 Generation of ECG*

The basic principle behind recording an ECG is an electromagnetic force, current or vector with both magnitude and direction. A moving wavefront of depolarization is produced (Fig. 1.7) when depolarization is transmitted to the adjoining cardiac myocytes. This generates electric current which is amplified and recorded as ECG.

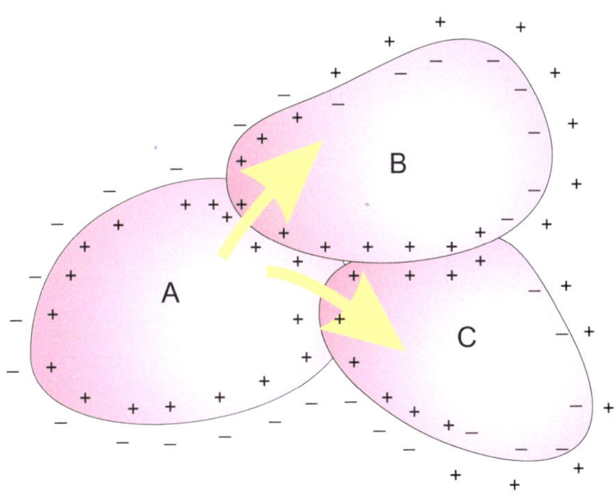


**Fig. 1.7** Depolarization wavefront moving from one cardiac myocyte to adjacent cardiac myocytes

Depolarization and repolarization occur in atrial as well as in ventricular muscles and the whole process is so well synchronized that the atria and ventricles contract and relax in a rhythmic way. However, depolarization and repolarization are electrical events and they are not equal to systole and diastole.

ECG actually records these two electrical events, depolarization and repolarization, while the impulse is traveling through the conducting system of heart. The summation of potential of phase 0 of both the atria results in P wave of ECG, i.e. P wave is produced by depolarization of both the atria. Similarly, all phase 0 potentials of both the ventricles produce the QRS complex; i.e. QRS complex represents depolarization of both the ventricles. S-T segment and T wave are produced by summation of potentials of phase 1, 2 and 3 of both the ventricles. Thus, S-T segment and T wave represent repolarization of both the ventricles. However, the routinely recorded 12-lead ECG fails to record any electrical activity while the impulse is traveling through the AV node and the bundle of His.

An electrode facing the wave of depolarization records a positive or an upright deflection while an electrode from which the wave of depolarization is moving away records a negative or downward deflection (Fig. 1.8). A partly positive and a partly negative (biphasic/equiphasic) deflection is recorded when an impulse moves perpendicularly to an electrode. Similarly, a current of repolarization traveling away from the positive electrode is seen as a positive deflection and towards a positive electrode as a negative deflection. A large positive wave will be observed over the larger muscle mass and a large negative deflection will be observed over the smaller muscle mass when two muscle masses of markedly different sizes are stimulated at the centre (Fig. 1.9).

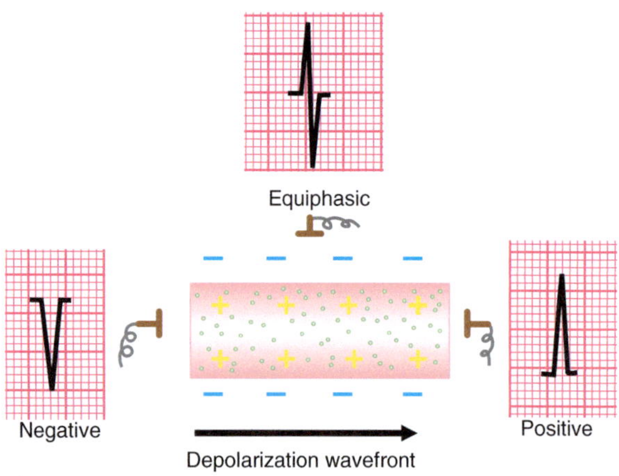


**Fig. 1.8** Fundamental principle of generation of negative, positive and equiphasic deflections

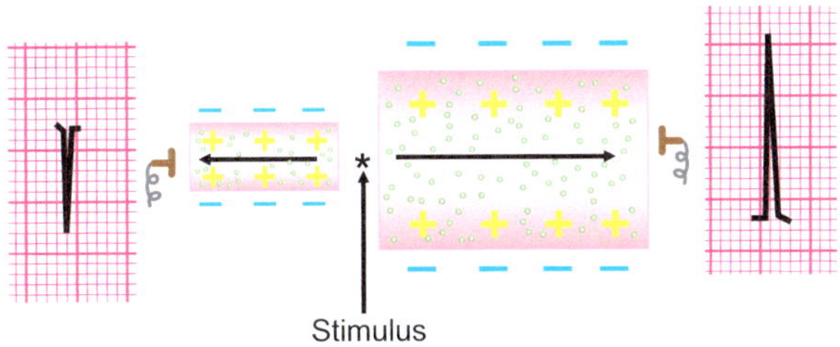


**Fig. 1.9** Generation of waves in two muscle strips of markedly different sizes

**Tips and Tricks**

- Strong electric activity leads to tall or large waveforms.
- Weak electric activity leads to small waveform.
- No electric activity leads to straight line.

### *1.2.3 Conduction of Electrical Impulse*

The electrical conduction system of the heart is the most important aspect of cardiac anatomy and physiology to master while learning the art of interpretation of ECG. To understand the conduction system of the heart, two types of cardiac tissue must be considered:

- Ordinary myocardium/cardiomyocytes (atrial and ventricular).
- Specialized cardiac conduction system, which includes sinoatrial (SA) or sinus node; anterior, middle and posterior internodal tracts; atrioventricular (AV) node; Bundle of His; right and left bundle branches; anterior and posterior divisions of the left bundle and the Purkinje fibre network.

The heart is a mechanical pump whose activity is governed by the electrical conduction system. The specialized conduction system is composed of myocardial tissue, whose primary function is to conduct electrical impulse rather than to contract. Both types of cardiac tissue can allow conduction of electrical impulses; but, cells in the specialized cardiac conduction system also depolarise spontaneously and act as cardiac pacemakers. However, there is a hierarchy of automaticity within the tissue of the heart. The tissue that possesses the greatest degree of automaticity (has the fastest rate of spontaneous depolarization) functions as the dominant pacemaker; it generates a spontaneous action potential that is conducted along the rest of the conduction system, activating the myocardium in a uniform fashion. The electrical impulse in heart is generated in the SA node (Fig. 1.10) located in upper part of right atrium near the opening of superior vena cava. It has the fastest rate of generation of electrical impulse as compared to any other part of the heart, and thus, acts as the main pacemaker of the heart.

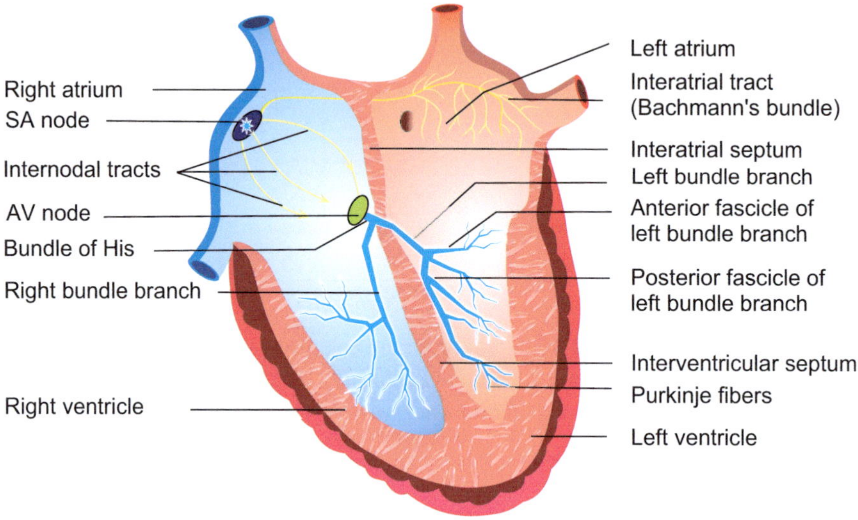


**Fig. 1.10** Conducting system of heart

The right atrium is the first part of the heart to be activated. The impulse travels longitudinally, and by contiguity through three intratrial pathways to the other parts of the right atrium. These intratrial pathways are also called internodal pathways because they conduct the impulse from SA node to the AV node. As the impulse travels from the SA node along the internodal tracts, the right atrium contracts and propels blood into the right ventricle. The impulse also travels to the left atrium by interatrial tract (Bachmann's bundle) resulting in contraction of left atrium. Contraction of left atrium propels blood into the left ventricle.

AV node is situated at the lower part of the right atrium on the interatrial septum. In AV node, the impulse is delayed which gives atria the time to contract, and empty into their respective ventricles, before the ventricles are activated for contraction. This AV nodal delay is the major contributor of P-R interval.

From AV node, the impulse passes on to the Bundle of His, which starts at the AV node and then divides into two parts, the left and right bundle branch. The left bundle branch is further divided into one anterior and one posterior fascicle. The anterior fascicle spreads over to the anterior and superior surface of the left ventricle, and the posterior fascicle spreads over the posterior and inferior surface of the left ventricle. These bundles further divide into their terminal ramifications the Purkinje fibres (Fig. 1.11). A small septal fascicle originates from the left bundle and activates the interventricular septum from left to right, and this is the first part of the ventricle to be activated. Next, the impulse passes on to the other parts of the fascicles and to Purkinje fibres. The right bundle branch does not divide and innervates the right ventricle. The Purkinje fibres conduct the electrical impulse to the ventricles which are then activated. The myocardium is activated from endocardium to epicardium.

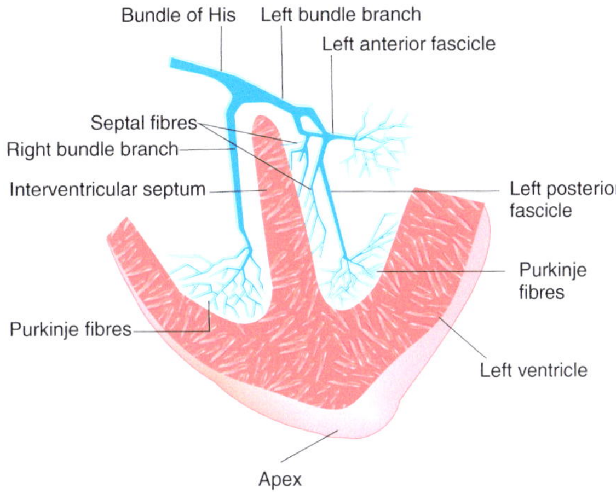


**Fig. 1.11** Diagram showing the Bundle of His, the bundle branches, the fascicles and the Purkinje fibres

#### 1.2.3.1 Velocity of Conduction

The velocity of conduction of action potential varies in the various parts of the heart. The velocity is maximum in the Purkinje fibres, and it is the minimum in the middle of AV node.

The average conduction velocity are:

- SA node: 0.05 m/s
- Atrial myocardium: 0.8–1 m/s
- AV node: 0.05 m/s
- Bundle of His: 0.8–1 m/s
- Purkinje fibres: 4 m/s
- Ventricular myocardium: 0.9–1 m/s.

**Self-Assessment Questions**

1. Willem Einthoven was awarded the Nobel Prize for his contribution in the field of ECG. True or false?
2. The resting membrane potential of cardiac myocyte is +90 mV. True or false?
3. Sodium ion enters the cell during phase 0 of action potential. True or false?
4. Right bundle divides into anterior and posterior fascicle. True or false?
5. The cardiac impulse is delayed at AV node. True or false?
6. **Which of the following pairs are correct?**

   a. P wave: Atrial depolarization
   b. QRS complex: Ventricular depolarization
   c. T wave: Ventricular repolarization
   d. All of the above

7. **Which of the following is the property of a cardiac cell to initiate and fire an action potential on its own without external stimulation?**
    a. Excitability
    b. Automaticity
    c. Contractility
    d. Conductance

8. **In which of the following depolarization is slow?**
    a. Atrial muscle
    b. AV node
    c. Ventricular muscle
    d. SA node

9. **Which of the following is usually the dominant pacemaker of the heart?**
    a. SA node
    b. AV node
    c. Bundle of His
    d. Purkinje fibres

10. **Which of the following is NOT a part of the specialized conduction system of the heart?**
    a. SA node
    b. Myocytes of mitral valve
    c. Bundle of His
    d. AV node

11. **The space in the middle of the thoracic cavity where the heart lies is the:**
    a. Pericardial cavity
    b. Pericardium
    c. Pleural cavity
    d. Mediastinum

12. **The velocity of conduction is maximum in:**
    a. SA node
    b. AV node
    c. Purkinje fibres
    d. Atrial myocardium

13. **During phase 0 of action potential, there is an abrupt increase in permeability of:**
    a. Sodium ion
    b. Potassium ion
    c. Calcium ion
    d. Magnesium ion

14. **The first part of heart to be activated is:**
    a. Left atrium
    b. Right atrium
    c. Left ventricle
    d. Right ventricle
15. **Resting membrane potential is due to gradient of:**
    a. Sodium ion
    b. Calcium ion
    c. Potassium ion
    d. Magnesium ion
16. Label the four chambers and the conducting system of heart in the given diagram. Trace the spread of impulse from atria to the ventricles (Fig. 1.12).
17. Label the five phases of action potential in the given diagram (Fig. 1.13). What are the movements of the ions during these phases of action potential?
18. Identify and label the depolarized and repolarized cardiac cell (Fig. 1.14).

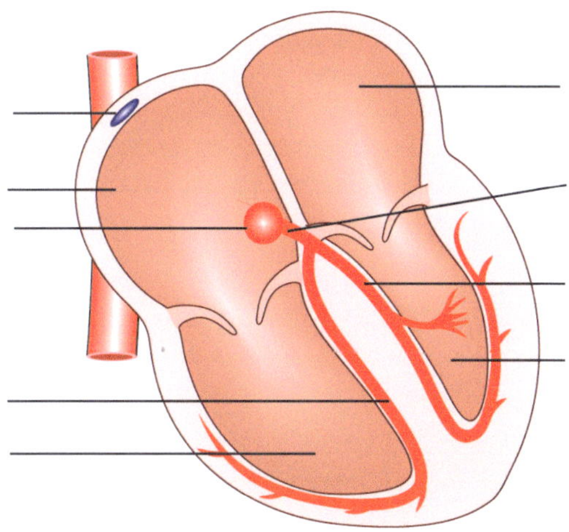

**Fig. 1.12** Label the diagram and trace the spread of impulse

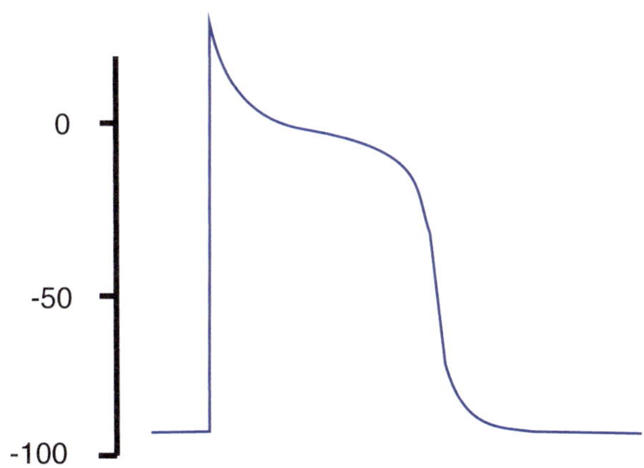


**Fig. 1.13** Label the five phases of action potential

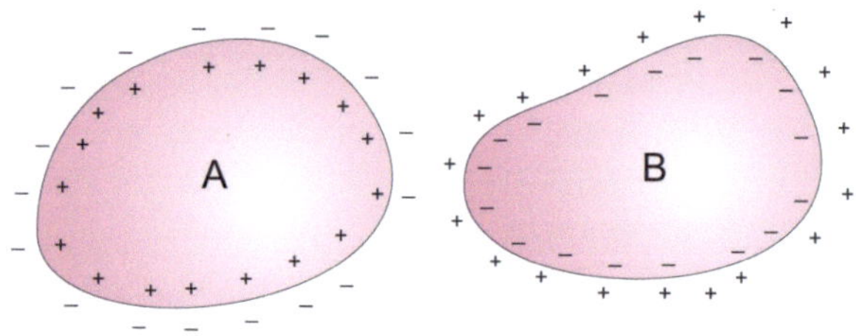


**Fig. 1.14** Identify the cardiac cells

## Answers

1. True 2. False 3. True 4. False 5. True 6. d 7. b 8. d 9. a 10. b 11. d 12. c 13. a 14. b 15. c.
16. The four chambers of the heart are right and left atrium and right and left ventricles (Fig. 1.15). The impulse originates at the SA node and travels via the conducting system, and its pathway is shown by yellow arrows in Fig. 1.15.
17. The five phases of action potential are labelled in Fig. 1.16. The movement of ions during the five phases are as follows:

| | |
|---|---|
| Phase 0 | Sodium ions move inside the cardiac cell |
| Phase 1 | Stoppage of inward sodium movement, potassium starts moving out of the cardiac cell |
| Phase 2 | Slow entry of calcium ions inside the cell |
| Phase 3 | Rapid extrusion of potassium ions from the cardiac cell |
| Phase 4 | Sodium ions are moved out and potassium ions are moved inside the cardiac cell |

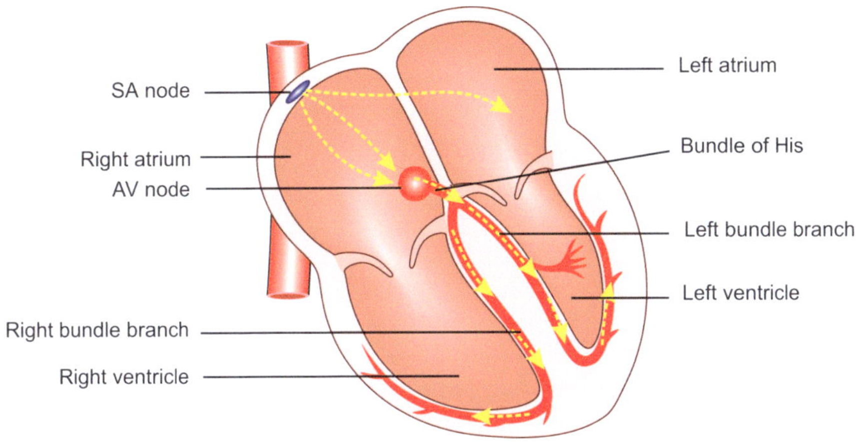


**Fig. 1.15** The four chambers of the heart and the conducting system. The origin and conduction of impulse via the conducting system is shown by yellow arrows

**Fig. 1.16** Five phases of action potential are labelled in the diagram

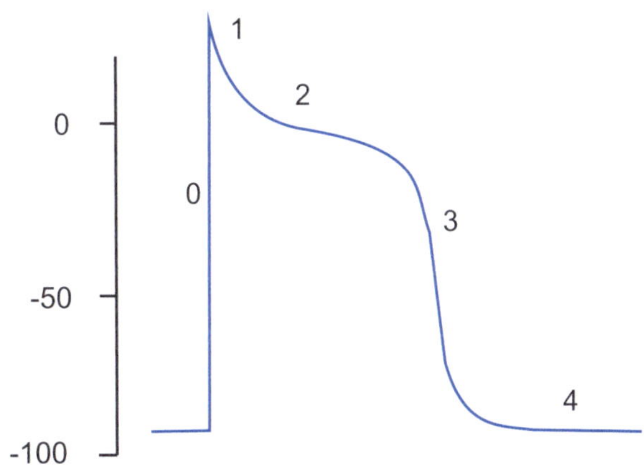


18. The cell A is depolarized and cell B is repolarized. Note the distribution of the positive and negative charges inside and outside the cells.

# Chapter 2
# ECG Paper and Leads

**Learning Objectives**
After studying this chapter, the reader will learn about:

- ECG paper
- Basic ECG conventions
- ECG leads
- Einthoven's equation
- Orientation of ECG leads

The ECG paper is made up of a grid in which the lines are separated by 1 mm in both horizontal and vertical direction. A heavier or dark line is present after every fifth line in both the directions. Each small square is 1 mm square and the large square is 5 mm square. The horizontal axis represents the time at 25 mm/s paper speed. 1 mm represents 0.04 s and 5 mm represent 0.2 s. The vertical axis represents the amplitude. At normal standardisation of 10 mm = 1 mV, each millimetre represents 0.1 mV (Fig. 2.1). The ECG conventions are enumerated in Box 2.1.

**Box 2.1 Basic ECG Conventions**

| | |
|---|---|
| Speed of paper | 25 mm/s |
| Each small square | 0.04 s in horizontal axis |
| Standardization | 10 mm = 1 mV |
| Each small square | 0.1 mV in vertical axis |



T. K. Koley, *Rapid Review of ECG*,
https://doi.org/10.1007/978-981-99-9116-7_2

**Fig. 2.1** Enlarged view of ECG paper showing time and voltage

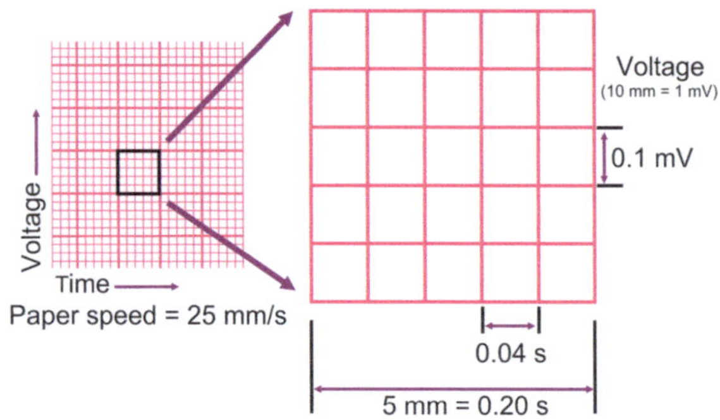


**Tips and Tricks**

- To calculate any interval or duration of ECG deflection, one has to multiply the number of small squares it occupies in horizontal axis with 0.04 s.
- To calculate the amplitude of an ECG deflection, the number of small squares along vertical axis, a positive wave or a negative wave occupies, is multiplied by 0.1 mV.

## 2.1 ECG Leads

The ECG leads consist of a pair of electrodes with a positive and negative terminal, across which the electrical potential is measured. Electrodes are positioned at predetermined locations on the body surface in accordance with guidelines to capture the electrical signal generated by heart. A lead captures the electrical activity of the heart from a specific direction only. A 12-lead ECG is created when these electrodes are electrically configured in such a way that the electrical activity of the heart may be seen and recorded from different angles. In modern ECG machines, these 12 leads are simultaneously recorded, allowing for the observation of the same electrical event in time from 12 different angles. Twelve conventional leads divided into frontal plane and horizontal plane leads are used to record ECG.

- Frontal plane leads: Standard leads I, II, III and lead aVR, aVL and aVF
- Horizontal plane leads: Precordial leads V1–V6

### 2.1.1 *Frontal Plane Leads*

#### 2.1.1.1 Standard Leads

In standard leads, the electrodes are placed at each of the extremities—the right arm, the left arm and the left leg (Fig. 2.2). The right leg electrode acts as earth or neutral electrode. No matter where the electrode is placed on the extremity, the electrical potential recorded from one extremity will be the same. If the limbs are

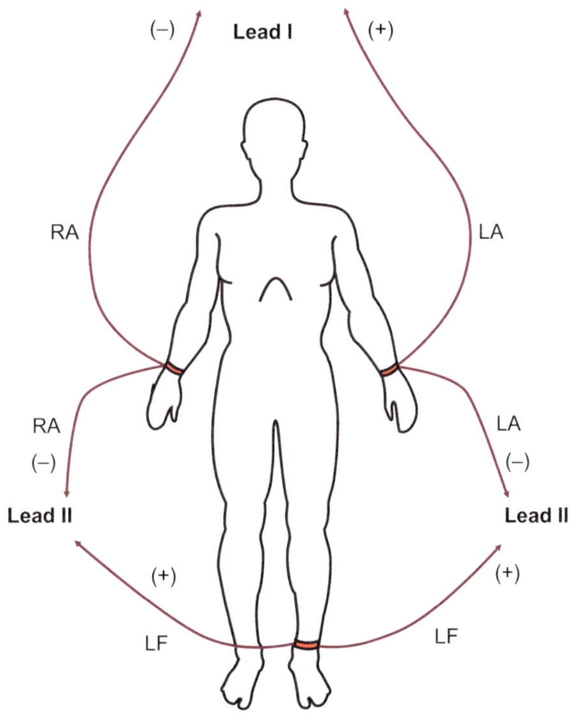


**Fig. 2.2** Diagram showing standard leads

amputated, then the electrodes are placed on the amputated stumps. Electrodes should be used on the proximal end of the limbs in patients with tremor or shivering.

The electrical signals of the heart are recorded by the two electrodes of a lead and it is recorded on ECG paper or displayed digitally. There are three standard leads.

1. Standard lead I: This lead is produced by placing the positive electrode on left arm and the negative electrode on the right arm.
2. Standard lead II: This lead is produced by placing the positive electrode on the left foot and the negative electrode on the right arm.
3. Standard lead III: This lead is produced by placing the positive electrode on left foot and negative electrode on the left arm.

**Tips and Tricks**

- To be noted that left foot is always positive and right arm is always negative as far as the placement of electrodes is concerned.
- Standard lead II is commonly used for cardiac monitoring as positioning of electrodes most commonly resembles the pathway of current flow during normal atrial and ventricular depolarization. It shows P wave most clearly as compared to other leads.
- Often only standard lead II is recorded to identify the rhythm. It is called rhythm strip. The rhythm strip should be strictly used to identify the rhythm only.

The axis of the lead is an imaginary line connecting the positively and negatively charged electrodes in a lead. The three lead axes of these three leads form an equilateral triangle with the heart at centre known as Einthoven's triangle (Fig. 2.3).

### Einthoven's Equation

The relation between the three leads is algebraically expressed by the Einthoven's equation. According to Kirchhoff's law, the sum of all currents in a closed circuit is equal to zero. Hence, if the polarity of lead two is reversed, then lead I, II and III will form a closed circuit and the potential difference will be zero. Since Einthoven has made a change in the polarity of lead II, the Einthoven's equation becomes $I - II + III = 0$. Thus, $II = I + III$.

**Tips and Tricks**

- The practical use of this equation is that the voltage of a waveform (e.g., the R wave) in lead I plus the same waveform in lead III is equal to voltage of the same waveform in lead II.

The limb leads are usually labelled and also colour coded. Lead colour coding and labelling are standardized among manufacturers. Commonly two types of colour codes are used for limb leads. In Europe, the IEC (International Electrochemical Commission) system uses the following colour code: red — right arm (RA), yellow — left arm (LA), green — left leg (LL), black — right leg (RL). In USA, the AHA (American Heart Association) system uses the following colour code: white — right arm, black — left arm, green — right leg, red — left leg. These two types of colour coding often cause confusion in countries like India, where both the colour codes are used. Hence, while recording ECG, first check the colour codes of the leads very carefully. The colour coding of these electrodes is mentioned in Box 2.2.

**Box 2.2 Colour Coding of Limb Leads**

| Colour | IEC (Europe) | USA (AHA) |
|---|---|---|
| Red | Right arm | Left leg |
| Yellow | Left arm | – |
| Green | Left leg | Right leg |
| Black | Right leg | Left arm |
| White | – | Right arm |

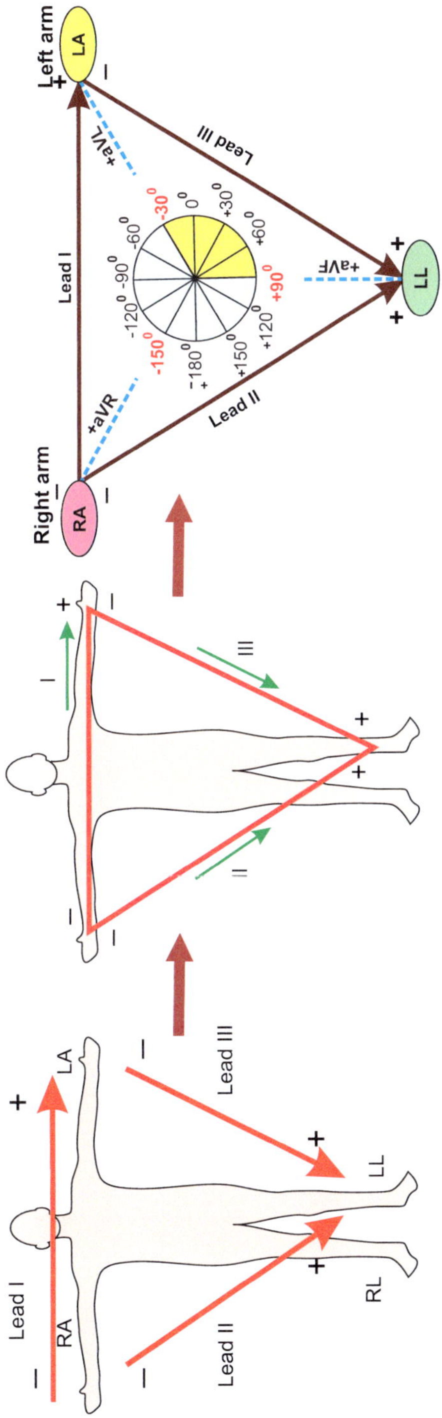


**Fig. 2.3** Diagrammatic representation of three lead axes and Einthoven's triangle

**Tips and Tricks**

- Mnemonics to memorize IEC coding system: '*Ride Your Green Bike*' — Starting from the red (*Ride*) electrode on the right arm, then move around patient's torso clockwise, yellow (*Your*), green (*Green*) and black (*Bike*).
- Mnemonics while using AHA's system:
  - White on right
  - Smoke over fire (black lead above the red lead)
  - Snow over grass (white lead above the green lead)

#### 2.1.1.2 Unipolar Augmented Limb Leads

Einthoven's law states that the sum of the potentials of the three lead axes is equal to zero. The central terminal (indifferent electrode) is created by connecting these three leads. The potential of this terminal is zero. The potential at any point in time relative to the indifferent electrode shall be recorded by an exploring electrode attached to a second pole of galvanometer. Disconnecting the indifferent electrode from a limb which has been examined increases voltage at the exploratory electrode. The 'a' stands for augmentation, i.e. the voltage is augmented by 50%. The three augmented leads were introduced by Goldberger and are also known as Goldberger leads.

The three augmented leads are leads aVR, aVL and aVF.

Lead aVR: This is the augmented unipolar right arm lead. The electrode on the right arm is positive, while the electrode on the left arm and left leg determines the neutral reference point (Fig. 2.4). The lead is oriented to the cavity of the heart or the right atrium All the complexes are negative in this lead because majority of the current goes away from the positive electrode of this lead.

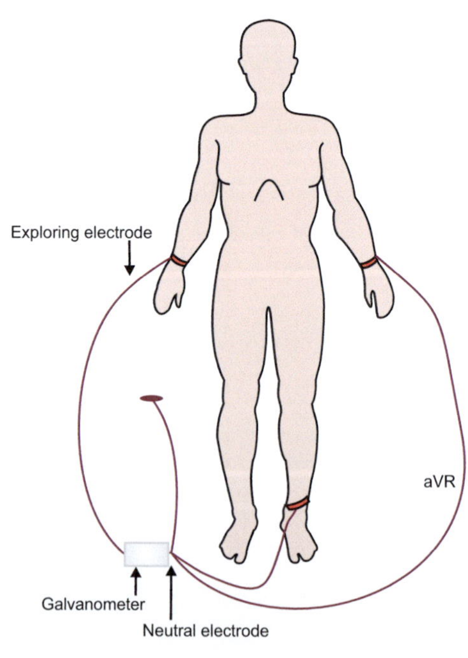


**Fig. 2.4** Diagram of lead aVR. Note the detached indifferent electrode from right arm

Lead aVL: This is the augmented unipolar left arm lead. The left arm electrode is positive, while the electrode on the right arm and left leg determines the neutral reference point (Fig. 2.5). This lead is oriented to the superior surface of left ventricle. The ECG complexes are usually positive.

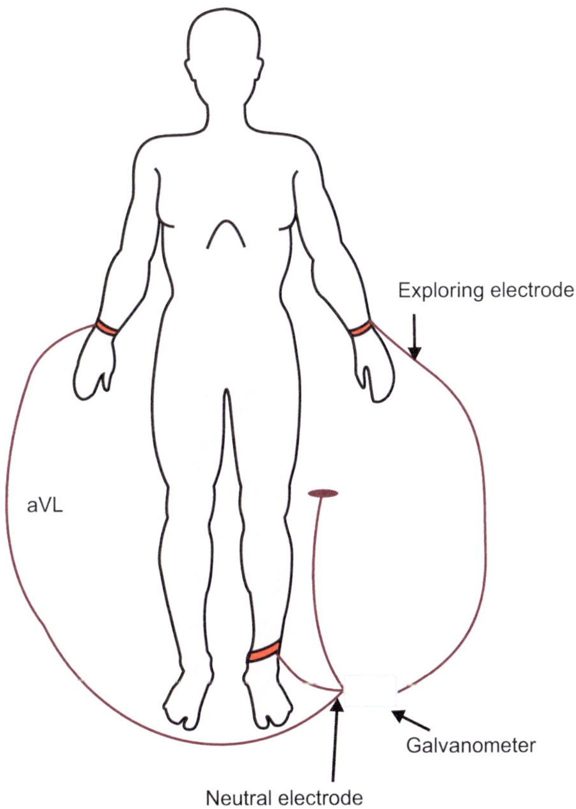


**Fig. 2.5** Diagram of lead aVL. Note the detached indifferent electrode from left arm

Lead aVF: This is the augmented unipolar left foot lead. The electrode on left leg is positive, while the electrode on the right and left arm determines the neutral reference point (Fig. 2.6). This lead is oriented to the inferior surface of the heart. The ECG complexes are usually positive.

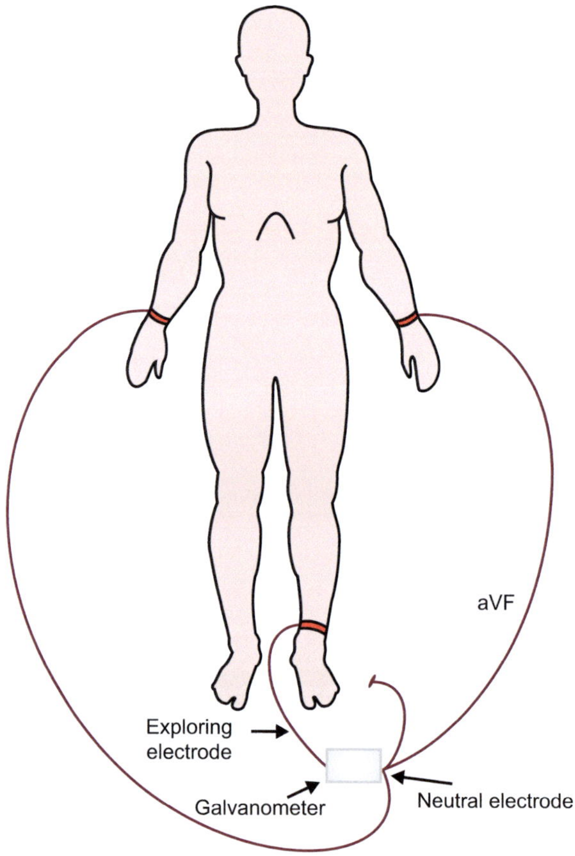


**Fig. 2.6** Diagram of lead aVF. Note the detached indifferent electrode from left foot

## 2.1.2 Horizontal Plane Leads

Horizontal plane leads are unipolar chest leads. The chest leads or precordial leads are represented by the letter 'V'. The chest leads look at the heart in the horizontal plane from the six positions as mentioned below. The leads are derived by placing the electrodes on the precordium in a semicircle around the heart (Fig. 2.7). The placement is as follows:

1. Lead V1: Placed at fourth intercostal space immediately to the right of sternum.
2. Lead V2: Placed at fourth intercostal space immediately to the left of sternum.
3. Lead V3: Placed in between V2 and V4.
4. Lead V4: Placed at left fifth intercostal space on midclavicular line.
5. Lead V5: Placed at same horizontal level as that of V4 on left anterior axillary line.
6. Lead V6: Placed at same horizontal level as that of V4 and V5 on left mid-axillary line.

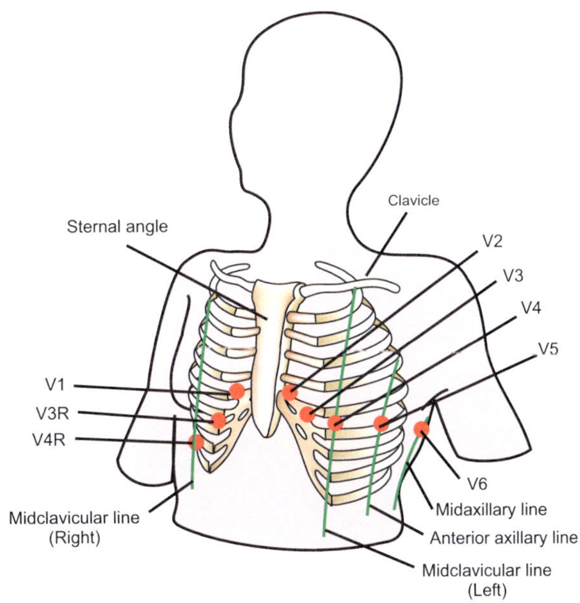


**Fig. 2.7** Diagram showing the position of chest leads

### 2.1.3 Orientation of ECG Leads

The position of the positive electrode can be considered like a camera or eye looking at the heart from that side. The view of each lead can be either committed to memory, or it can be reasoned easily by remembering the location of the positive electrode of each lead.

The standard 12 lead ECG evaluates the left ventricle mainly. If there is a need to evaluate the right ventricle, for example, right ventricular myocardial infarction, then right-sided chest leads are required. Six leads are placed on the right side of the chest in a mirror image of the standard chest leads. The location is identical to placement of standard chest leads except they are placed on right side. Sometimes, posterior lead ECG is required to evaluate the posterior surface, to record damage of myocardium. These three are leads V7, V8 and V9. These are placed in the same horizontal line as the standard chest leads on the back of the patient. The placement of leads is summarized in Box 2.3. The orientation of the various leads to the various parts of heart is as mentioned below:

Leads I and aVL: High left lateral wall of the heart (often called lateral leads).
Leads II, III and aVF: Inferior surface of the heart.
Leads aVR and V1: Cavity of the heart.
Leads V1–V6: Anterior wall of the heart. The anteroseptal leads are leads V1–V4 (more precisely leads V2 and V3) and the apical leads are leads V5 and V6.
Leads V1 and right-sided chest leads: Right ventricle.

**Box 2.3 Lead Placement**

| | |
|---|---|
| Lead I | Left arm positive, right arm negative |
| Lead II | Left foot positive, right arm negative |
| Lead III | Left foot positive, left arm negative |
| aVR | Right arm |
| aVL | Left arm |
| aVF | Left foot |
| V1 | Right fourth intercoastal space by the side of sternum |
| V2 | Left fourth intercoastal space by the side of sternum |
| V3 | Between leads V2 and V4 |
| V4 | Left fifth intercoastal space on midclavicular line |
| V5 | Same horizontal plane as V4 on anterior axillary line |
| V6 | Same horizontal plane as V4 and V5 on mid-axillary line |
| V7 | Same horizontal plane as V4 on posterior axillary line |
| V8 | Same horizontal plane as V4 on posterior scapular line |
| V9 | Same horizontal plane as V4 on posterior left border of spine |
| V3R to V9R | Same position as V3–V9 but on right side of chest |

## Self-Assessment Questions

1. On the ECG graph paper, one small square represents 0.04 s, and one large square is equal to 0.20 s. True or false?
2. The vertical axis of ECG paper represents amplitude of the ECG waves. True or false?
3. On ECG paper, ECG is produced by a black ink. True or false?
4. The ECG paper normally moves at a speed of 50 mm/s. True or false?
5. If the ECG paper is moved at a speed of 50 mm/s, the ECG waves will be broad. True or false?
6. **At 25 mm/s paper speed, in 1 min the number of large squares are:**

   a. 200 b. 300 c. 30,000 d. 100
7. **The number of electrodes in an ECG lead are:**

   a. 1 b. 2 c. 3 d. 4
8. **The augmented leads increase the voltage by:**

   a. 25% b. 40% c. 50% d. None of the above
9. **Spot the false statement:**

   a. Lead aVR is directed to cavity of the heart.
   b. Lead aVL is directed to inferior surface of the heart.
   c. Lead aVF is directed to high lateral wall of the heart.
   d. Both b. and c.
10. **Which one of the following lead is oriented towards right ventricle?**

    a. V2 b. V3R c. V5 d. V8
11. Measure the time duration represented by the arrows placed over the ECG paper (Fig. 2.8) considering that paper speed is 25 mm/s.

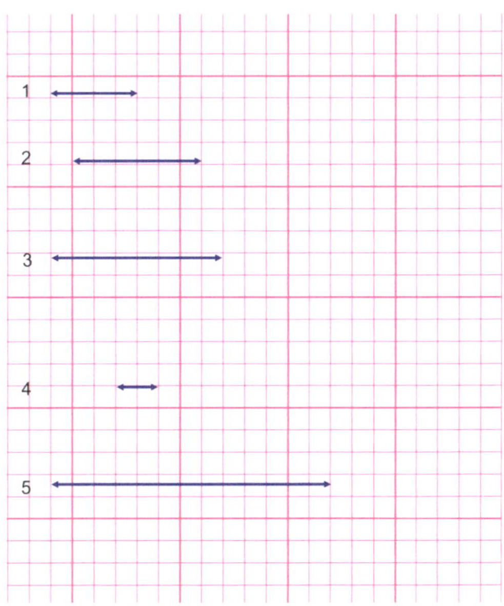


**Fig. 2.8** Measure the time duration

12. Measure the voltage represented by the arrows placed over the ECG paper (Fig. 2.9) considering that 10 mm = 1 mV.
13. Examine Fig. 2.10 carefully. There are several mistakes regarding the direction of the arrows and labelling of the limb leads. Identify all of them and rectify them.
14. Place the chest leads at appropriate places in the diagram of Fig. 2.11.

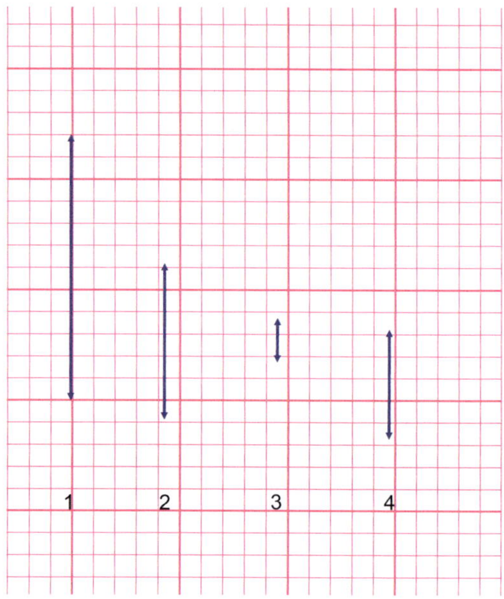


**Fig. 2.9** Measure the voltage

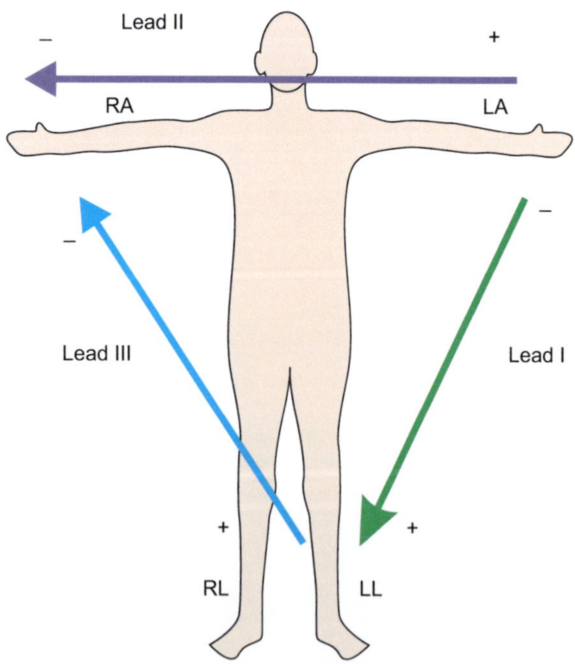


**Fig. 2.10** Identify the mistakes and rectify them

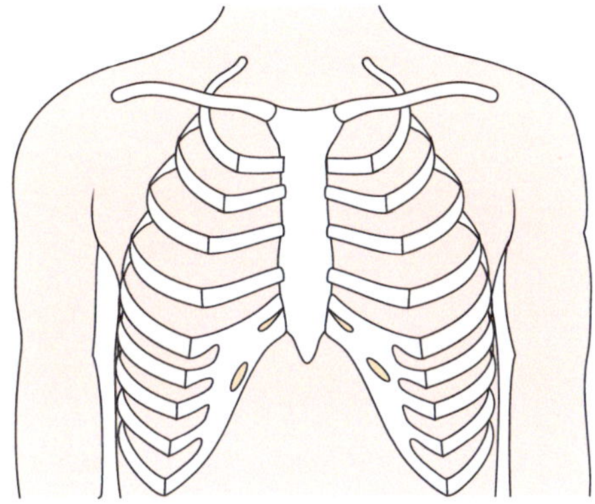

**Fig. 2.11** Place the chest leads

## Answers

1. True 2. True 3. False 4. False 5. True 6. b 7. b 8. c 9. d 10. b.
11. Arrow number 1 represents 0.16 s (4 × 0.4 = 0.16). Arrow number 2 represents 0.24 s (6 × 0.4 = 0.24). Arrow number 3 represents 0.32 s (8 × 0.4 = 0.32). Arrow number 4 represents 0.08 s (2 × 0.4 = 0.08). Arrow number 5 represents 0.52 s (13 × 0.04 = 0.52).
12. Arrow number 1 represents 1.2 mV (12 × 0.1 = 1.2). Arrow number 2 represents 0.7 mV (7 × 0.1 = 0.7). Arrow number 3 represents 0.2 mV (2 × 0.1 = 0.2). Arrow number 4 represents 0.5 mV (5 × 0.1 = 0.5).
13. All the three limb leads have been labelled in correct manner in Fig. 2.12. The direction of arrows of all the three leads are shown in correct manner in Fig. 2.12 as well.
14. The chest leads have been placed at appropriate places as shown in Fig. 2.13.

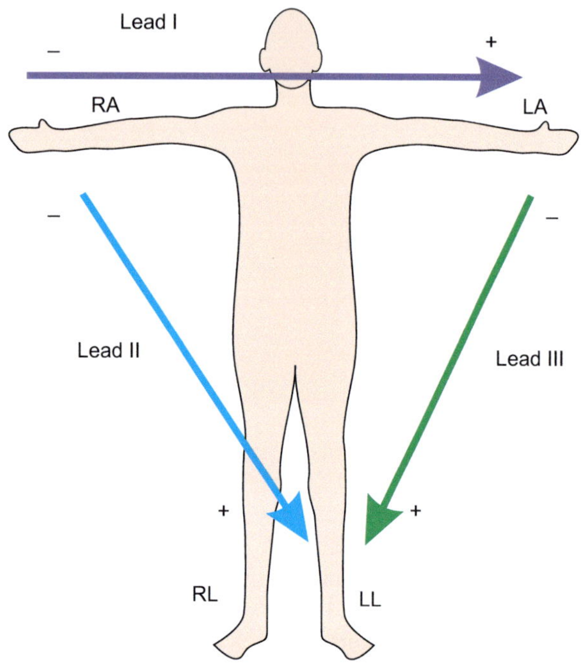


**Fig. 2.12** Answer of Question 13

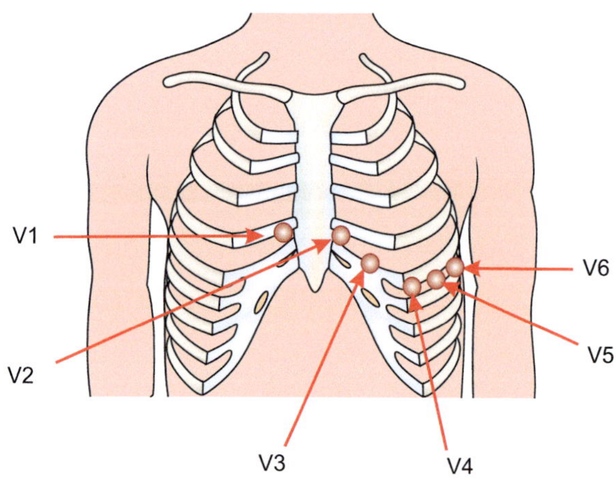


**Fig. 2.13** Answer of Question 14

# Chapter 3
# ECG Waveforms

**Learning Objectives**
After studying this chapter, the reader will learn about:

- Waves and complexes
- Genesis of QRS complex

One of the most fundamental aspects of learning ECG is to know about the components of a normal ECG and its range of normal attributes. The moment one takes a look at an ECG, instantaneously the mind starts comparing it with the memory of normal ECG stored in the mind, to look for abnormalities. Hence, it is very important to know about the normal morphology of various waves and complexes of ECG.

The nomenclature of the waves of ECG is arranged in alphabetic order as P, Q, R, S, T and U waves (Fig. 3.1). Small letters denote smaller waves (less than 5 mm), while capital letters denote larger waves or complexes (greater than 5 mm). The amplitude of the wave depends upon the thickness of the myocardium, the amount of intervening tissue, the magnitude and direction of the electric current and the distance between the heart and the electrodes. In absence of any waves, an isoelectric line is produced (Fig. 3.2).



T. K. Koley, *Rapid Review of ECG*,
https://doi.org/10.1007/978-981-99-9116-7_3

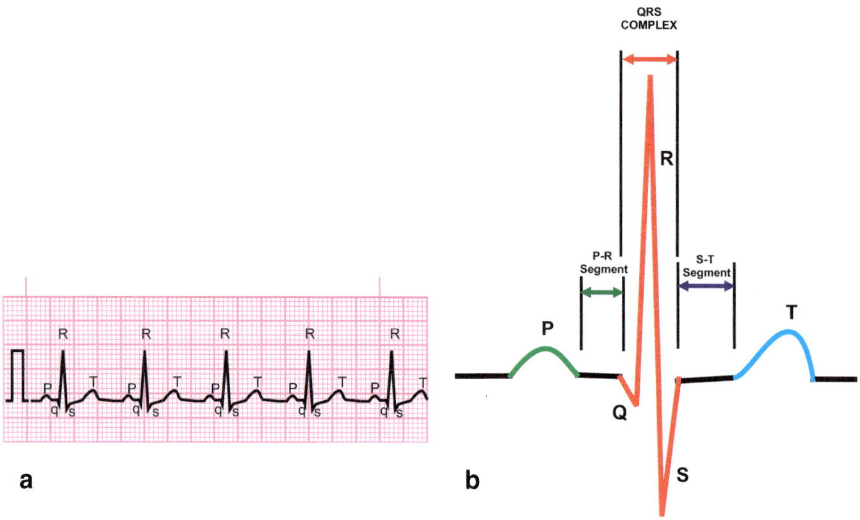


**Fig. 3.1** Nomenclature of waves of ECG. (**a**) Nomenclature of waves and complexes on ECG paper. (**b**) Diagrammatic representation of the various waves and complexes

**Fig. 3.2** Isoelectric line and relation of various waves of ECG

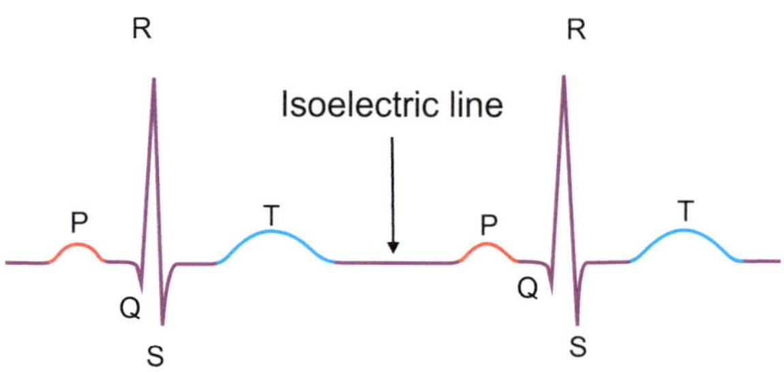


## 3.1 Waves and Complexes

### *3.1.1 Components of ECG*

The deflections P, Q, R, S, T and U are called waves. The Q, R and S together form a complex. In this chapter, various waveforms and complexes of ECG will be discussed. ECG intervals and segments are covered in next chapter.

The various components of an ECG are the following:

- Waveforms: P, T, U waves.
- Intervals: P-R, R-R, Q-T, P-P intervals and QRS duration.
- Junction: QRS-T junction, called J point.
- Segments: S-T segment, T-Q segment.
- Complex: QRS complex

#### 3.1.1.1 P Wave

P wave is the first wave of the ECG which is produced by atrial depolarization. The first part of P wave is produced by the depolarization of the right atrium and the second part reflects the depolarization of left atrium. It is smooth and rounded with a maximum amplitude and duration of 2.5 mm (Figs. 3.3 and 3.4). The P wave is always positive in leads I and II and negative in lead aVR. In lead III and lead V1, it may be positive, biphasic or inverted. The presence of smooth and upright P wave before every QRS complex especially in lead II indicates that the rhythm is originating from SA node. This normal rhythm generated at the SA node is called sinus rhythm.

Ectopic P waves may be either positive or negative in lead II. If the ectopic P wave originates in the atria, it will be upright, and if it originates in the AV junction, it will be negative. The various causes of abnormal P waves, including absent P wave, tall p wave and inverted p wave are mentioned in Box 3.1.

**Fig. 3.3** P wave (arrow)

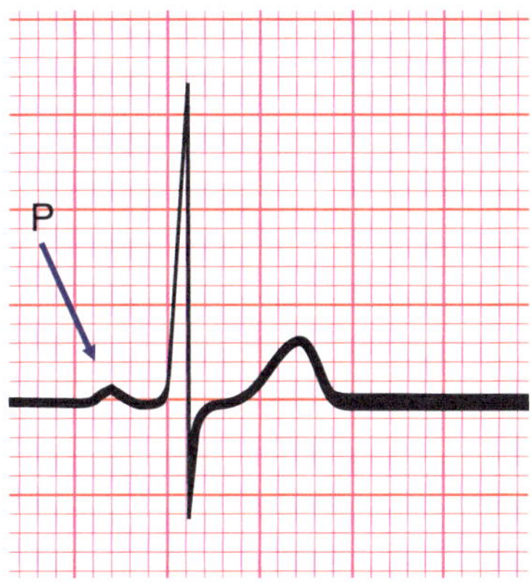


**Fig. 3.4** P waves (arrows)

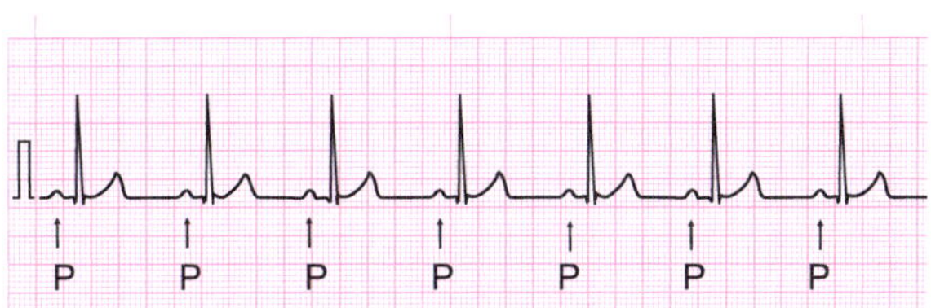


**Box 3.1 P Wave Abnormalities**

| Abnormality | Causes |
|---|---|
| Tall P wave (amplitude >2.5 mm) | Pulmonary hypertension, right atrial enlargement, pulmonary stenosis, mitral stenosis, COPD, tricuspid stenosis |
| Wide P wave | Left atrial enlargement, mitral stenosis, hyperkalaemia |
| Inverted P wave | Atrioventricular junctional/nodal rhythm, premature atrial complex |
| Absent P wave | Atrial fibrillation, atrioventricular junctional/nodal rhythm, ventricular tachycardia, hyperkalaemia, SA block/arrest |

**Tips and Tricks**

- P wave is best seen in lead II.
- Normal P wave is always inverted in lead aVR.
- Normal P wave in lead V1 may be positive, biphasic or inverted.
- Tall P wave is seen in right atrial enlargement and broad and bifid P wave is seen in left atrial enlargement.

#### 3.1.1.2 Ta or Pt Wave

Ta wave is produced by atrial repolarization. It is usually not visible. It is a small, asymmetric, negative wave after the P wave. It is obscured by the QRS complex which occurs at the same time. It may be visible during sinus tachycardia, when it manifests as a negative rounded wave at the beginning of the QRS complex and well extending into the S-T segment. The duration of Ta wave is about 300 ms.

#### 3.1.1.3 QRS Complex

QRS complex, the major ECG deflection, is produced by synchronous depolarization of both the ventricles. This is the largest deflection of ECG because the ventricles contain the largest mass of cardiac myocytes. Unlike the rounded contour of P wave, the contour of QRS complex is peaked or pointed (Fig. 3.5). The QRS complex is positive in all leads except lead aVR. The normal QRS complex has smooth limbs with no notch or slurring. The positive and negative deflections of QRS complexes have specific nomenclature, unlike the positive or negative deflections of the P wave. The positive deflection is called R wave and the negative deflections are called Q and S waves. If additional positive wave is present, it is called R′ (R prime) wave. If additional negative wave is present, it is called S′ (S prime) wave. Further additional waves are called R″ (R double prime) and S″ (S double prime) waves.

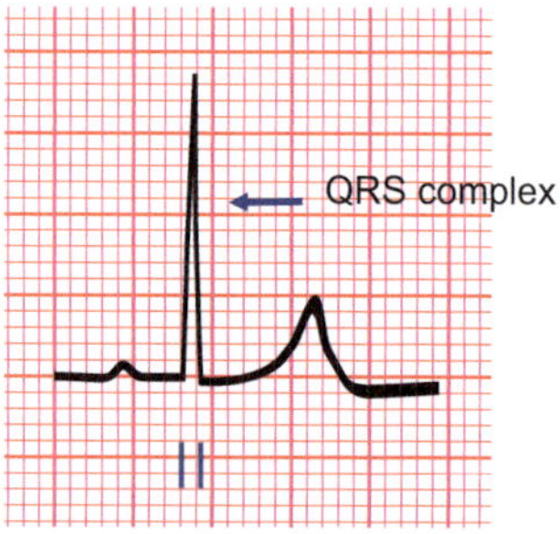


**Fig. 3.5** Normal QRS complex

**Tips and Tricks**

- Normally not every QRS complex contains a Q wave, a R wave or a S wave. If R wave is absent, it is called QS complex.
- Low QRS voltage is a condition in which the QRS (R + S) amplitude is less than 5 mm in limb leads. In chest leads, the QRS (R + S) amplitude is less than 10 mm.
- If you come across low voltage, at first check the standardization.
- Think of the common conditions in which low voltage is seen such as pericardial effusion, obesity, pleural effusion, emphysema and hypothyroidism.
- The atria have less muscle mass as compared to the large ventricles. Hence, the depolarization current is less in atria after activation as compared to that of ventricles. As a result, the P wave is small and the QRS complex is big.
- If QRS complex is broad, think of bundle branch block or WPW syndrome.
- If there is increased amplitude of QRS complex, think of left and right ventricular hypertrophy.

#### 3.1.1.4 Q Wave

Q wave is the first negative deflection after P wave (Fig. 3.6). It occurs before the first positive deflection (R wave). Depolarization of the interventricular septum from left to right leads to generation of Q wave. Normal Q wave is less than 0.04 s in duration, less than 25% of the height of R wave in the same complex. It is normally visible in leads I, aVL, V5 and V6. Presence of Q wave in leads V1, V2 and V3 should be considered abnormal. The normal Q wave is represented by q. Pathological Q waves, seen in myocardial infarction, have large amplitude (Fig. 3.7). Large Q waves may be seen normally in leads III and aVR.

**Fig. 3.6** Q waves (arrows)

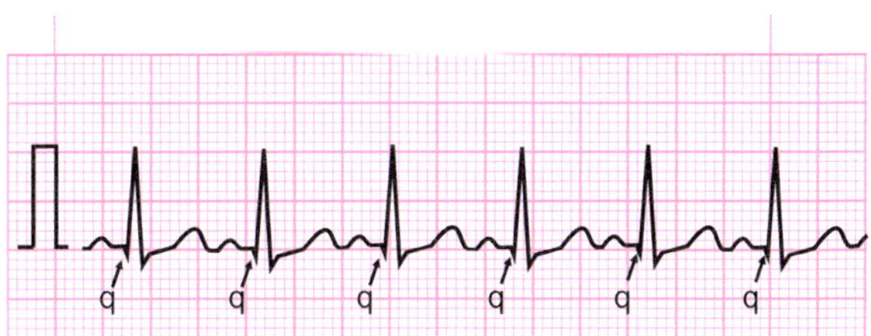


**Fig. 3.7** Q wave (arrow)

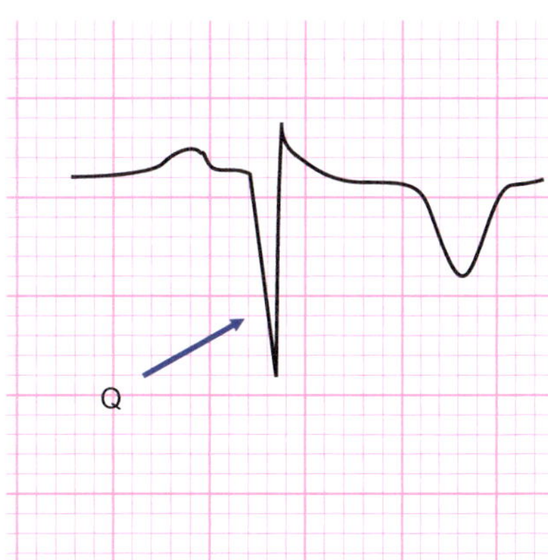

#### 3.1.1.5 R Wave

The first positive deflection of the QRS complex is the R wave (Figs. 3.8 and 3.9). It may or may not be preceded by Q wave. The amplitude of the R wave varies in different leads. Usually in the limb leads, the height of the R wave is at least 5 mm and in the chest leads the height is at least 10 mm. In leads V1 and V2, the height of R wave is small which gradually increases from lead V1 to lead V6. This is known as progression of the R wave amplitude (Fig. 3.10). Loss of progression of R wave amplitude is seen in anterior wall myocardial infarction. However, it may be a normal finding in young persons, especially in young women. R wave may be absent in lead V1 and a QS complex may be recorded in normal persons.

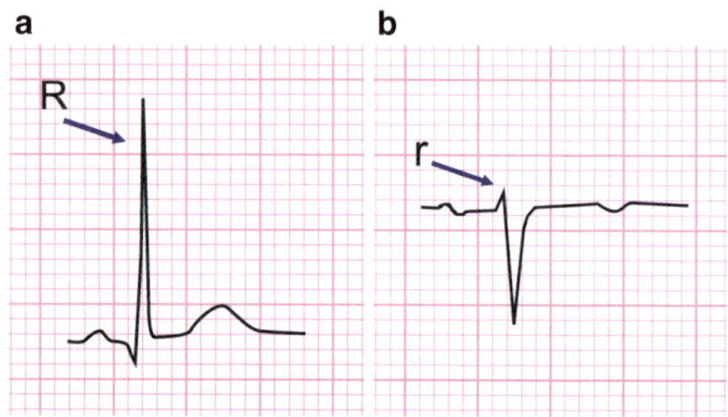


**Fig. 3.8** R wave (arrow). Panel **a** shows large R wave and panel **b** shows small r wave

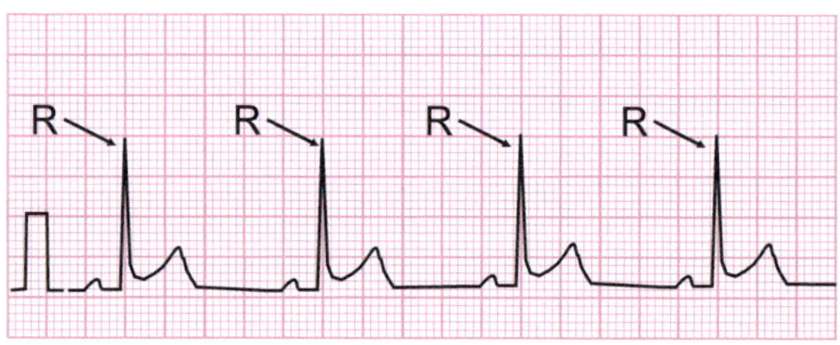


**Fig. 3.9** R waves (arrows)

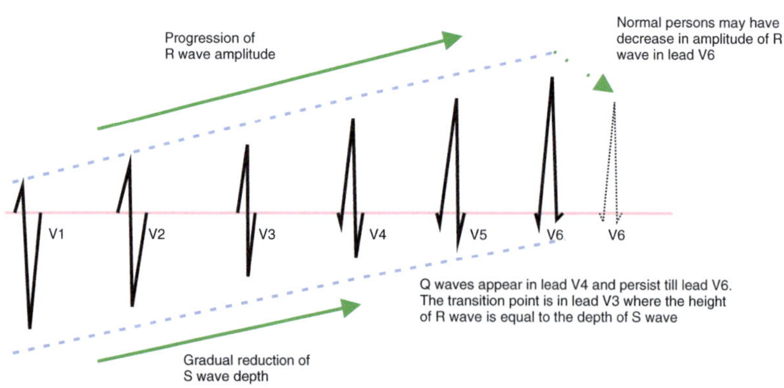


**Fig. 3.10** Progression of R waves in chest leads. Note the gradual increase in the height of R waves from lead V1 to V6. The height of R wave in lead V6 may be more or may be less than the height of R wave in lead V5 in normal persons

### 3.1.1.6 S Wave

The first negative deflection of QRS complex after R wave is the S wave. It is the terminal part of ventricular depolarization (Figs. 3.11 and 3.12). The S wave is large in lead V1 and gradually become smaller from lead V3 to lead V6. S wave may be absent in leads V5 and V6 in normal persons. The depth of S wave in lead V1 is more than the height of R wave and in lead V6 the depth of S wave is much less than the height of R wave.

**Fig. 3.11** S wave (arrow)

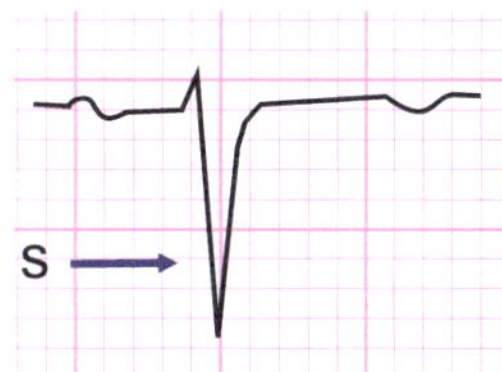


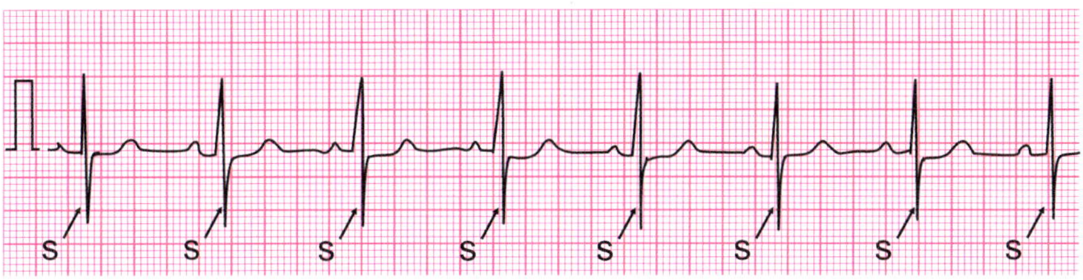


**Fig. 3.12** S waves (arrows)

#### 3.1.1.7 R′ Wave (R Prime)

The second positive deflection after R wave in the QRS complex is known as R′ wave (Fig. 3.13). It is seen during bundle branch block.

#### 3.1.1.8 S′ Wave (S Prime)

The second negative deflection after S wave in the QRS complex is known as S′ wave. It is also seen during bundle branch block.

#### 3.1.1.9 T Wave

T wave is seen after QRS complex. It is produced by ventricular repolarization. It has got asymmetric limbs with blunt apex and it is in the same direction as that of the QRS complex (Fig. 3.14). The slope of the ascent of T wave is more gradual than that of the terminal portion. The suggested criteria for the typical T wave include the amplitude less than two-thirds of the size of the R wave and a height of less than 10 mm. The absolute refractory period is present during the beginning of the T wave and at the peak of the T wave the relative refractory period begins.

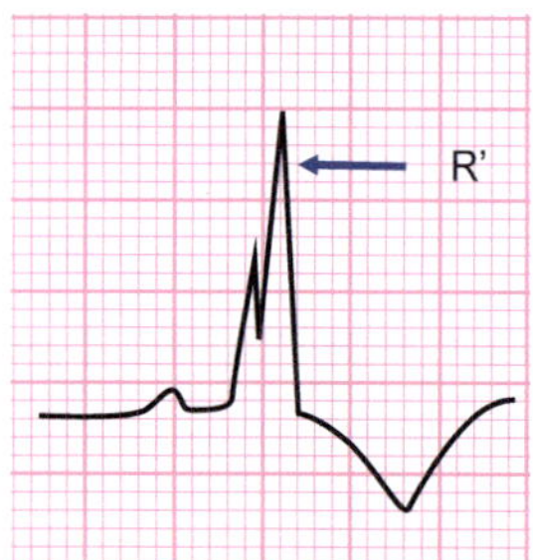


**Fig. 3.13** R′ wave (arrow)

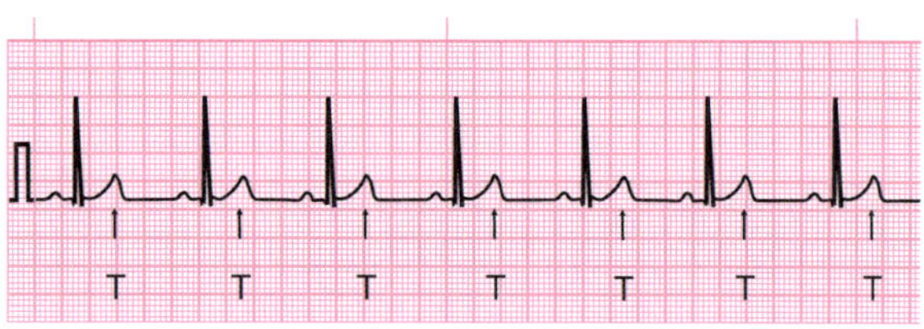


**Fig. 3.14** T waves (arrows)

**Tips and Tricks**

- Normal T wave is always inverted in lead aVR and it is often inverted in lead V1 also.
- T wave is normally inverted in leads V1, V2 and V3 in infants and children due to right ventricular dominance.
- In normal ECG, the direction of T wave is the same as that of QRS complex. If the QRS complex is positive, the T wave will be positive, and if the QRS is negative, the T wave will be negative.
- An inverted T wave in lead III is normal, if T wave is upright in lead aVF.
- If there is a tall and peaked T wave, think of hyperkalaemia.

The various causes of abnormal T waves are mentioned in Box 3.2.

**Box 3.2 T Wave Abnormalities**

| Abnormalities | Causes |
|---|---|
| Tall T wave | Hyperkalaemia, early repolarization syndrome, myocardial infarction, Prinzmetal's angina, cerebrovascular accident, left bundle branch block, ventricular hypertrophy, vagotonia, athletes, acute pericarditis |
| Inverted T wave | Normal variant, myocardial ischaemia, hyperventilation, anxiety, myocarditis, left ventricular hypertrophy, pericarditis, pulmonary embolism, drinking hot or cold beverages, digoxin effect or toxicity, myxoedema, hypertrophic cardiomyopathy (apical type), conduction abnormalities, WPW syndrome, hypokalaemia |

### 3.1.1.10 U Wave

The genesis of U wave is uncertain and it is disputed. Probably, it represents the slow repolarization of the Purkinje fibres or the papillary muscles. It follows T wave and is in the same direction as that of T wave (Fig. 3.15) and it is best seen in leads V2–V4. U wave more than 2 mm is considered abnormal and may be due to hypokalaemia or digitalis effect.

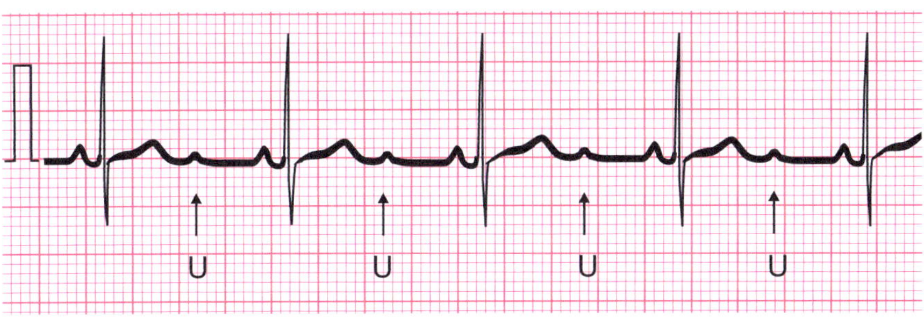


**Fig. 3.15** U waves (arrows)

**Tips and Tricks**

- U wave is often not seen in any of the leads in a normal ECG.
- An upright U wave after a flat T wave is usually pathological.

## 3.2 Genesis of QRS Complex

The ventricular activation begins at the interventricular septum with the activation force moving from left to right. This results in a small positive wave (r wave) in lead V1, i.e. the lead facing the wavefront and a small negative wave (q wave) in lead V6, i.e. the lead from which the wavefront is receding (Fig. 3.16).

Next the activation of free walls of both the ventricles occurs transversely from endocardium to epicardium. This leads to a large right to left wavefront (vector) because of thicker left ventricular myocardium and a small wavefront from left to right because of thinner right ventricular myocardium. These two vectors are opposite to each other and therefore the resultant vector is directed from right to left. This leads to recording of a deep negative wave in lead V1 (S wave) as the wavefront is moving away from this electrode and a large positive wave in V6 (R wave) as the wavefront is going towards the electrode (Fig. 3.17).

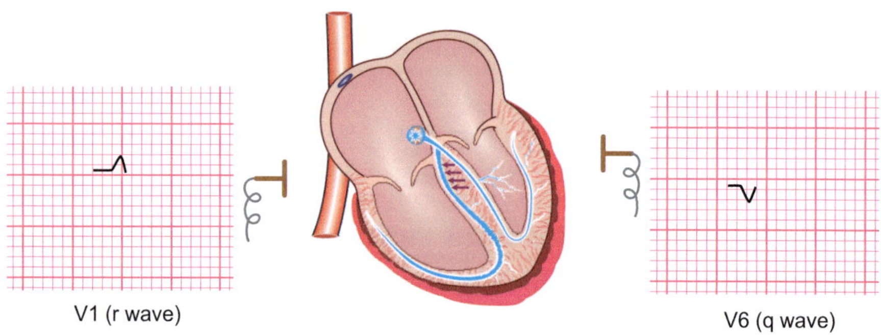


**Fig. 3.16** Genesis of 'q' wave

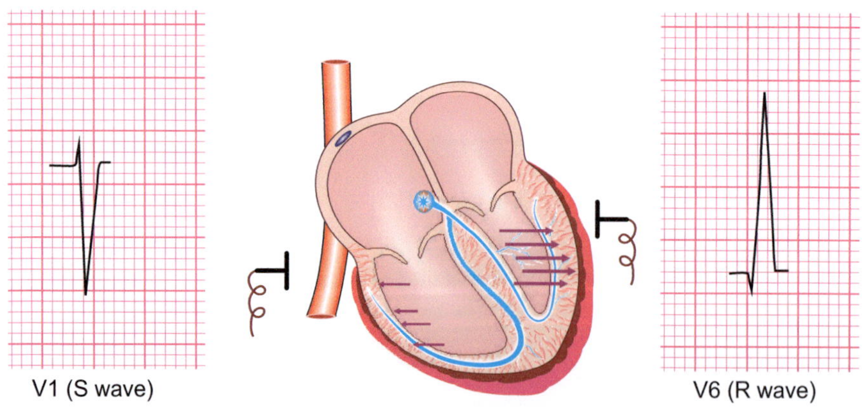


**Fig. 3.17** Genesis of R and S waves

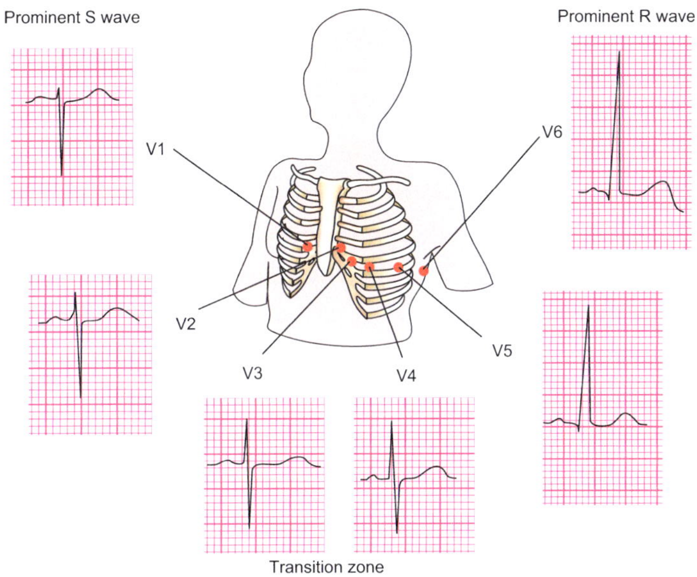


**Fig. 3.18** ECG configuration in chest leads

The transition zone is the area that records the transition of QRS complex from rS to qR pattern. It is usually in lead V3 or V4 where the R and S waves are of same height and depth, respectively (Fig. 3.18). The genesis of the waves is summarized in Box 3.3.

**Box 3.3 Genesis of ECG Waves**

| | |
|---|---|
| P wave | Atrial depolarization |
| Ta wave | Atrial repolarization |
| QRS complex | Ventricular depolarization |
| T wave | Ventricular repolarization |
| U wave | Uncertain |

**Self-Assessment Questions**

1. The first part of P wave is due to depolarization of left atrium. True or false?
2. The normal Q wave is more than 25% of the R wave. True or false?
3. The second positive deflection after R wave in the QRS complex is known as R′ wave. True or false?
4. T wave precedes QRS complex. True or false?
5. U wave is twice the height of T wave in lead II. True or false?
6. **Which of the following can cause a wide P wave in an ECG?**

   a. Mitral stenosis b. Ventricular tachycardia c. Bundle branch block d. Aortic stenosis

7. **What does the T wave represent in an ECG?**

   a. Depolarization of the atria b. Repolarization of the ventricles c. Atrial contraction d. Ventricular contraction

8. **What does the QRS complex represent in an electrocardiogram (ECG)?**

   a. Depolarization of the atria b. Repolarization of the ventricles c. Contraction of the atria d. Depolarization of the ventricles

9. **Which of the following is a common cause of a pathological Q wave in an ECG?**

   a. Atrial fibrillation b. Ventricular tachycardia c. Myocardial infarction d. Atrial flutter

10. **Which of the following is true regarding the R wave in the QRS complex?**

    a. It represents depolarization of the atria b. It precedes P wave c. It is absent lead III d. The amplitude of R wave is less than the amplitude of S wave in lead V1

**Case Studies**

1. Carefully examine the electrocardiograms in Figs. 3.19, 3.20, 3.21, 3.22, 3.23 and 3.24 and label the waves. For all ECGs in this book, consider paper speed of 25 mm/s and standardization of 10 mm = 1 mV.
2. Identify two abnormalities in the ECG of Fig. 3.25.
3. Identify the abnormality in the ECG of Fig. 3.26. Identify the S-T segment by placing arrow.
4. Identify the abnormal wave in the ECG of Fig. 3.27. Name one condition in which you get it.
5. Identify the abnormal wave in the ECG of Fig. 3.28. Mark the J point with arrow.

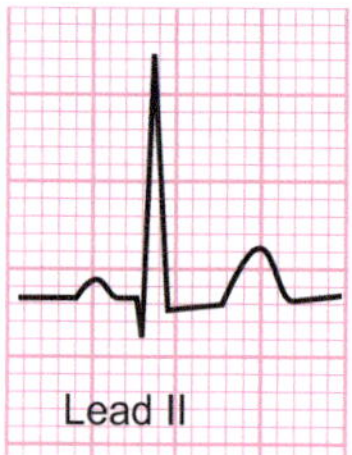


**Fig. 3.19** Label the ECG waves

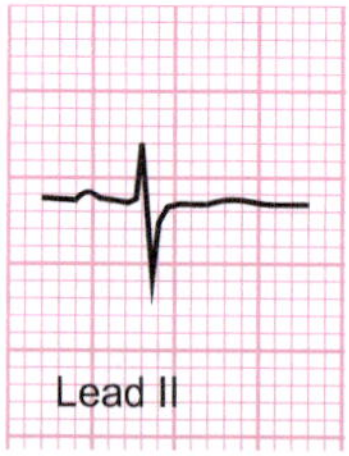


**Fig. 3.20** Label the ECG waves

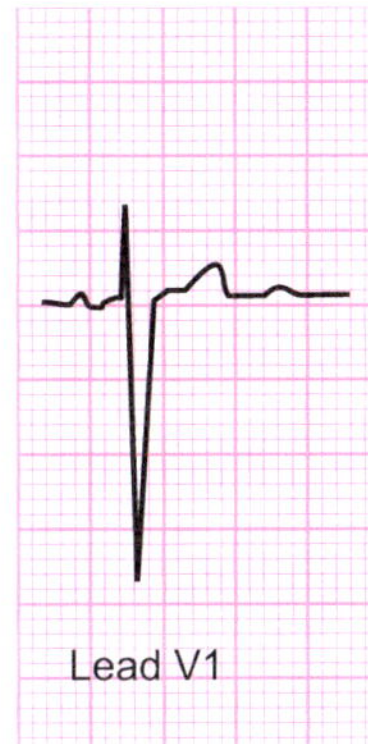


**Fig. 3.21** Label the ECG waves

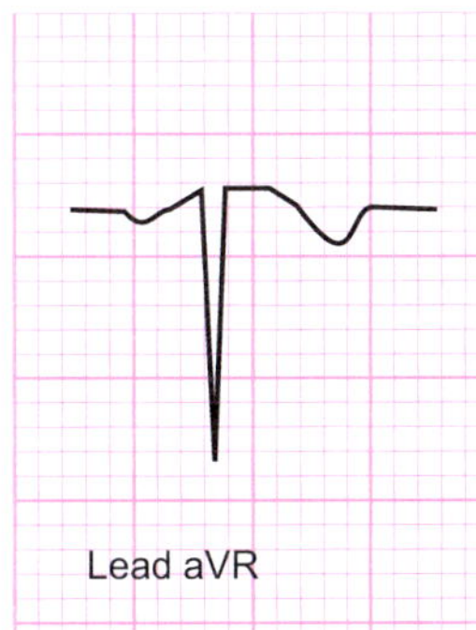


**Fig. 3.22** Label the ECG waves

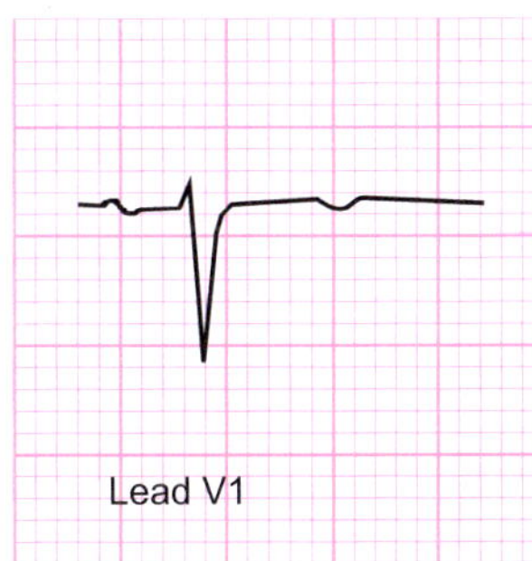


**Fig. 3.23** Label the ECG waves

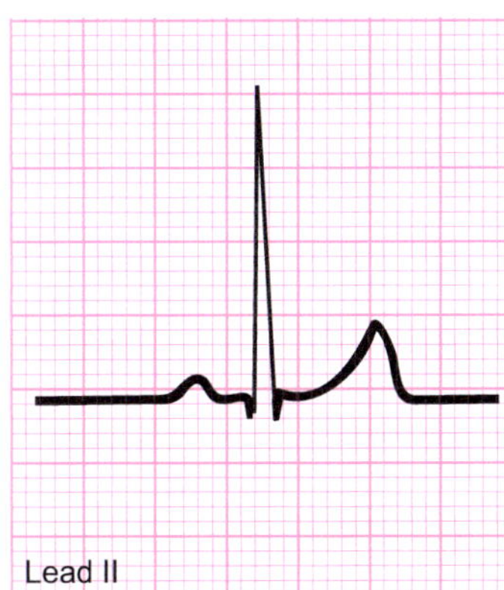


**Fig. 3.24** Label the ECG waves

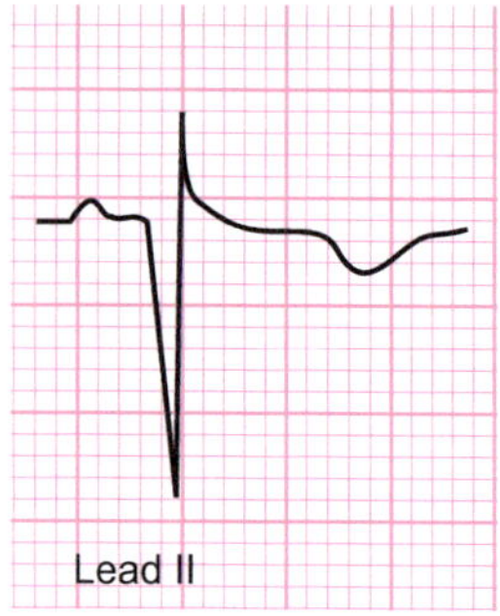


**Fig. 3.25** Identify two abnormalities

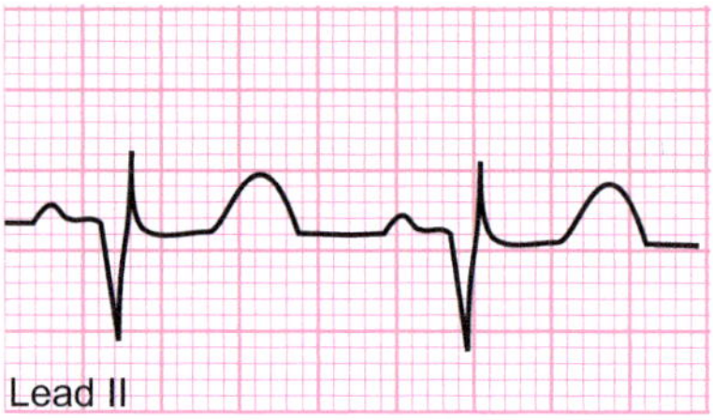


**Fig. 3.26** Identify the abnormality

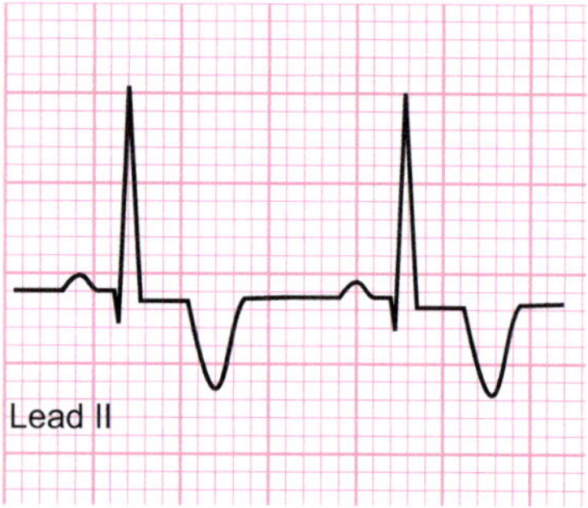


**Fig. 3.27** Identify the abnormal wave

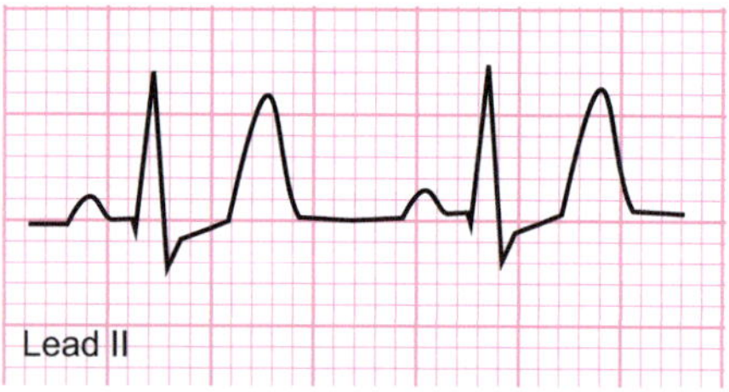


**Fig. 3.28** Label the abnormal wave

6. Label the abnormal wave in the ECG of Fig. 3.29. Describe the abnormality and name one condition in which you get this type of abnormal wave.
7. Measure the amplitude of R and S waves in the ECG of Fig. 3.30.
8. Measure the amplitude of R and S waves in the ECG of Fig. 3.31. Mark the U wave by placing arrow.

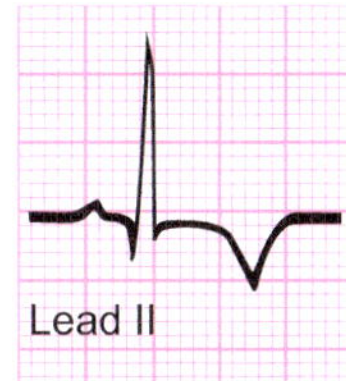


**Fig. 3.29** Label the abnormal wave

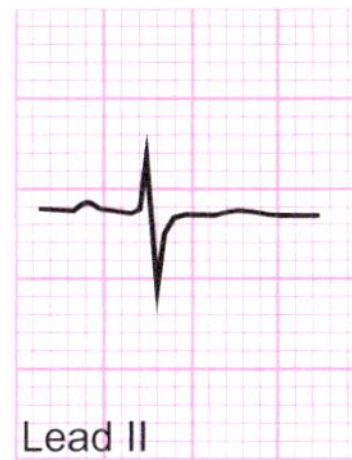


**Fig. 3.30** Measure the amplitude of R and S waves

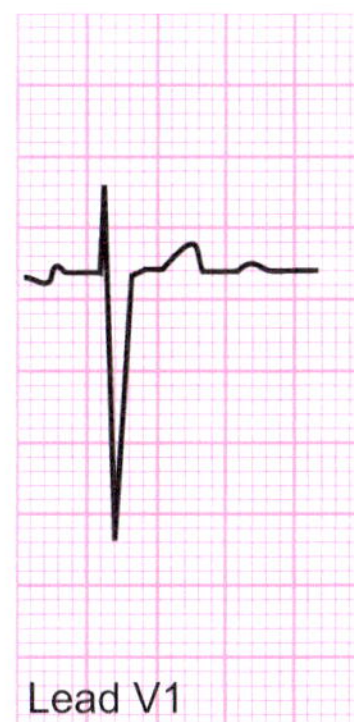


**Fig. 3.31** Measure the amplitude of R and S waves and mark the U wave

## Answers

1. False 2. False 3. True 4. False 5. False 6. a 7. b 8. d 9. c 10. d

## Case Studies

1. The answer of this question is given in Figs. 3.32, 3.33, 3.34, 3.35, 3.36 and 3.37.
2. The two abnormalities are pathologic Q waves and inversion of T wave (Fig. 3.38).
3. The abnormality in this ECG is presence of pathologic Q waves. The Q waves and S-T segments are marked by arrows (Fig. 3.39).
4. The abnormality in the ECG is inversion of T wave (Fig. 3.40). It is seen in myocardial ischaemia.

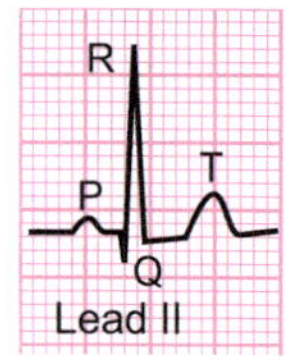


**Fig. 3.32** Answer of Case Study Question 1 (Fig. 3.19)

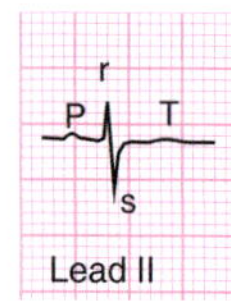


**Fig. 3.33** Answer of Case Study Question 1 (Fig. 3.20)

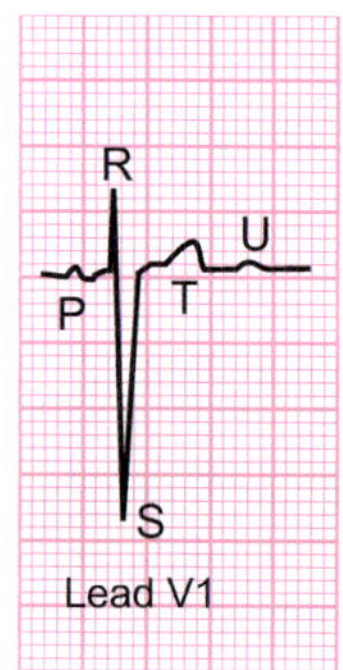


**Fig. 3.34** Answer of Case Study Question 1 (Fig. 3.21)

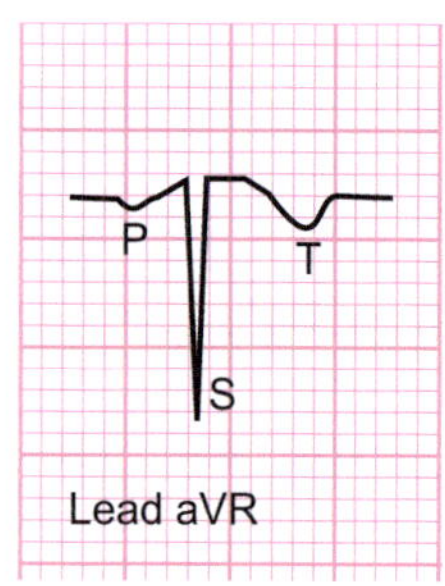


**Fig. 3.35** Answer of Case Study Question 1 (Fig. 3.22)

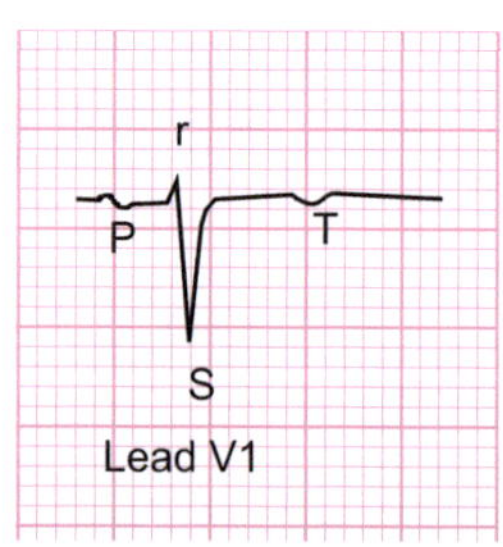


**Fig. 3.36** Answer of Case Study Question 1 (Fig. 3.23)

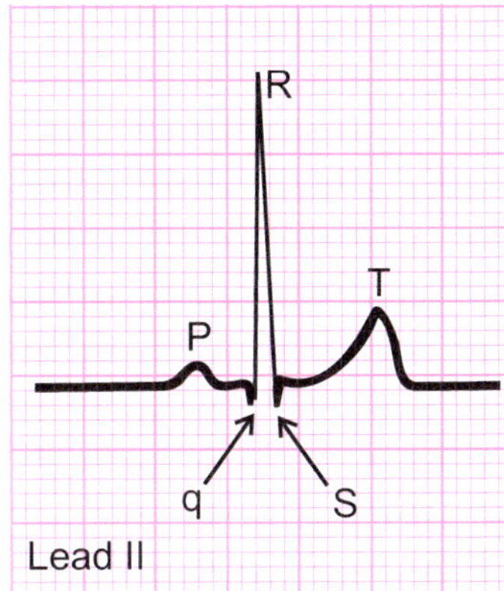


**Fig. 3.37** Answer of Case Study Question 1 (Fig. 3.24)

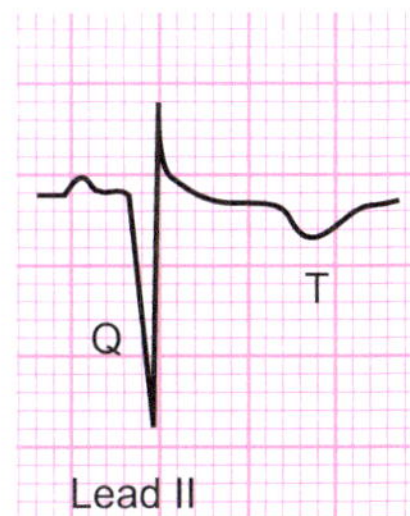


**Fig. 3.38** Answer of Case Study Question 2

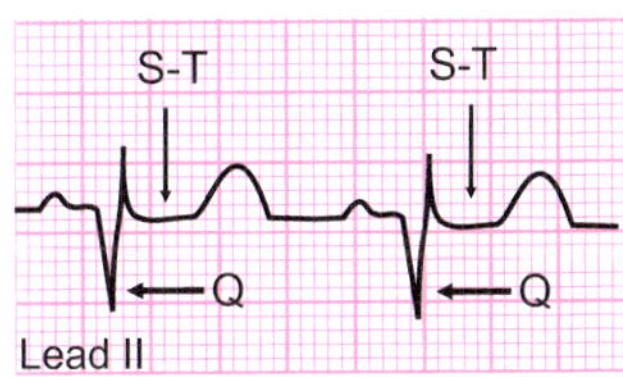


**Fig. 3.39** Answer of Case Study Question 3

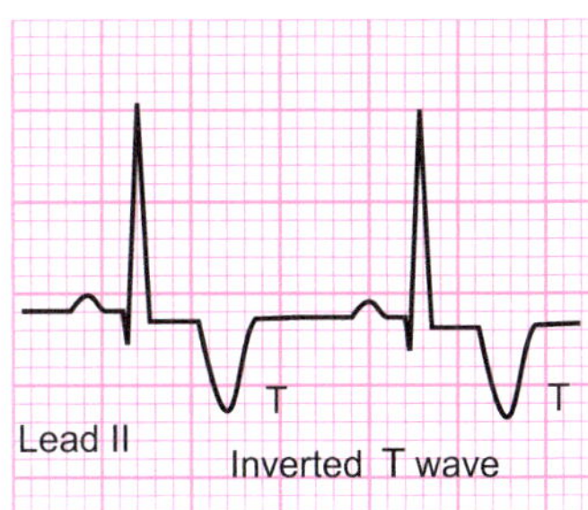


**Fig. 3.40** Answer of Case Study Question 4

5. The abnormality in the ECG is tall T waves. The J points are marked with arrows (Fig. 3.41).
6. The abnormal wave is marked by arrow (Fig. 3.42). This is a symmetrical, deep and pointed T wave inversion. This is seen in myocardial infarction.
7. To calculate the amplitude of R and S waves, P-R segment is used as isoelectric line. The horizontal blue line represents the P-R segment, which is prolonged over the isoelectric S-T segment for calculation of amplitude of waves (Fig. 3.43).

   The amplitude of r wave is 4 × 0.1 mV = 0.40 mV. Similarly, the amplitude of S wave is 5 × 0.1 mV = 0.50 mV.
8. The amplitude of R wave is 6 × 0.1 s = 0.6 mV (Fig. 3.44). The amplitude of S wave is 23 × 0.1 mV = 2.3 mV. The U wave is marked by arrow.

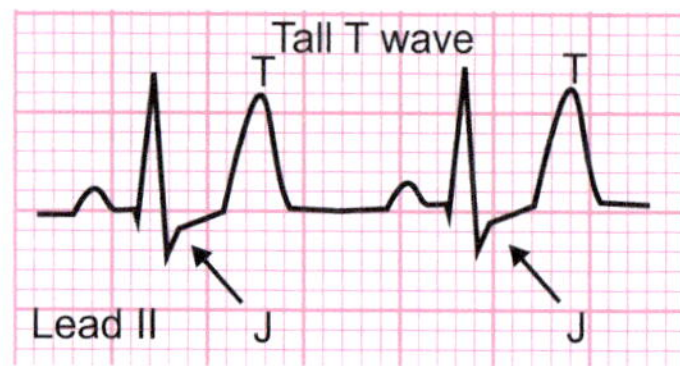


**Fig. 3.41** Answer of Case Study Question 5

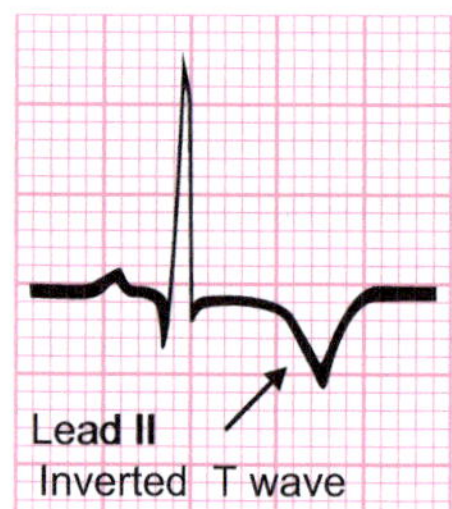


**Fig. 3.42** Answer of Case Study Question 6

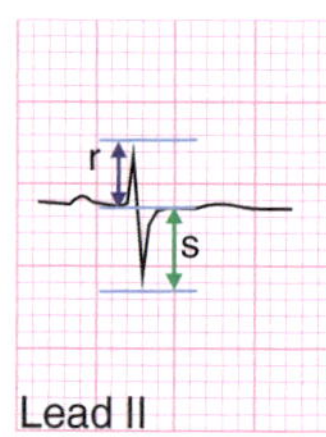


**Fig. 3.43** Answer of Case Study Question 7

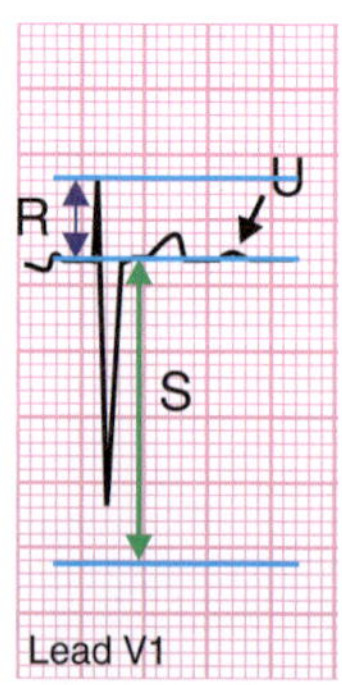


**Fig. 3.44** Answer of Case Study Question 8

# Chapter 4
# ECG Intervals and Segment

**Learning Objectives**
After studying this chapter, the reader will learn about:

- P-R interval
- P-R segment
- P-P interval
- R-R interval
- QRS interval
- S-T segment
- Q-T interval
- T-Q segment
- Ventricular activation time

Various time intervals and segments are studied while reading an ECG. A segment in ECG is the area between two waves. Segment is usually isoelectric in normal ECG. Elevation or depression and lengthening or shortening of segments are of great significance while studying segments. An interval in ECG is a time duration that includes one segment and one or more waves. While studying intervals morphology or depression or elevation is not considered. The important intervals and segments are the following:

- P-R interval
- P-R segment
- P-P interval
- R-R interval
- QRS interval
- S-T segment
- Q-T interval


T. K. Koley, *Rapid Review of ECG*,
https://doi.org/10.1007/978-981-99-9116-7_4

## 4.1 P-R Interval

In a QRS complex, P-R interval is the time interval between the beginning of P wave to beginning of Q wave or R wave (in absence of Q wave) (Fig. 4.1). It denotes the time interval between atrial and ventricular depolarization and is mainly contributed by AV nodal delay in conduction of the impulse.

It includes the time for atrial depolarization, normal conduction delay of the AV node (0.07 s) and time for the passage of impulse through bundle of His and bundle branches to the onset of ventricular depolarization.

The normal P-R interval is 0.12–0.20 s. Prolonged P-R interval is seen in the first degree heart block and shortened P-R interval is seen in Wolff–Parkinson–White syndrome and Lown–Ganong–Levine syndrome.

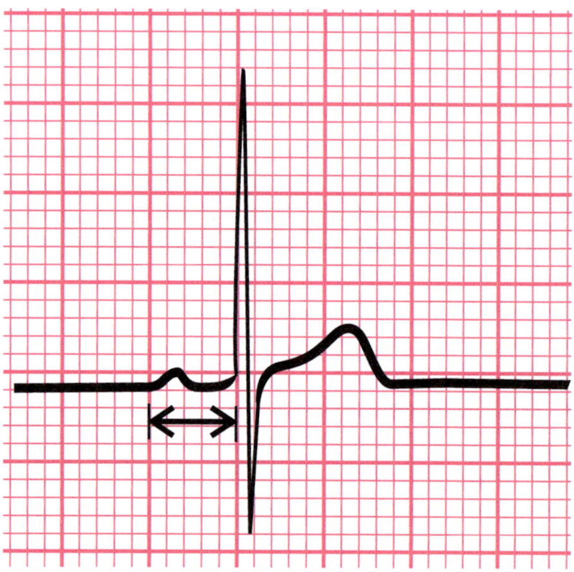

**Fig. 4.1** P-R interval. In this ECG the number of small boxes between beginning of P wave and beginning of R wave is 5 (as shown with arrow). Hence, P-R interval is 5 × 0.04 s = 0.20 s

**Tips and Tricks**

- Often mild P-R interval prolongation is found in athletes and normal persons. No treatment is required.
- Normal P-R interval is 3–5 small squares in horizontal axis in ECG.

## 4.2 P-R Segment

P-R segment starts from the end of the P wave to the beginning of the QRS complex (Fig. 4.2). It is an isoelectric line. It does not include the P wave and is part of the P-R interval. It allows time for the atria to empty blood into the ventricles before ventricular contraction begins. It represents the time taken by electrical impulse to travel through the AV node, bundle of His, bundle branches and Purkinje system. P-R segment is frequently used as isoelectric baseline for calculating the amplitude of the waves of ECG.

**Fig. 4.2** P-R segment

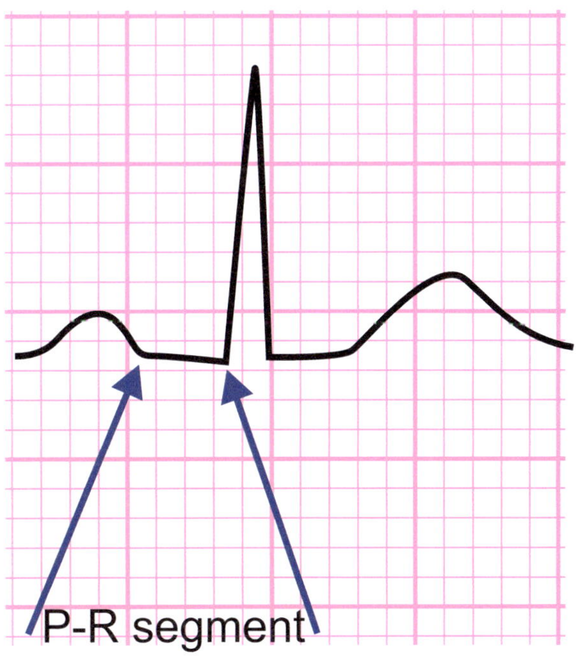

## 4.3 P-P Interval

P-P interval is the time interval between two consecutive P waves. It is calculated from the beginning of any P wave to the beginning of the subsequent P wave. It helps in calculation of atrial rate. In normal sinus rhythm, P-P interval is equal to the R-R interval. Varying P-P interval is seen in sinus arrhythmia.

## 4.4 R-R Interval

R-R interval is the time interval between two consecutive R waves (Fig. 4.3). It helps in calculation of ventricular rate (heart rate). Slight variation of R-R interval may be normal due to effect of respiration.

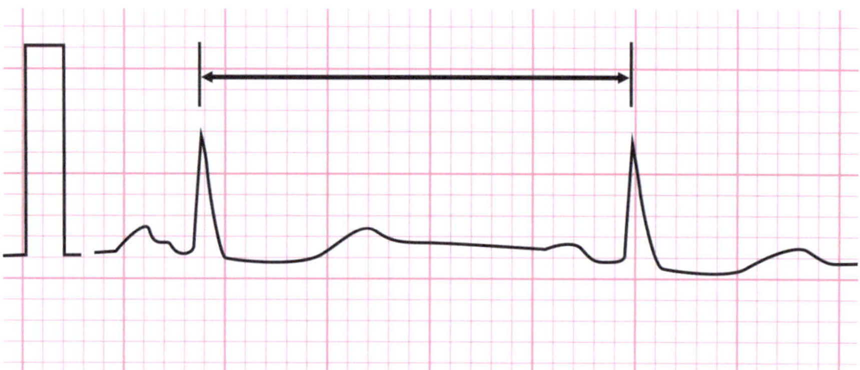

**Fig. 4.3** R-R interval. In this ECG, there are 21 small boxes between the peak of one R wave to the peak of next R wave (as shown with arrow). Hence, the R-R interval is 21 × 0.04 s = 0.84 s

## 4.5 QRS Interval

QRS interval or duration denotes the total time taken for ventricular depolarization. It is calculated from beginning of Q wave to end of S wave or J point (junction point—it is junction between end of S wave and beginning of S-T segment, Figs. 4.4 and 4.5). The normal QRS interval is less than 0.12 s. It is prolonged in various conditions enumerated in Box 4.1.

**Box 4.1 Causes of Wide QRS Complex**
Bundle branch block
WPW syndrome
Intraventricular conduction delay
Idioventricular rhythm
Hyperkalaemia
Ventricular premature beat
Ventricular tachycardia

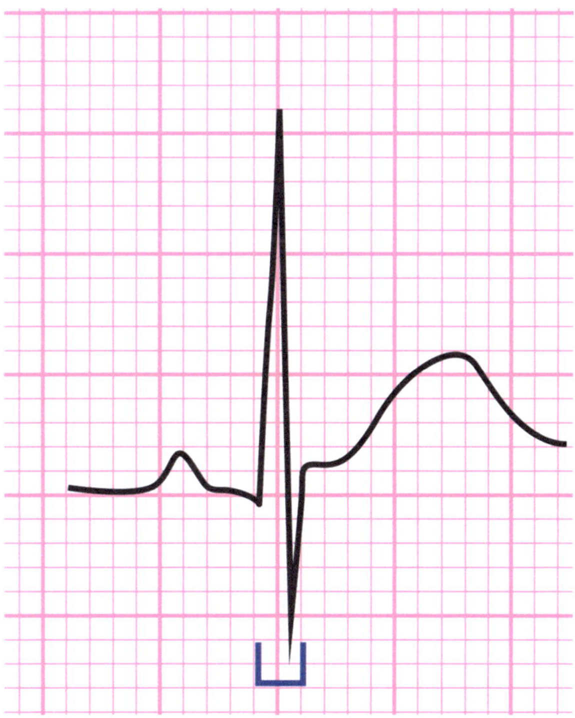

**Fig. 4.4** QRS interval. There are two small boxes between the beginning of R wave to the end of S wave. Hence, the QRS duration is 0.04 s × 2 = 0.08 s

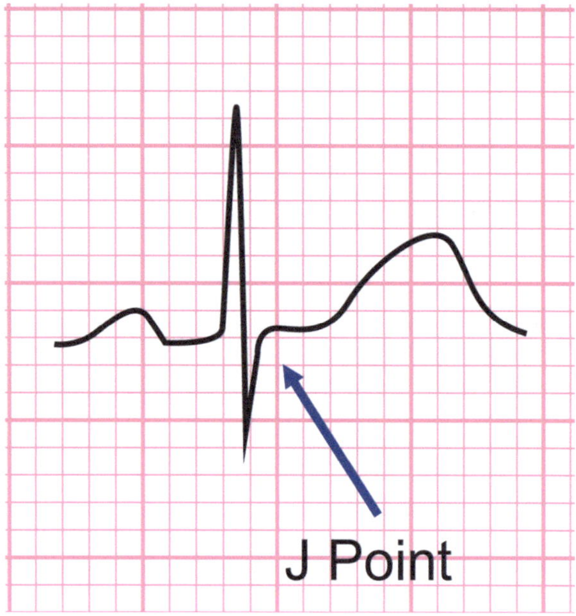


**Fig. 4.5** J point

## 4.6 S-T Segment

S-T segment starts at the end of S wave (J point) and ends at the beginning of T wave (Fig. 4.6). S-T segment is isoelectric. The average duration of the S-T segment is less than 2 to 3 small squares (0.08–0.12 s). It represents ventricular repolarization (phase 2 of repolarization, i.e. plateau phase). 1 mm S-T segment elevation in leads I, II and III and up to 2 mm elevation is normal in some precordial leads (in absence of clinical features of myocardial infarction). S-T segment elevation in only one lead is not diagnostic of any disease.

**Tips and Tricks**

- The shape and deviation of S-T segment help us to diagnose life threatening diseases like myocardial infarction, ischaemia and pericarditis.
- Often a dangerous looking S-T segment may be normal, and the reverse is equally true.
- If S-T segment is elevated, think of myocardial infarction and pericarditis.
- If S-T segment is depressed, think of myocardial ischaemia, ventricular hypertrophy, abnormal intraventricular conduction and digitalis effect.
- Often minor degree of S-T segment deviation in absence of any symptoms is seen in normal healthy persons.

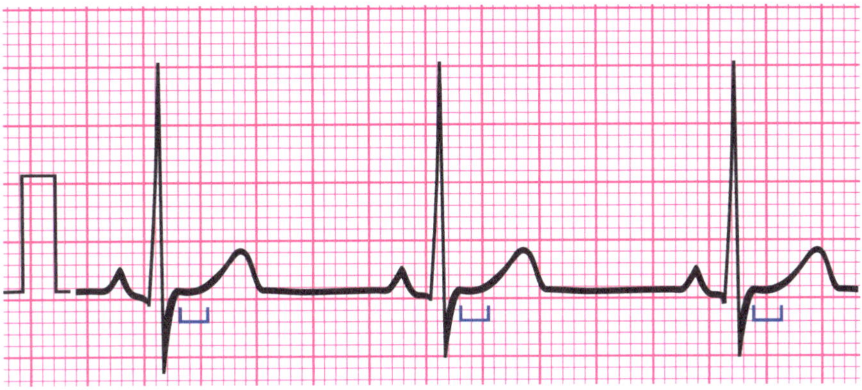

**Fig. 4.6** S-T segment (normal)

## 4.7 Q-T Interval

Q-T interval is calculated from the beginning of Q wave to end of T wave (Fig. 4.7). If Q wave is absent, the Q-T interval is measured from the beginning of R wave to the end of T wave. It represents the duration of ventricular systole, both depolarization and repolarization. Normally, it comprises about 40% of the complete cardiac cycle. Q-T interval varies with heart rate. It prolongs during bradycardia and shortens during tachycardia. Q-T interval corrected for heart rate is called Q-Tc.

Q-Tc = $Q\text{-}T/\sqrt{\text{R-R}}$ interval (Bazett's formula)

The normal range of Q-Tc is 0.35 s to 0.44 s (men) and 0.45 s (women). It is longer in females and in old age. Prolonged Q-T interval (more than about 0.48 s) may lead to a special type of ventricular tachycardia, called Torsades de Pointes.

**Tips and Tricks**

- At heart rate of 60/min, Q-T is the same as Q-Tc.
- Within heart rate of 60–100/min, Q-T interval should not be more than half of R-R interval.

The various causes of abnormal Q-Tc are enumerated in Box 4.2, and the various time intervals are enumerated in Box 4.3.

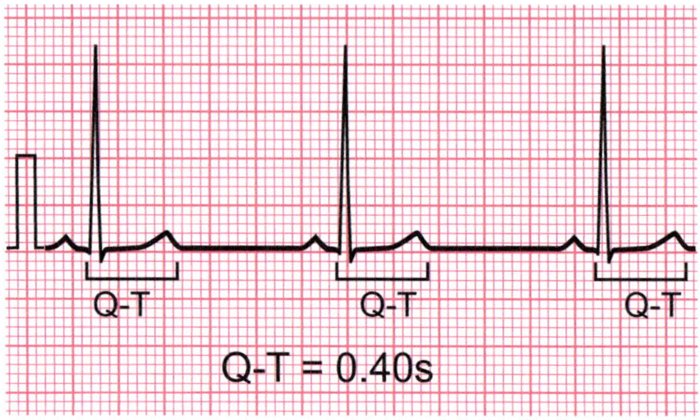


**Fig. 4.7** Q-T interval. There are 10 small boxes between the beginning of q wave to end of T wave. In this ECG the Q-T interval is 10 × 0.4 = 0.40 s

**Box 4.2 Abnormal Q-Tc**

***Prolonged Q-Tc***

Hypocalcaemia
Quinidine and procainamide effect
Acute myocardial infarction
Acute myocarditis
Congenital—Prolonged Q-T syndrome, Romano Ward syndrome
CVA
Torsades de Pointes
Tricyclic antidepressant drugs
Electrolyte imbalance
(a) Hypokalaemia
(b) Hypomagnesaemia
Hypothermia
Deep sleep
Idiopathic

***Shortened Q-Tc***

Hypercalcaemia
Digitalis effect
Hyperthermia
Phenytoin sodium therapy

**Box 4.3 Various Time Intervals**

| | |
|---|---|
| QRS interval | Less than 0.12 s |
| P-R interval | 0.12–0.20 s |
| Q-Tc | 0.35–0.44 s |
| Heart rate | 1500/R-R interval |

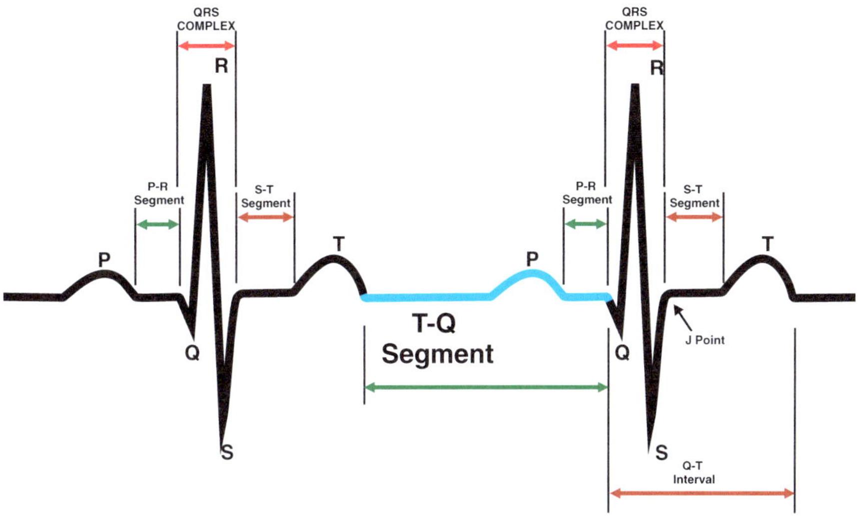


**Fig. 4.8** T-Q segment

## 4.8 T-Q Segment

T-Q segment represents phase 4 of action potential and corresponds to electrical diastole. It starts from the end of T wave to the beginning of the next QRS complex (Fig. 4.8). This segment is used as isoelectric baseline for deviations of J point or S-T segment. However, more precisely it is the T-P segment (end of T wave to beginning of P wave) which is used as isoelectric baseline for measurement of deviations of J point or S-T segment. T-P segment is a part of T-Q segment.

## 4.9 Ventricular Activation Time

The time taken by an impulse to travel from endocardium to epicardium is known as ventricular activation time (VAT). It is also known as time of onset of intrinsicoid deflection. It is calculated from the beginning of Q wave to the peak of the R wave (Fig. 4.9). If Q wave is absent, then it is calculated from the beginning of R wave to the peak of R wave. Normally, it is 0.02 s in lead V1 and 0.04 s in lead V6. VAT increases in ventricular hypertrophy.

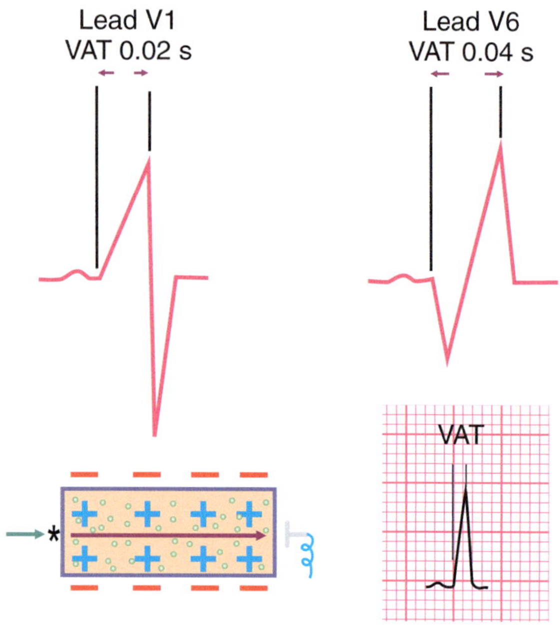


**Fig. 4.9** Ventricular activation time

**Self-Assessment Questions**

1. J point is the junction of Q wave and R wave. True or false?
2. P-P interval helps in calculation of atrial rate. True or false?
3. Prolonged Q-T interval can lead to Torsades de pointes. True or false?
4. R-R interval helps in calculation of ventricular rate. True or false?
5. QRS interval indicates time taken for ventricular repolarization. True or false?
6. **Which of the following is the wrong statement?**

   a. P-R interval is calculated from the beginning of P wave to beginning of R wave.
   b. S-T segment starts from the J point and ends at the beginning of T wave.
   c. Q-T interval starts from the beginning of Q wave to the end of T wave.
   d. Usually, Q-T interval is more than half of R-R interval.

7. **P-R interval is mainly contributed by:**

   a. AV nodal delay b. Ventricular depolarization c. Atrial depolarization d. Ventricular repolarization

8. **S-T segment is used to diagnose:**

   a. First degree heart block b. Heart rate c. WPW syndrome d. Myocardial infarction

9. **Bazett's formula is used to calculate:**

   a. Atrial rate b. Ventricular rate c. Corrected Q-T interval d. P-R interval

10. **Ventricular activation time is increased in:**

    a. Atrial dilatation b. Complete heart block c. Electrolyte disturbance d. Ventricular hypertrophy

**Case Studies**

1. Measure the duration of QRS complex and P-R interval in the ECG of Fig. 4.10.
2. Measure the P-P and R-R intervals in the ECG of Fig. 4.11.
3. Measure the duration of QRS complex and P-R interval in the ECG of Fig. 4.12. Mark the J point by placing arrow.
4. Measure the duration of QRS complex in the ECG of Fig. 4.13. Mark all the waves of the PQRST complex and the S-T segment.

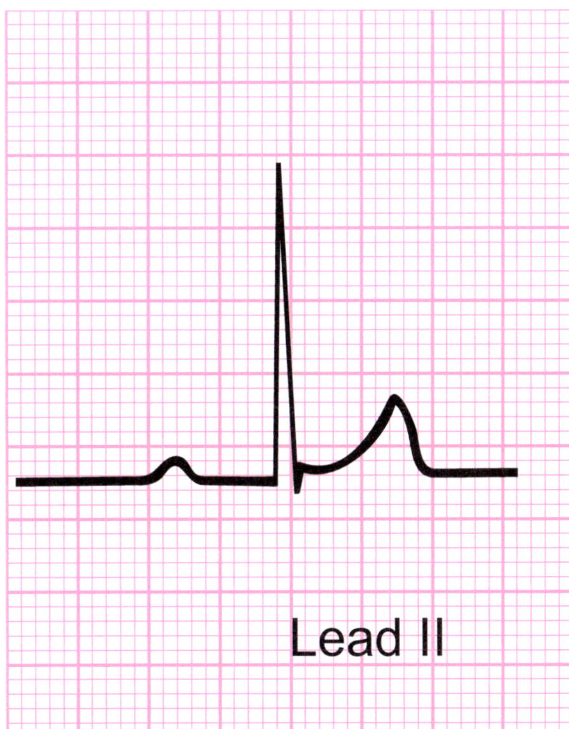


**Fig. 4.10** Measure the duration of QRS complex and P-R interval

5. Measure the Q-T interval in the ECG of Fig. 4.14 and name one important condition where you will get this abnormality.
6. Measure the Q-T interval in the ECG of Fig. 4.15 and name one important condition where you will get this abnormality.

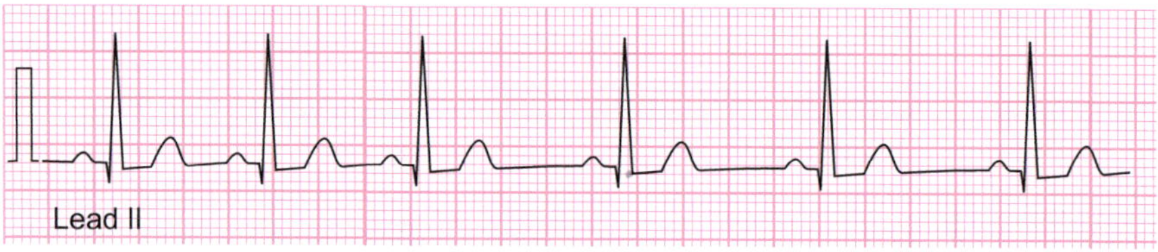


**Fig. 4.11** Measure the P-P and R-R intervals

**Fig. 4.12** Measure the duration of QRS complex and P-R interval and mark the J point

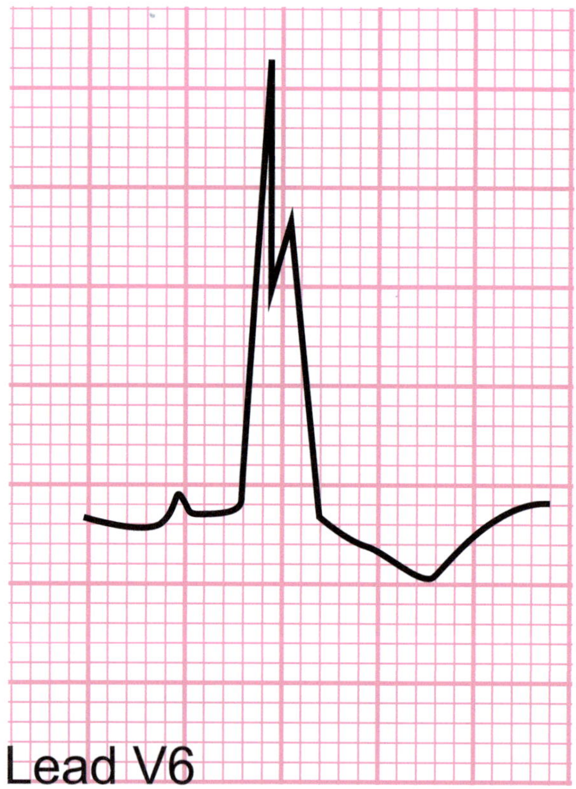

**Fig. 4.13** Measure the duration of QRS complex and mark all the waves

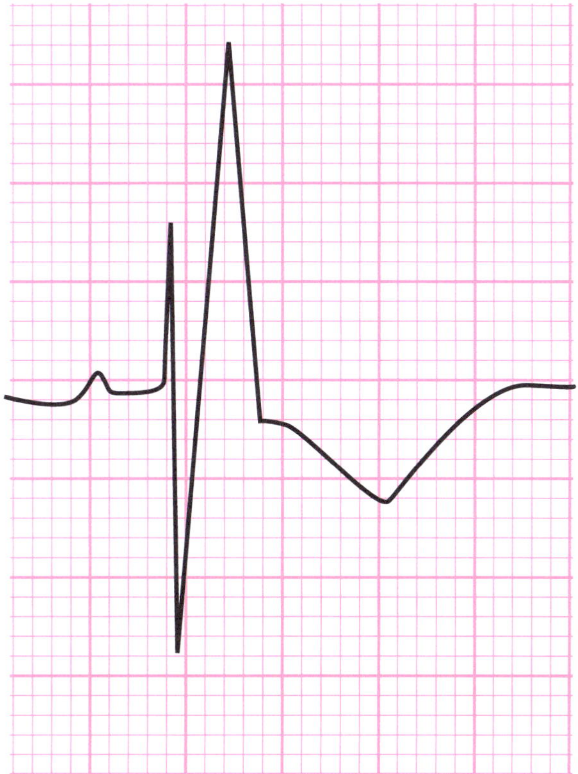

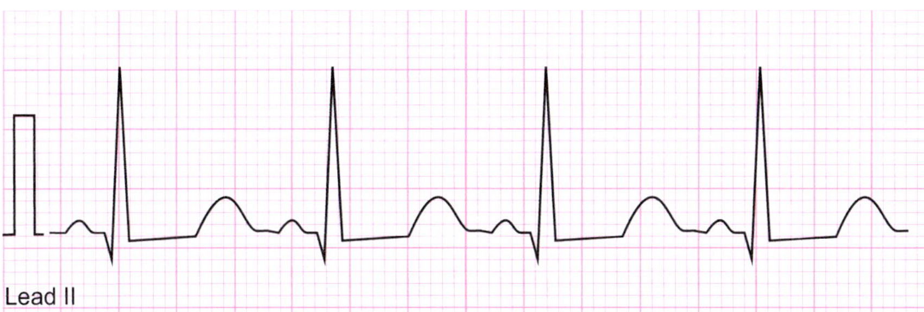


**Fig. 4.14** Measure the Q-T interval

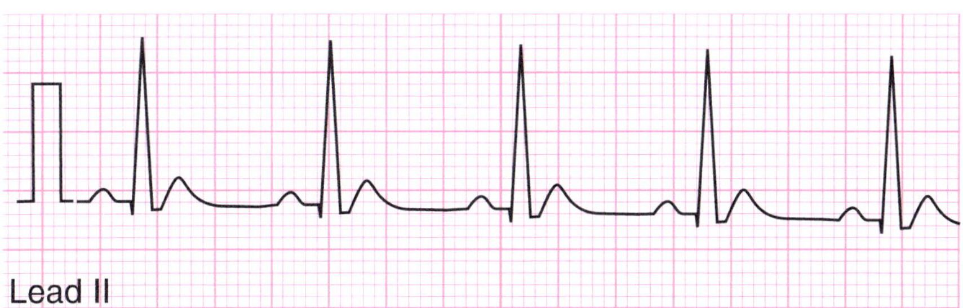


**Fig. 4.15** Measure the Q-T interval

7. A 32-year-old gentleman had an electrocardiogram as part of a medical check-up. Examine his 12-lead ECG given in Fig. 4.16 and answer the following questions:

    a. Calculate the P-R interval.
    b. Calculate the QRS duration.
    c. Is normal sinus rhythm present?
    d. Calculate the Q-T interval.

8. A 28-year-old gentleman got his ECG done during renewal of medical insurance policy. He has no chest pain, palpitation or dyspnoea. He does not smoke or drink alcohol. He is not suffering from hypertension or diabetes. His lipid profile is normal. Examine his 12-lead ECG given in Fig. 4.17 and answer the following questions:

    a. Calculate the P-R interval.
    b. Calculate the QRS duration.
    c. Is normal sinus rhythm present?
    d. What is the shape of the S-T segment?
    e. Calculate the Q-T interval.

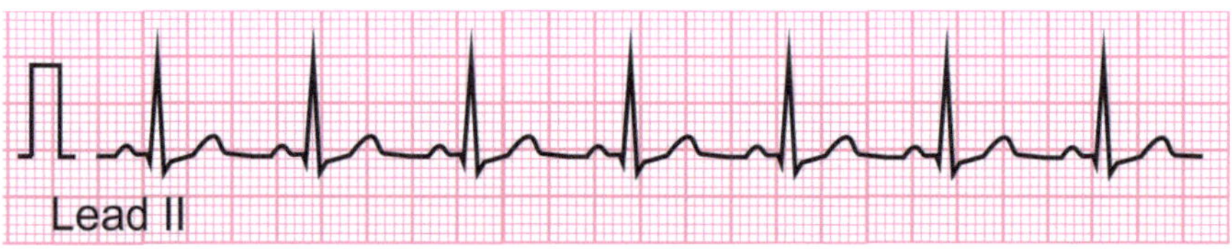


**Fig. 4.16** Calculate the P-R, QRS and Q-T interval

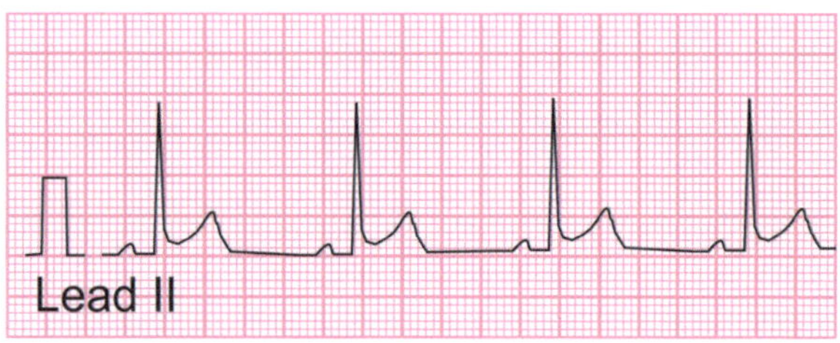


**Fig. 4.17** Calculate the P-R, QRS and Q-T interval. Identify the rhythm

**Answers**

1. False 2. True 3. True 4. True 5. False 6. d 7. a 8. d 9. c 10. d

**Case Studies**

1. The QRS duration (interval) is measured from the beginning of Q wave (R wave in absence of Q wave) to end of S wave. Here, there are two small squares between the beginning R wave (Q wave is absent) and end of s wave (Fig. 4.18). Hence, the QRS duration is 2 × 0.04 s = 0.08 s.

   The P-R interval is 9 × 0.04 s = 0.36 s. This is prolonged P-R interval, also known as first degree heart block.
2. This is a rhythm strip. You must calculate all the P-P and R-R intervals (Fig. 4.19). The first P-P interval is 17 × 0.04 s = 0.68 s.

   The second P-P interval is 17 × 0.04 s = 0.68 s.
   The third P-P interval is 22 × 0.04 s = 0.88 s.
   The fourth P-P interval is 22 × 0.04 s = 0.88 s.
   The fifth P-P interval is 22 × 0.04 s = 0.88 s.
   The first R-R interval is 17 × 0.04 s = 0.68 s.
   The second R-R interval is 17 × 0.04 s = 0.68 s.
   The third R-R interval is 22 × 0.04 s = 0.88 s.
   The fourth R-R interval is 22 × 0.04 s = 0.88 s.

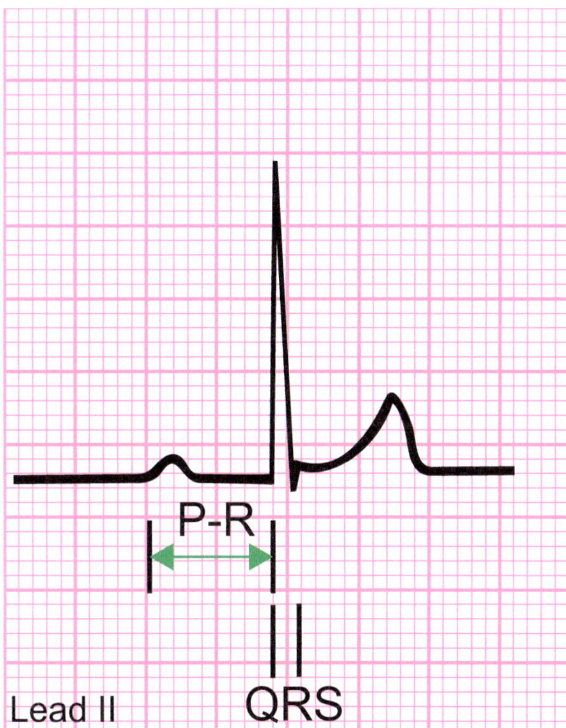


**Fig. 4.18** Answer of Case Study Question 1 (Fig. 4.10)

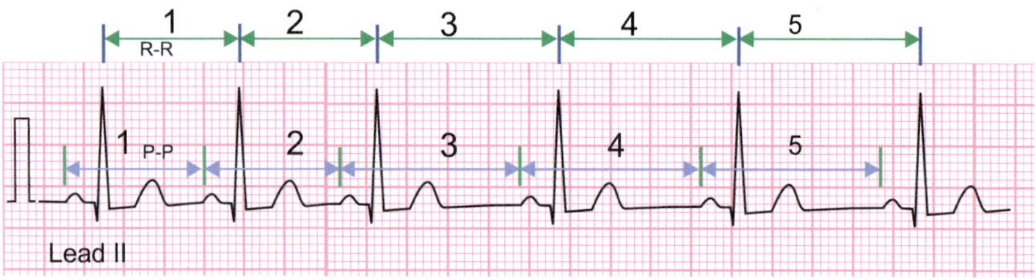


**Fig. 4.19** Answer of Case Study Question 2 (Fig. 4.11)

The fifth R-R interval is 22 × 0.04 s = 0.88 s.

Hence, it can be seen that there is varying R-R intervals (as well as P-P intervals). This is seen in sinus arrhythmia, where the heart rate varies with the various phases of respiration. The most important point to be noted is that one must not stop after calculating only the first P-P and R-R interval. One has to calculate all the intervals. You will read about sinus arrhythmias in Chapter 18.

3. The QRS duration is 4 × 0.04 s = 0.16 s. This is a wide QRS interval. It is seen in bundle branch block. Also note the notch in the descending limb of R wave (Fig. 4.20). The P-R interval is 4 × 0.04 s = 0.16 s. The J point is marked with arrow.

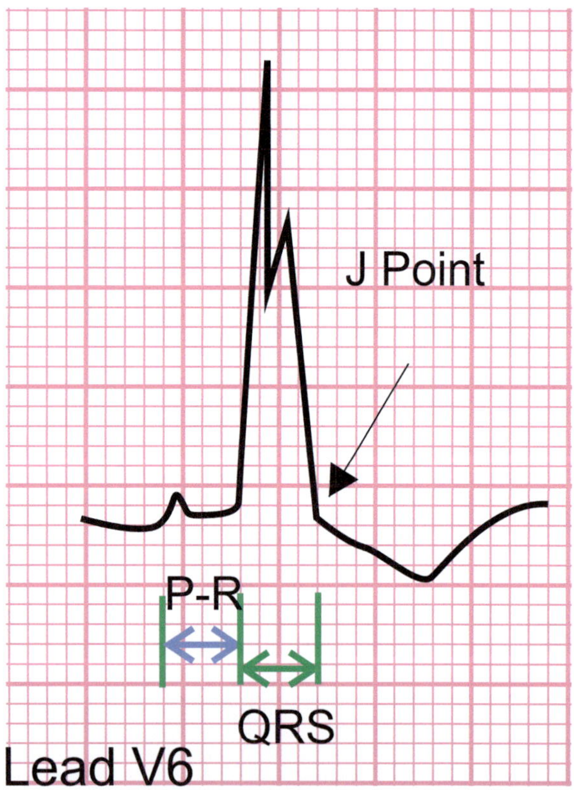


**Fig. 4.20** Answer of Case Study Question 3 (Fig. 4.12)

4. The QRS duration is 5 × 0.04 s = 0.20 s (Fig. 4.21). This is another example of wide QRS interval, which is seen in bundle branch block. Actually this is a RSR' pattern, which is typically seen in bundle branch block.
5. The Q-T interval is 13 × 0.04 s = 0.52 s (Fig. 4.22). This is prolonged Q-T interval. At a glance one can detect, that, Q-T interval is prolonged, because the Q-T interval is more than half of R-R interval (T wave ends closer to next P wave). This condition is typically seen in hypocalcaemia.

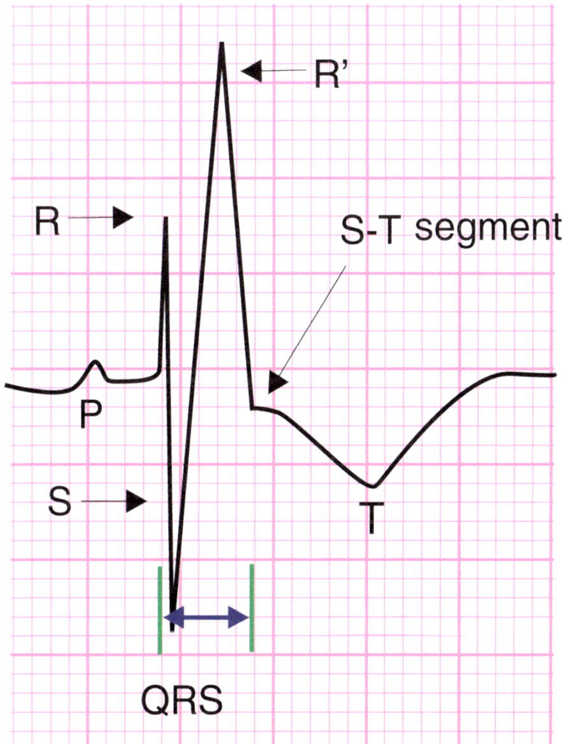


**Fig. 4.21** Answer of Case Study Question 4 (Fig. 4.13)

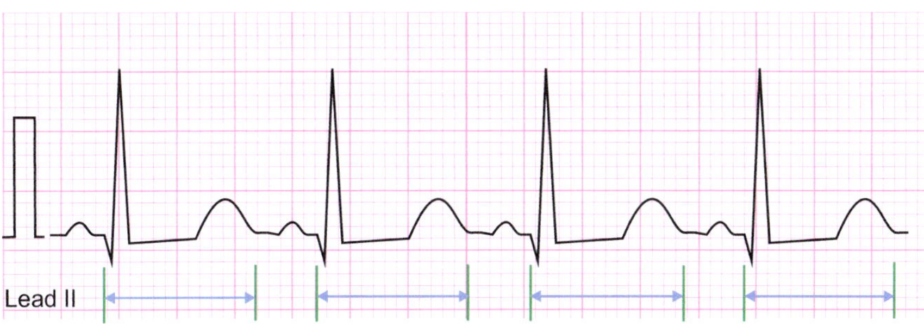


**Fig. 4.22** Answer of Case Study Question 5 (Fig. 4.14)

6. The Q-T interval is 7 × 0.04 s = 0.28 s (Fig. 4.23). This is shortened Q-T interval. At a glance one can detect, that, Q-T interval is shortened, because the Q-T interval is much less than half of R-R interval (T wave ends closer to QRS complex). This condition is typically seen in hypercalcaemia.
7. a. The P-R interval is 3.5 × 0.04 s = 0.14 s.
   b. The QRS duration is 2.5 × 0.04 s = 0.10 s.
   c. P wave: Smooth, round, upright and every P wave is followed by QRS complex. Hence, sinus rhythm is present.
   d. Q-T interval: 9 × 0.04 s = 0.36 s.
8. a. The P-R interval is 4.5 × 0.04 s = 0.18 s.
   b. The QRS duration is 2 × 0.04 s = 0.08 s.
   c. Every QRS complex is preceded by P wave. The P wave is smooth, round and upright. Hence, normal sinus rhythm is present.
   d. The S-T segment is elevated with concavity upwards.
   e. Q-T interval: 9 × 0.04 s = 0.36 s.

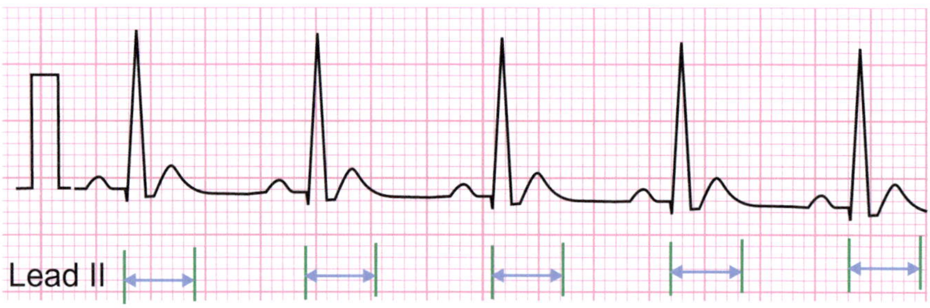


**Fig. 4.23** Answer of Case Study Question 6 (Fig. 4.15)

# Chapter 5
# Calculation of Heart Rate

**Learning Objectives**
After studying this chapter, the reader will learn about:

- Card method of checking cardiac rhythm
- Caliper method of checking cardiac rhythm
- Six second method of calculation of heart rate

Calculation of heart rate in ECG means calculation of ventricular rate. This is done by calculating the number of QRS complexes per minute. Ventricular rate can be calculated from R-R interval and atrial rate can be calculated from P-P interval. In sinus rhythm both are same, but, during arrhythmia they have to be calculated separately. Before proceeding to the actual calculation of heart rate, one must check whether the rhythm is regular or irregular. To check rhythm, two methods are used: card method and caliper method.

## 5.1 Card Method (Paper and Pencil Method)

In card method, the ECG strip is placed on a flat surface. Next, the straight edge of a card is placed along the baseline of the ECG strip. Gradually, the card is moved up near the peak of the R wave and peak of three consecutive R waves is marked on the card. Next, the card is moved and placed over the next three R waves and so on. If the rhythm is regular, the marks on the card will coincide with the peak of the R waves. If the rhythm is irregular, the marks on the card will not coincide with the peak of the R waves.



T. K. Koley, *Rapid Review of ECG*,
https://doi.org/10.1007/978-981-99-9116-7_5

## 5.2 Caliper Method

In this method, the two points of ECG caliper are placed on the peak of two consecutive R waves (Fig. 5.1). This is the R-R interval. Next, by pivoting the first point of the caliper towards the third R wave, it is checked if it falls on the peak of that wave. By proceeding from left to right, the succeeding R-R intervals are checked. If they are all the same, the ventricular rhythm is regular, otherwise irregular.

### *5.2.1 Regular Rhythm*

Heart rate is calculated by calculating the R-R interval in presence of regular rhythm. Heart rate = 1500/R–R interval. This is true when the paper speed is at 25 mm/s. For example, if the R-R interval is 10 (10 smallest squares), then heart rate is 1500/10 = 150 bpm (beats per minute).

There are 5 large squares per second and 300 per minute. Hence, simply count the number of larger squares (5 mm squares) in the R-R interval and divide 300 by the number of bigger squares if the R-R interval is such that the peak of the R wave corresponds with the dark lines on the ECG paper. This is true when the rhythm is regular and paper speed is 25 mm/s (Figs. 5.2 and 5.3). For example, if the number of bigger squares in the R-R interval is 5, then heart rate is 300/5 = 60 bpm.

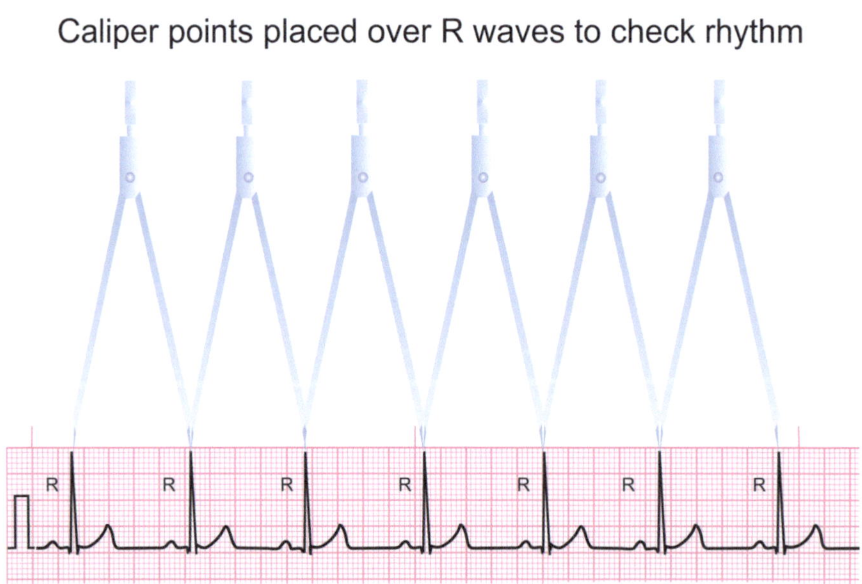


**Fig. 5.1** ECG caliper is used to see regularity of R waves. This helps in checking the rhythm of the ECG waves

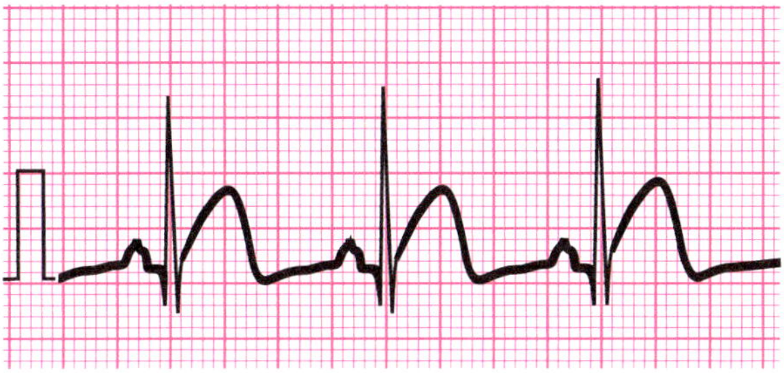

**Fig. 5.2** Calculation of heart rate. In this ECG, the number of small squares between the two successive R waves is 20. Hence, the heart rate (ventricular rate) is 1500 ÷ 20 = 75 bpm. In the other method, the calculation will be 300 ÷ 4 = 75 bpm, because there are four big squares between the two 'R' waves

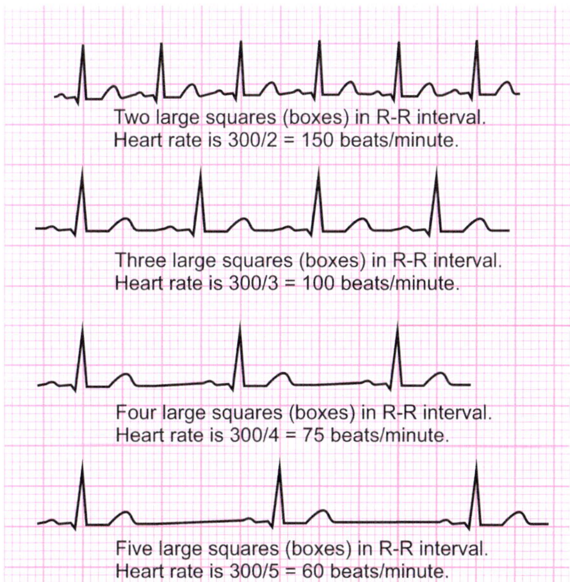


**Fig. 5.3** Calculation of heart rate by counting the number of large squares between two successive R waves

### 5.2.2 *Irregular Rhythm*

During irregular rhythm, rapid rate calculation is done by 6-second method. While using this method, the number of QRS complexes in a 6 second strip (thirty 5 mm squares) is counted, and, then it is multiplied by 10. This will give the heart rate per minute. It is easy to calculate the 6 s period, as majority of the ECG papers are scored with a vertical mark every 3 s (Fig. 5.4). The 6 second strip is equal to 15 cm (at 25 mm/s paper speed, 1 s = 2.5 cm, thus, 6 s = 6 × 2.5 cm = 15 cm). For example, if the number of QRS complexes is 15 in a 6 second strip, heart rate is 15 × 10 = 150 bpm. See Fig. 5.5 also.

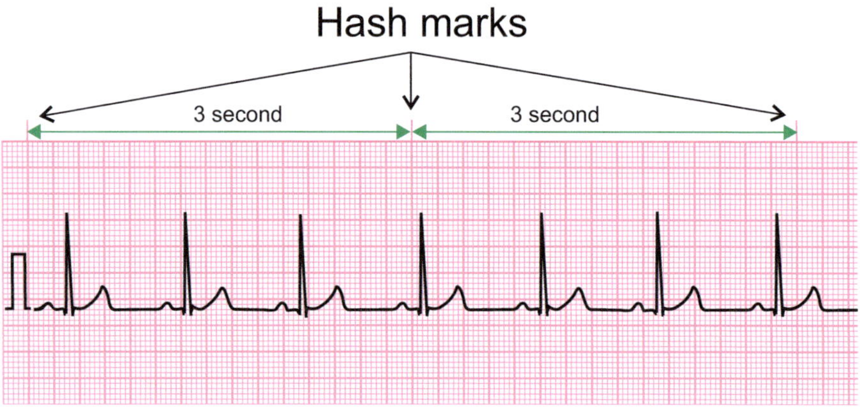


**Fig. 5.4** ECG paper with hash mark at the top of the ECG paper. These hash marks help to mark time. The distance from one hash mark to the next represents 3 s; the distance from the first to the third hash mark represents 6 s. 15 big boxes take up the space between two hash marks

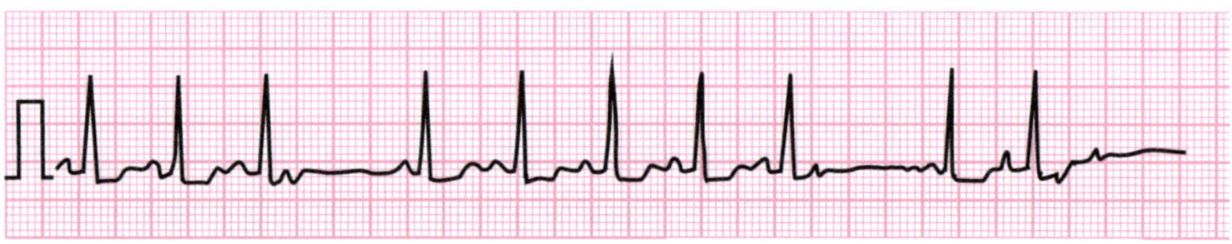

**Fig. 5.5** 6-second method of calculation of heart rate. In this strip, the number of QRS complexes in 6 s (thirty 5 mm squares) is 10. Thus, heart rate is 10 × 10 = 100 bpm

## Tips and Tricks

- First check the R-R interval to determine whether the rhythm is regular or irregular.
- If regular, count the number of small boxes between two R waves and divide 1500 by this number to get the heart rate.
- If irregular, use the 6-second method.

## Self-Assessment Questions

1. The heart rate can be calculated by counting the number of QRS complexes in a 6-second strip of ECG and multiplying it by 10. True or false?
2. The heart rate calculation is affected by irregular heart rhythms such as atrial fibrillation. True or false?
3. The heart rate can also be calculated by dividing 1500 by the number of small squares between two R waves. True or false?
4. If the R-R interval in an ECG is 0.8 s, the heart rate is 75 bpm. True or false?
5. To calculate the heart rate from an ECG, one must count the number of P waves on an ECG strip over a 10-s interval and multiply by 6. True or false?

6. **While calculating heart rate, 300 is divided by:**

    a. The number of large boxes between two R waves, when the R waves fall on the dark vertical lines.
    b. The number of small boxes between two R waves, when the R waves fall on the dark vertical lines.
    c. The number of small boxes between beginning of P wave and end of T wave.
    d. The number of large boxes between beginning of P wave and end of T wave.

7. **While calculating heart rate, by 6-second method, which of the following is multiplied by 10?**

    a. Total number of QRS complexes in 6 s.
    b. Total number of P waves in 6 s.
    c. Total number of P waves and QRS complexes in 6 s.
    d. Total number of T waves in 6 s.

**Case Studies**

1. Calculate the heart rate in the ECG of Fig. 5.6. The paper speed is 25 mm/s and 10 mm = 1 mV.
2. Calculate the heart rate in the ECG of Fig. 5.7. The paper speed is 25 mm/s and 10 mm = 1 mV.
3. Calculate the heart rate in the ECG of Fig. 5.8. The paper speed is 25 mm/s and 10 mm = 1 mV.
4. Calculate the heart rate in the ECG of Fig. 5.9. The paper speed is 25 mm/s and 10 mm = 1 mV.
5. Calculate the heart rate in the ECG of Fig. 5.10. The paper speed is 25 mm/s and 10 mm = 1 mV.

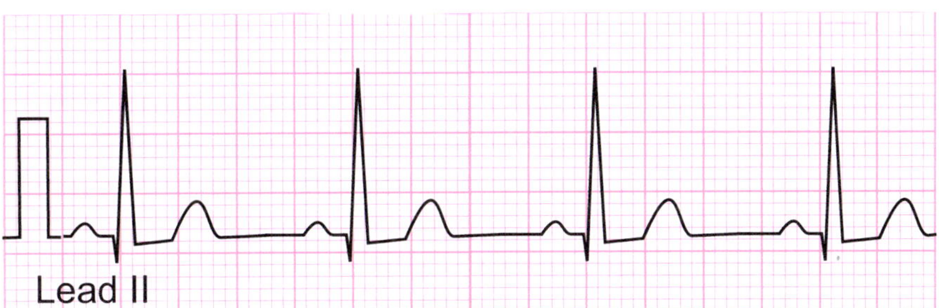


**Fig. 5.6** Calculate the heart rate

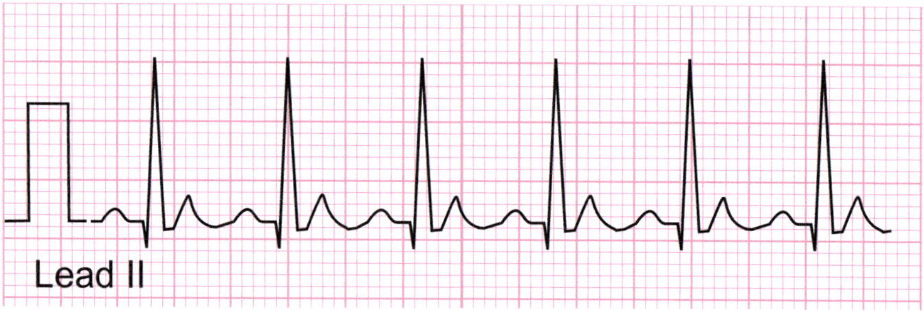


**Fig. 5.7** Calculate the heart rate

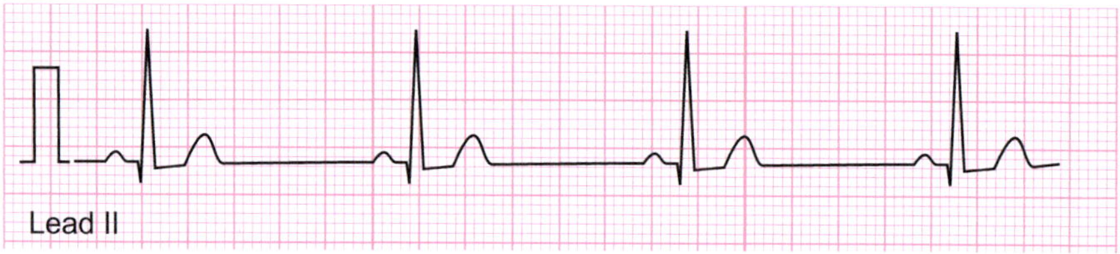


**Fig. 5.8** Calculate the heart rate

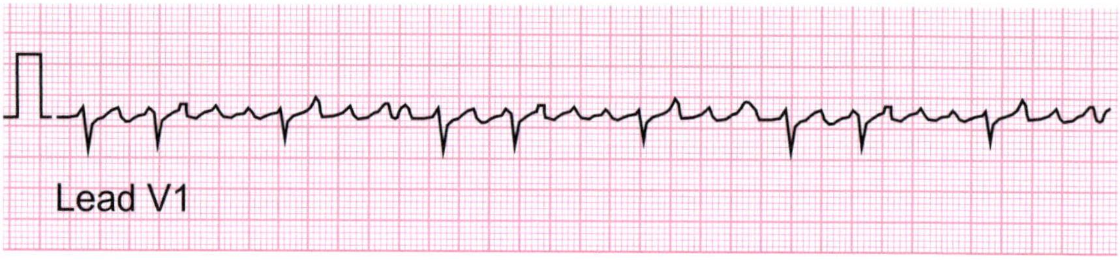


**Fig. 5.9** Calculate the heart rate

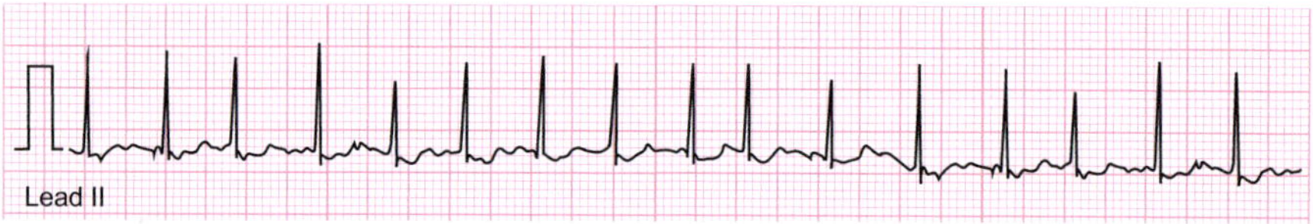


**Fig. 5.10** Calculate the heart rate

**Answers**

1. True 2. True 3. True 4. True 5. False 6. a. 7. a

**Case Studies**

1. Figure 5.6 is a rhythm strip. To calculate the heart rate, first check whether the rhythm is regular or irregular. In this strip, the rhythm is regular (R-R intervals are equal).

   Next, calculate the number of small squares between two successive R waves. Here, the number of small squares is 20.

   Next, divide 1500 by 20 to get the heart rate per minute, i.e. 1500 ÷ 20 = 75 bpm. This is normal heart rate.
2. Figure 5.7 is another rhythm strip. First check the regularity of the rhythm. In this strip, the rhythm is regular and the number of small squares is 11.5 between two successive R waves. Next, divide 1500 by 11.5 to get the heart rate per minute, i.e. 1500 ÷ 11.5 = 130.43 bpm. This may be considered as heart rate 130 bpm.
3. Figure 5.8 is also a rhythm strip. To calculate the heart rate, the first step is to check the regularity of the rhythm. In this strip, the rhythm is regular (equal R-R intervals) and the number of small squares is 29 between two successive R waves. Next, divide 1500 by 29 to get the heart rate per minute, i.e. 1500 ÷ 29 = 51.72 bpm. This may be considered as heart rate 52 bpm.
4. Figure 5.9 is a rhythm strip as well. Here also at the first step check the regularity of the complexes. In this strip, the rhythm is irregular (unequal R-R intervals). Hence, you have to use the 6-second method. Look at the hash marks present at the top of the ECG paper at intervals of 15 big squares. This is a 3 s interval. So to get a 6 s interval, you have to consider three hash marks, which in turn mean 30 big squares. Next, calculate the number of QRS complexes in these 30 big squares. In this strip, there are 8 QRS complexes inside the 30 big squares. Carefully note that the ninth QRS complex is beyond the third hash mark. The next step is to multiply the number of QRS complexes by 10 to get the heart rate per minute. Hence, the heart rate is 8 × 10 = 80 bpm.
5. To calculate the heart rate in the rhythm strip given in Fig. 5.10, first check the regularity of the QRS complexes. Here, the rhythm is irregular (unequal R-R interval). Hence you have to use the 6-second method. The number of QRS complexes in the 6 s interval is 16. Hence, the heart rate is 16 × 10 = 160 bpm.

# Chapter 6
# Rotation of Heart

**Learning Objectives**

After studying this chapter, the reader will learn about:

- Vertical position of heart
- Horizontal position of heart
- Intermediate position of heart
- Clockwise rotation of heart
- Anticlockwise rotation of heart

Rotation of heart refers to rotation of the electrical forces. There is no anatomical rotation. Theoretically, the heart rotates along two axes: the anteroposterior axis and the longitudinal axis. Rotation around the anteroposterior axis reflects the rotation along the frontal plane, whereas rotation around the longitudinal axis reflects rotation in the horizontal plane.

## 6.1 Rotation Around the Anteroposterior Axis

The rotation of electrical forces of heart across an anteroposterior axis, that runs through the interventricular septum from anterior to the posterior surface of the heart, leads to three different positions of heart:

- Vertical position
- Horizontal position
- Intermediate position


T. K. Koley, *Rapid Review of ECG*,
https://doi.org/10.1007/978-981-99-9116-7_6

### 6.1.1 Vertical Position

The depolarization wavefront of ventricles is directed mainly downward in vertical position of the heart. Left ventricular complex (qR type of complex) is recorded in lead aVF, as the positive pole of lead aVF is oriented exactly vertically downward. Hence, PQRS complex of lead aVF resembles that of lead V6 (Figs. 6.1 and 6.2). The mean QRS axis is directed inferiorly (+75° or more). This is commonly seen in tall and thin persons.

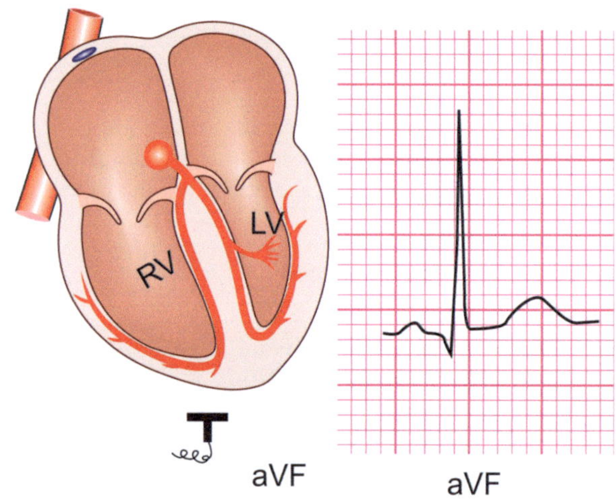


**Fig. 6.1** Diagram of vertical heart. RV, right ventricle; LV, left ventricle

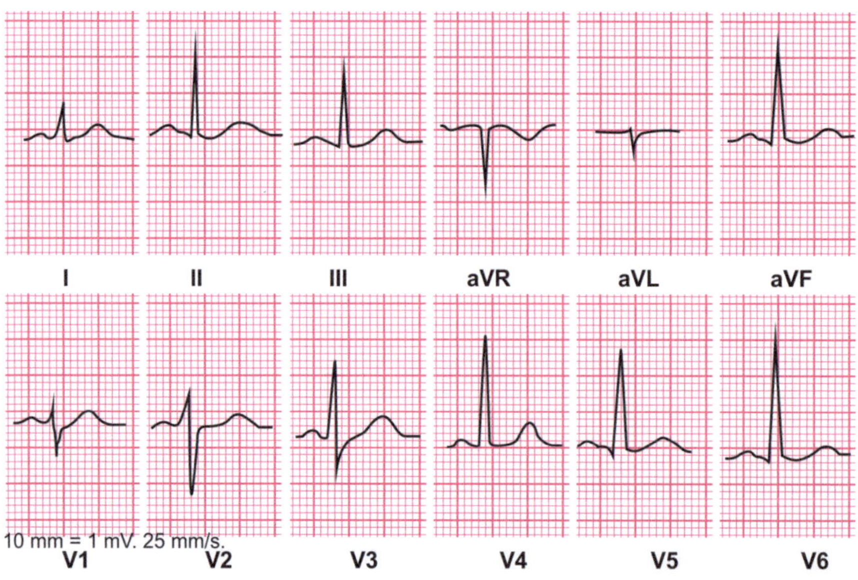


**Fig. 6.2** ECG of vertical heart position. QRS complex of aVF resembles that of V6

### 6.1.2 Horizontal Position

The depolarization wavefront of ventricles is directed mainly horizontally and to the left in horizontal position of heart. Left ventricular complex (qR type of complex) is recorded in leads I and aVL, as the positive poles of these leads are directed horizontally and to the left. The QRS complexes in leads I and aVL resemble that of lead V6 (Figs. 6.3 and 6.4). The mean QRS axis is between 0° and −30°. Horizontal position of heart is seen in obese persons with broad chests.

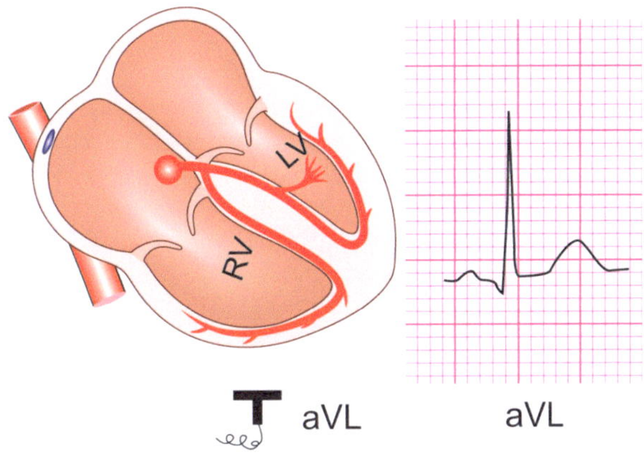


**Fig. 6.3** Diagram of horizontal heart

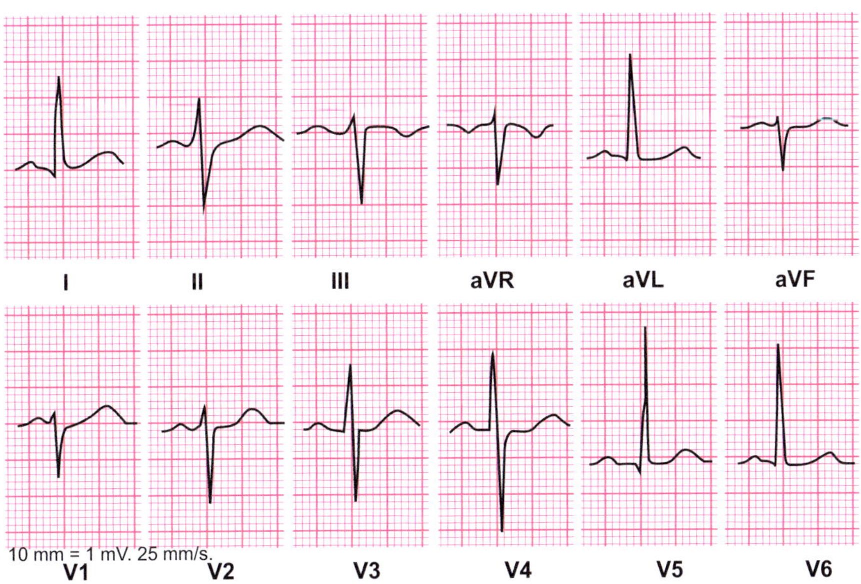


**Fig. 6.4** ECG showing horizontal position of heart. PQRS complex of lead aVL resembles that of lead V6

### 6.1.3 Intermediate Position

Intermediate position of heart is midway between the vertical and horizontal position. In this condition, QRS complexes of both lead aVL and lead aVF resemble that of lead V6 (Fig. 6.5). The mean QRS axis is approximately +30°.

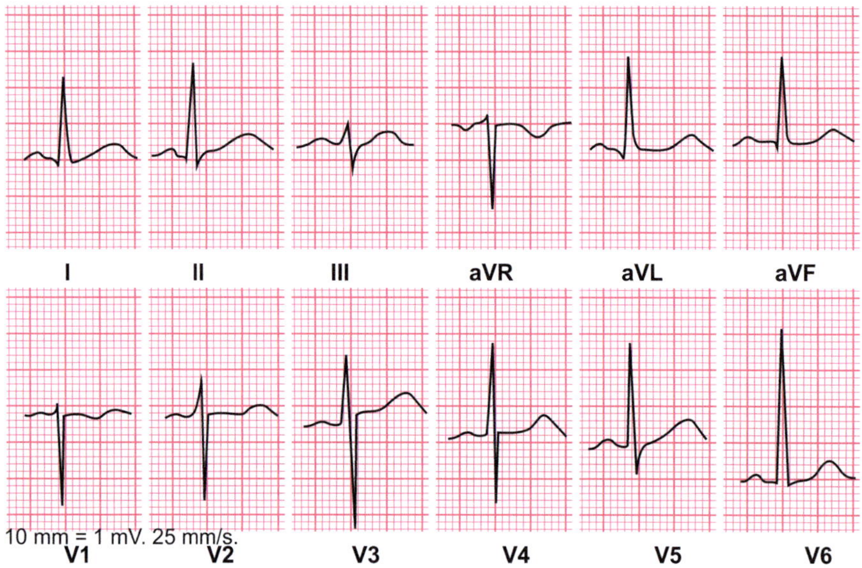


**Fig. 6.5** ECG showing intermediate position of heart. PQRS complex of both lead aVL and lead aVF resembles that of lead V6

**Tips and Tricks**

- If PQRS complex in lead aVF resembles that of lead V6, it is vertical heart.
- If PQRS complex in lead aVL resembles that of lead V6, it is horizontal heart.
- If PQRS complex in lead aVF and aVL both resemble that of lead V6, it is intermediate heart.

## 6.2 Rotation Around the Longitudinal Axis

The longitudinal axis of heart runs through the interventricular septum from apex to the base. Rotation is conventionally viewed from below the heart (through the diaphragm) looking upwards. Rotation around this axis results in clockwise and counterclockwise rotation (Fig. 6.6).

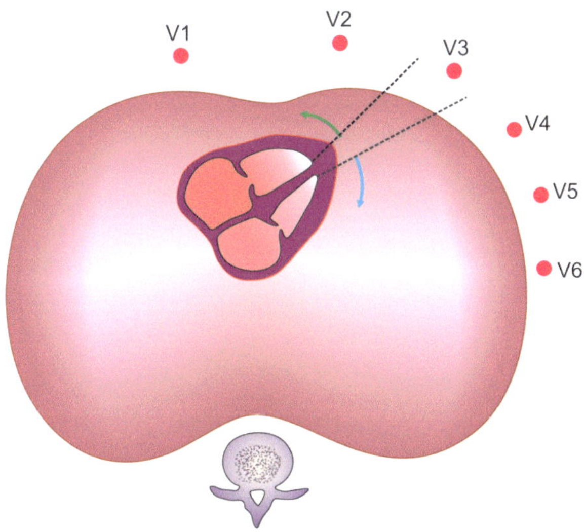


**Fig. 6.6** Diagram showing rotation of heart. Rotation along green coloured arrow leads to counterclockwise rotation, and rotation along blue coloured arrow leads to clockwise rotation. Look at heart from foot end (through the diaphragm)

### 6.2.1 Clockwise Rotation

During clockwise rotation, the right ventricle is thought to come anteriorly and the interventricular septum becomes parallel to the chest wall. As a result, most of the chest leads will record a rS or RS complex, and the transition zone will shift to lead V5 or V6 (Fig. 6.7). However, no such anatomical change occurs. There is merely the deviation of the electrical forces.

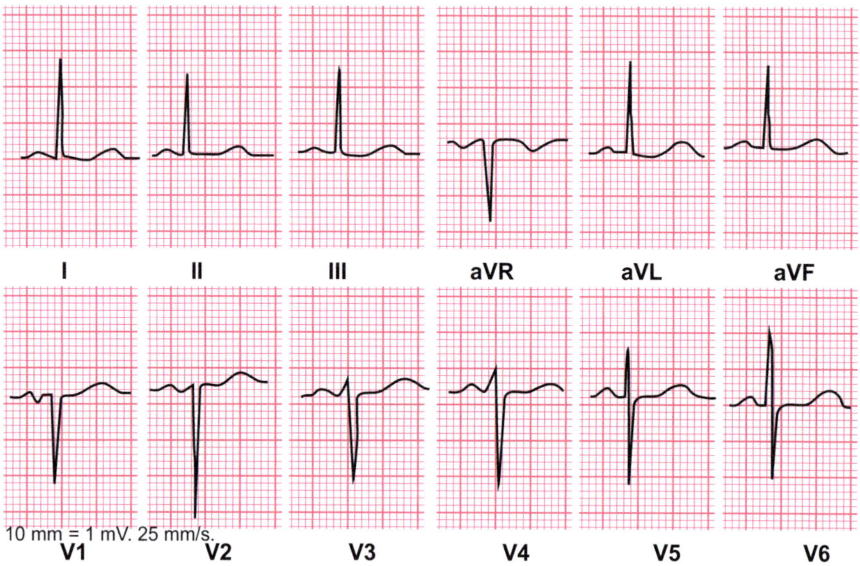


**Fig. 6.7** ECG of clockwise rotation of heart. Transition zone is shifted to lead V5 in which the height of R wave and the depth of S wave are more or less equal

### *6.2.2 Counterclockwise Rotation*

Counterclockwise rotation brings the left ventricle more anteriorly. As a result, the changes will be opposite to that described in clockwise rotation. The transition zone is shifted to lead V1 or V2 (Fig. 6.8).

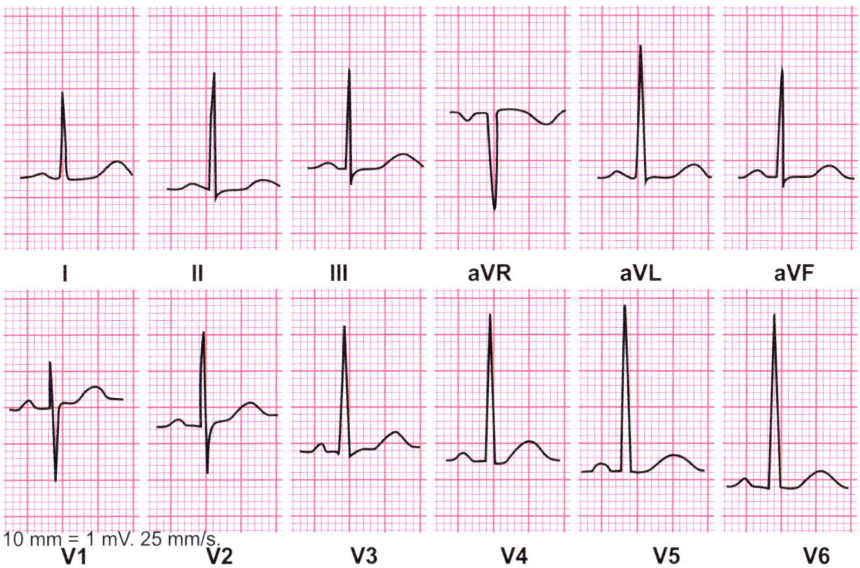


**Fig. 6.8** ECG showing counterclockwise rotation of heart. Transition zone is shifted to lead V1 in which the height of R wave and the depth of S wave are more or less equal

**Tips and Tricks**

- RS complex in lead V5 or V6 indicates clockwise rotation of heart.
- RS complex in lead V1 or V2 indicates counterclockwise rotation of heart.

**Self-Assessment Questions**

1. The vertical position of the heart can affect the amplitude and duration of the QRS complex on an ECG. True or false?
2. The horizontal position of the heart does not affect the timing of the P wave on an ECG. True or false?
3. In counterclockwise rotation, the transition zone shifts to lead V1. True or false?
4. A vertical heart position can cause a rightward shift of the QRS axis on an ECG. True or false?
5. A horizontal heart position can cause a leftward shift of the QRS axis on an ECG. True or false?

**Answers**

1. True 2. True 3. True 4. False 5. True

# Chapter 7
# Electrical Axis

**Learning Objective**
After studying this chapter, the reader will learn about:

- Axial reference system
- Basic concept of mean QRS axis
- Calculation of QRS axis

It is often very difficult, for a beginner, to understand the concept of electrical axis. However, it becomes easy, if the basic aspects of the leads and generation of waves and complexes are understood well. Electrical axis means the direction of the net electrical force of the heart. Mean QRS axis represents the overall direction in which the wave of ventricular depolarization travels.

Ventricular activation starts at the upper part of the interventricular septum. From left to right, a small initial electric wavefront (vector) is generated. Next the free walls of the ventricles are activated, generating a series of vectors that vary in magnitude and direction. These vectors add up if they are in the same direction and cancel each other if they are in opposite direction. They may increase or decrease in size and change direction if they are at an angle to each other (Fig. 7.1). The vectors, exactly opposite to each other and of equal magnitude, neutralize each other totally. The larger vectors dominate and, because of maximum muscle mass, the largest electric force is produced close to the apex of the left ventricle and adjacent wall of the left ventricle. It is directed mainly to the left and downwards. The mean vector is the dominant vector, out of all these multiple vectors and the direction of the mean vector is called the mean QRS axis (Fig. 7.2).



T. K. Koley, *Rapid Review of ECG*,
https://doi.org/10.1007/978-981-99-9116-7_7

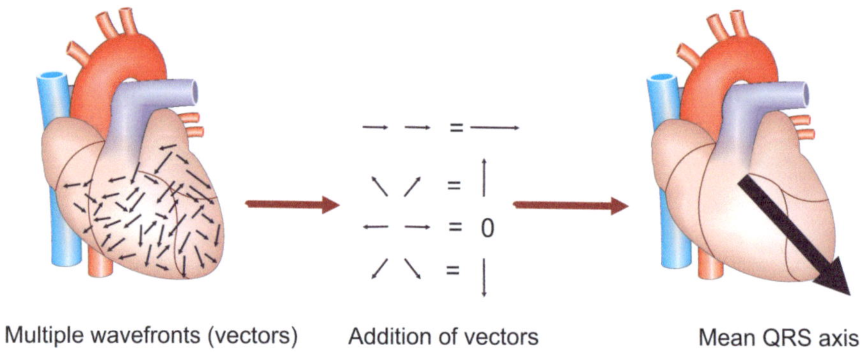


**Fig. 7.1** Genesis of mean QRS axis. Multiple wavefronts (vectors) generated during ventricular depolarization add up and the resultant mean vector is equal to the mean QRS axis

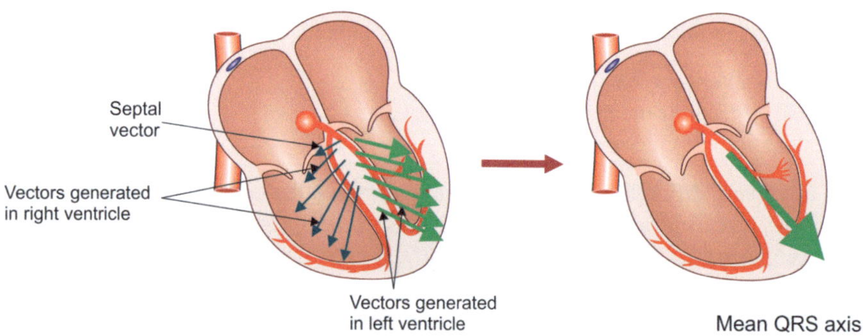


**Fig. 7.2** Mean QRS axis. The first vector generated is the septal vector at the top of the interventricular septum. After this, numerous vectors are generated in both the ventricles (green in left ventricle and blue in right ventricle). The vectors generated in left ventricle are dominant vectors which neutralize the vectors generated in right ventricle. The direction of the mean vector is the mean QRS axis

## 7.1 Axial Reference System

### *7.1.1 Triaxial Reference System*

The three standard limb lead axes are aligned in a way, that they form an equilateral triangle with the heart at its centre. This is known as Einthoven's triangle. By redrawing the lead axes (the three axes are passing through a common point), a triaxial reference system can be constituted with each axis separated from the other by 60° (Fig. 7.3). However, the polarity and the orientation of the lead axes are not changed.

Similarly, another triaxial reference system is constituted by the three lead axes of the augmented unipolar leads (Fig. 7.4).

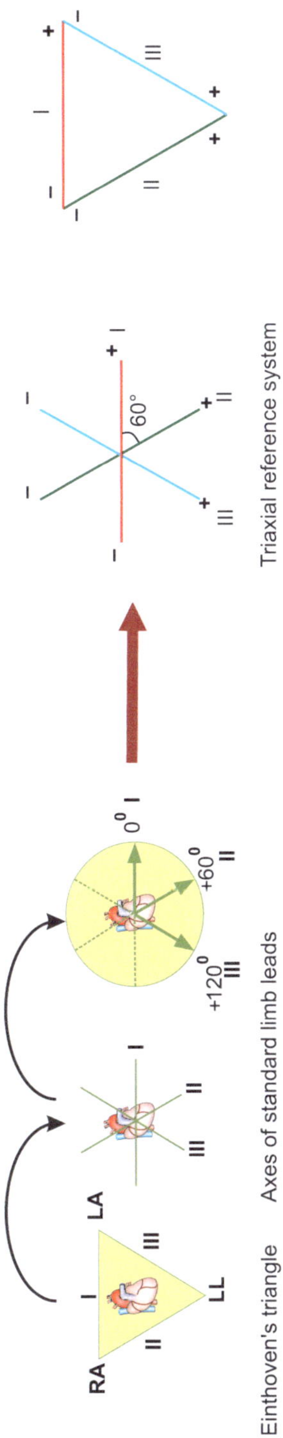


**Fig. 7.3** Diagram showing triaxial reference system formed by axes of standard limb leads

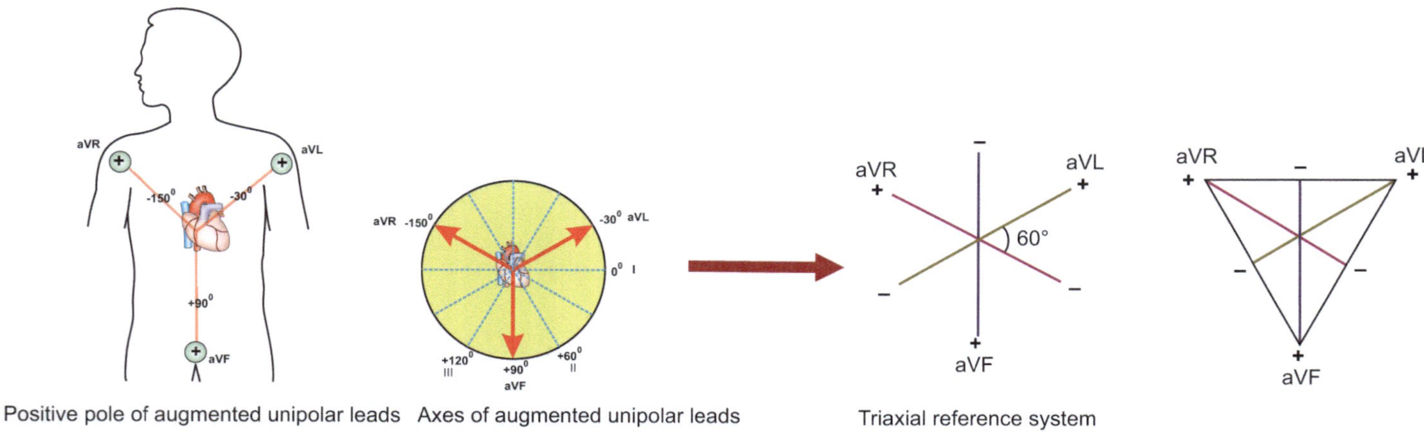


**Fig. 7.4** Diagram showing triaxial reference system formed by axes of augmented limb leads

### 7.1.2 *Hexaxial Reference System*

The hexaxial reference system is constituted and the lead axes are separated from each other by 30° (Fig. 7.5) by combining and superimposing the two triaxial reference system. In this reference system, all the lead axes maintain their polarity and direction. By convention, all the degrees in the lower half are labelled as positive (0° to +180°) and all the degrees in the upper half are labelled negative degrees (0° to −180°). It is very important to understand some basic facts before we move onto the actual calculation of the QRS axis.

## 7.2 Basic Concept of QRS Axis

- The QRS axis is expressed in the form of degrees on the hexaxial reference system and it represents the mean direction of the electrical force on the frontal plane.
- An electrical force traveling perpendicular to a lead produces nil or equiphasic deflection in that lead and when the electrical force travels parallel to a lead it produces maximum deflection in that lead. For example, if the QRS axis is 0°, then the maximum deflection will be seen in lead I and least deflection is recorded in lead aVF which is at right angle to lead I (Fig. 7.5). Keep in mind that lead I and lead aVF are perpendicular to each other. Similarly, lead II and lead aVL are perpendicular to each other, and lead III and lead aVR are perpendicular to each other.
- In the lead showing the maximum deflection, the axis corresponds to the major deflection in that lead. For example, if in lead II the major deflection is positive, then the axis is towards +60°. See Fig. 7.5 and note that the positive pole of the lead II axis points to +60°. Similarly if the major deflection in lead aVF is −7 mm, then the axis is −90°. See Fig. 7.5 and note that the negative pole of the lead aVF axis points to −90°.
- The net or resultant deflection in any lead is the algebraic sum of the positive and negative deflection in that lead. For example, if in lead I the height of R wave is 10 mm (+10) and the depth of S wave is 4 mm (−4), then the net deflection is +10 + (−4) = +6.

The mean QRS vector points downwards and to the left. It is aligned to the direction of current flow, from base of heart towards the apex. Thus, it can be observed that the direction is towards +40° to +60° if we take into account the hexaxial reference system. This is towards the positive pole of lead II (Fig. 7.6). This in turn means the deflection in lead II will be upward (positive) and R wave will be recorded in lead II.

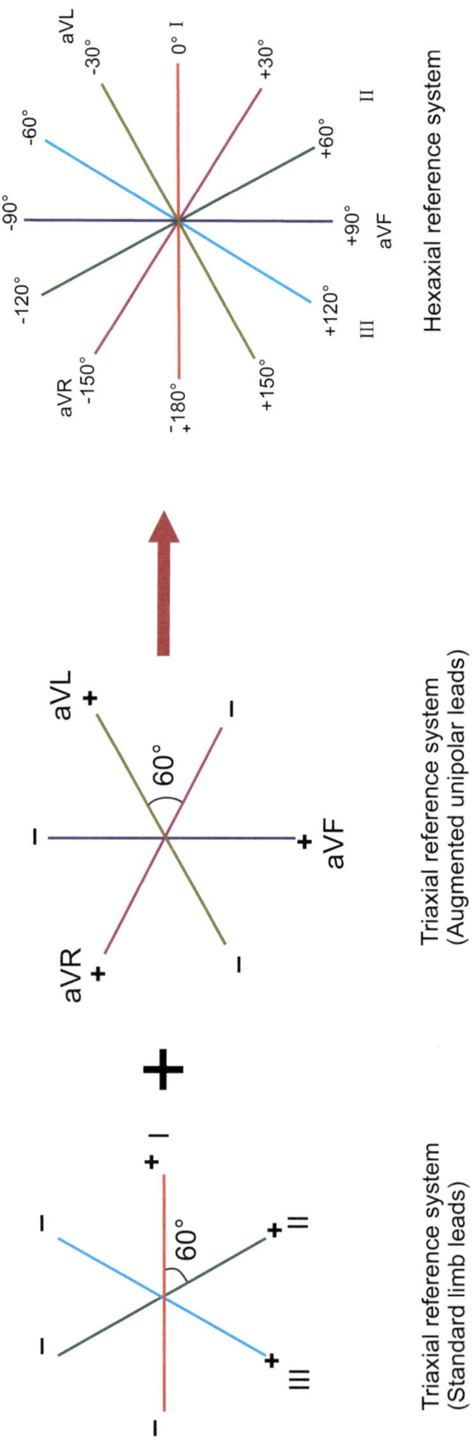


**Fig. 7.5** Diagram showing hexaxial reference system formed by combination of two triaxial reference systems

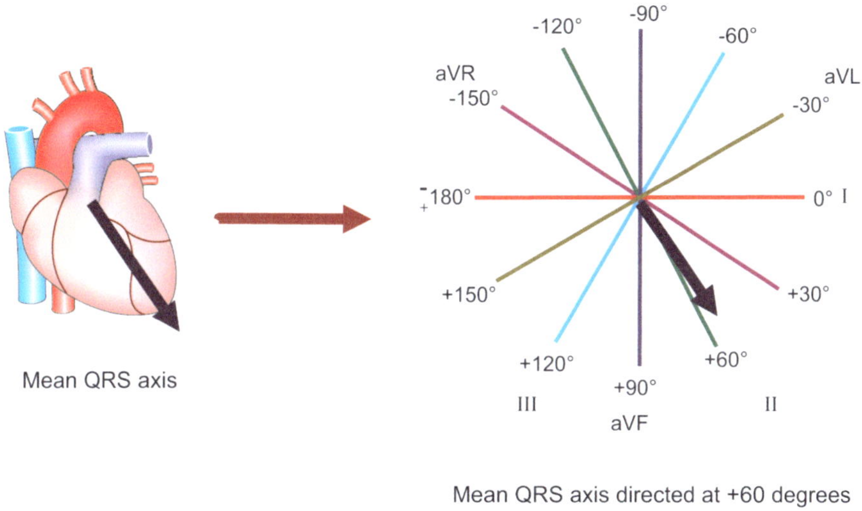


**Fig. 7.6** Mean QRS axis is directed towards positive pole of lead II (+60°)

## 7.3 Calculation of QRS Axis

No unanimity exists on the range of normal QRS axes. It has been described as between 0° and +90° by many authors, while some others have taken the view that it ranges from −30° to +110°. In this book, the normal range of QRS axis will be considered as −30° to +90° (Fig. 7.7). In most of the cases, the normal axis lies between +40° and +60°.

QRS axis beyond the normal range indicates deviation of electrical axis. QRS axis beyond −30° (more negative, anticlockwise) is called left axis deviation (LAD), and if it lies beyond +90° (more positive, clockwise), it is called right axis deviation (RAD) (Fig. 7.8). If the QRS axis happens to fall between −90° and 180°, this would be referred to as extreme axis deviation or northwest axis whereby the ventricular vector is directed upward and to the right. Axis in northwest region is very rare. It may be a manifestation of extreme right or left axis deviation.

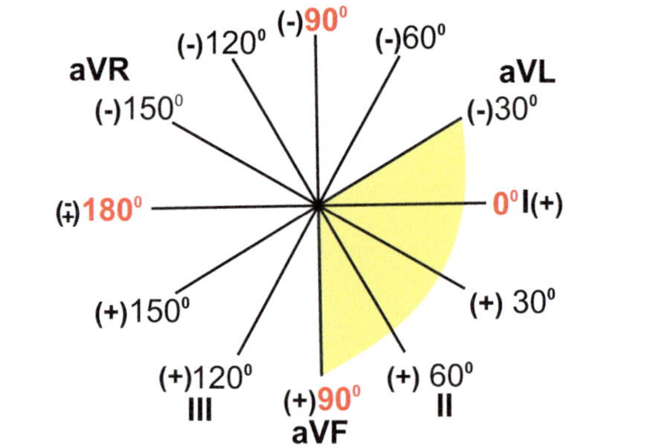


**Fig. 7.7** Normal QRS axis. The area shaded light green is the normal QRS axis, which is directed between −30° and +90°

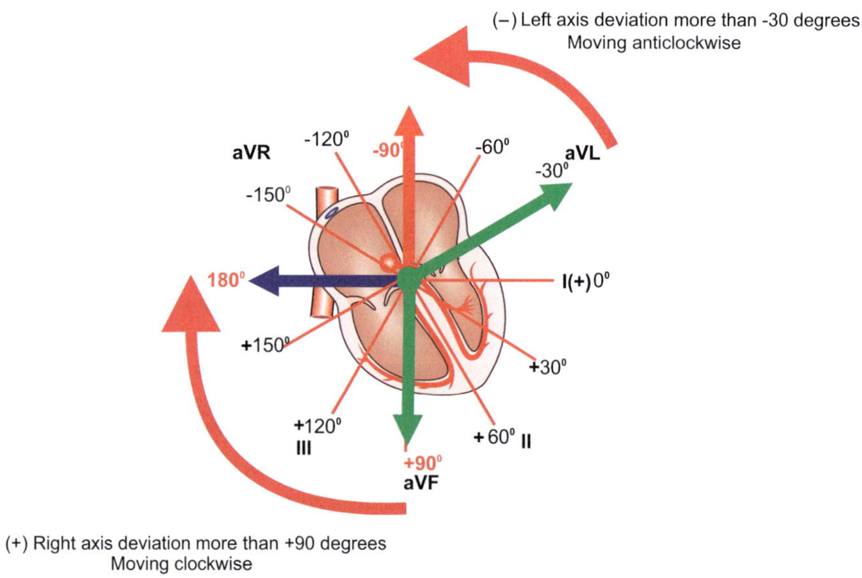


**Fig. 7.8** Axis deviation. In right axis deviation QRS axis is in between +90° and +180° and in left axis deviation the QRS axis is in between −30° and −90°

## Tips and Tricks

- Minor degrees of axis deviation is common in tall thin persons as well as in short obese persons.
- One should look for hypertrophy of ventricles, conduction defect and pulmonary embolism if an axis deviation is present.

Hexaxial reference system is used for calculation of QRS axis. Out of several methods described in various books, some of which are confusing for beginners, only two simple methods will be described here.

### 7.3.1 Method 1

The first method is the quadrant approach or two-lead method. A rough estimation of the QRS axis can be obtained by this rapid method. This method is for the beginners, for whom it is important to determine whether the QRS axis is in normal range or not. In this method, the dominant QRS deflections in lead I and lead aVF are considered. After this the interpretation is as follows (Fig. 7.9):

| Lead I | Lead aVF | QRS axis |
|---|---|---|
| Positive (R wave) | Positive (R wave) | Normal (−30° to +90°) |
| Negative (S wave) | Positive (R wave) | Right axis (+90° to +180°) |
| Positive (R wave) | Negative (S wave) | Left axis (−30° to −90°) |
| Negative (S wave) | Negative (S wave) | Northwest axis (−90° to −180°) |

The main drawback of this method is it only gives a close approximation to the true axis. It narrows the normal axis range. This can result in an inaccurate interpretation of the true electrical axis. For example, if using this approach with a positive lead I and negative lead aVF, the axis would be interpreted as left axis deviation. However, if the true axis were −10°, it would still be within the normal axis range. In spite of this drawback, this method is easy to learn and sufficient in most cases.

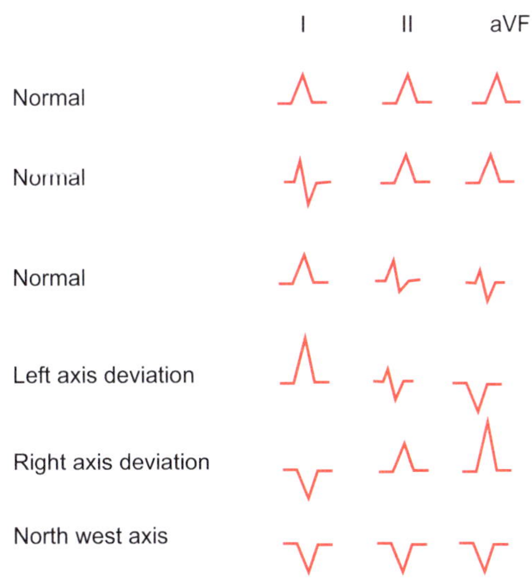


**Fig. 7.9** Method 1 of QRS axis determination

### 7.3.2 *Method 2*

This is a more precise method of calculation of QRS axis. In the methods described above, axis calculation is an estimate or near approximation. Generally, further accuracy is not clinically significant, yet, it is always important to know the precise calculation to gain complete understanding about QRS axis calculation.

The following steps are to be followed to calculate the QRS axis of the ECG shown in Fig. 7.10.

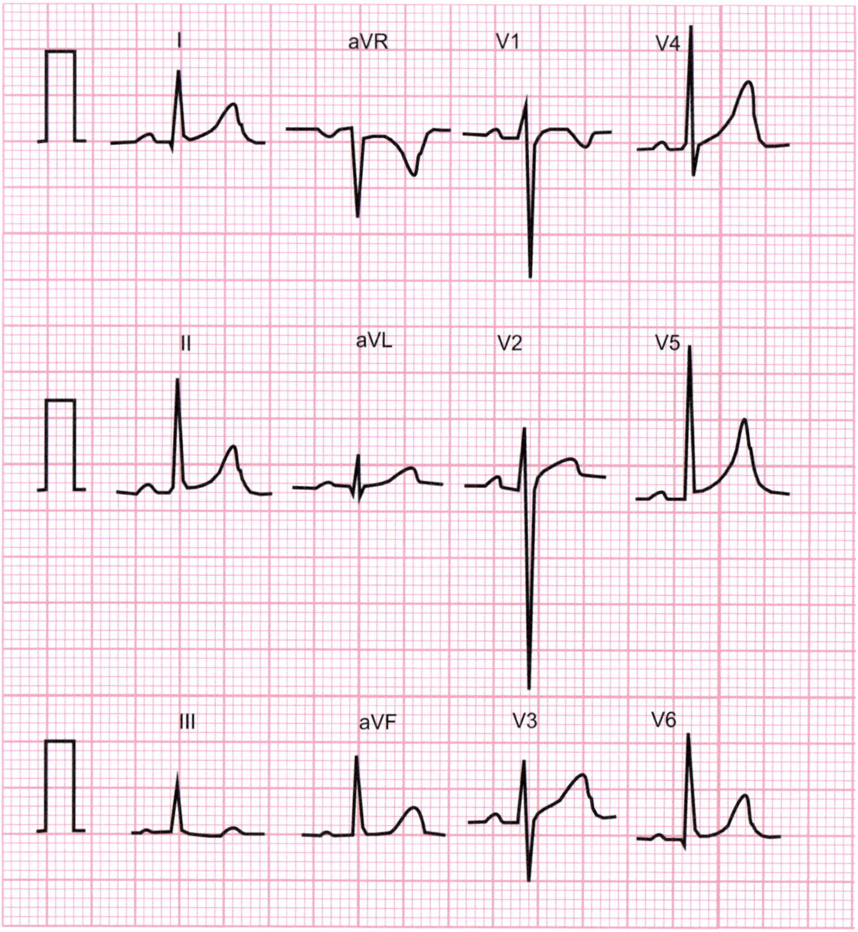


**Fig. 7.10** 12-Lead ECG

### Step I

Plot the lead axis of lead I and lead aVF.

### Step II

Next calculate the total positive and total negative deflection of the QRS complex in lead I. For example, it is +9 (R wave) and −1 (s wave) in the given ECG. So, the net resultant is +8 (+9 + [−1] = +8).

Now, plot +8 in the lead axis of lead I (Fig. 7.11).

### Step III

Next draw a perpendicular through the plotted point on lead I axis (Fig. 7.12).

### Step IV

Now calculate the net resultant in lead aVF. In the given ECG, the net resultant is +10 (+10 + 0) = +10). Plot +10 in the lead axis of lead aVF (Fig. 7.13).

**Fig. 7.11** Plotting of +8 on axis of lead I

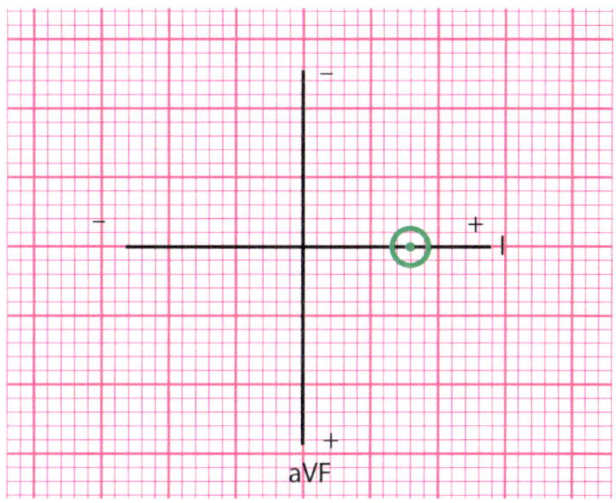


**Fig. 7.12** Perpendicular drawn on lead I axis through +8

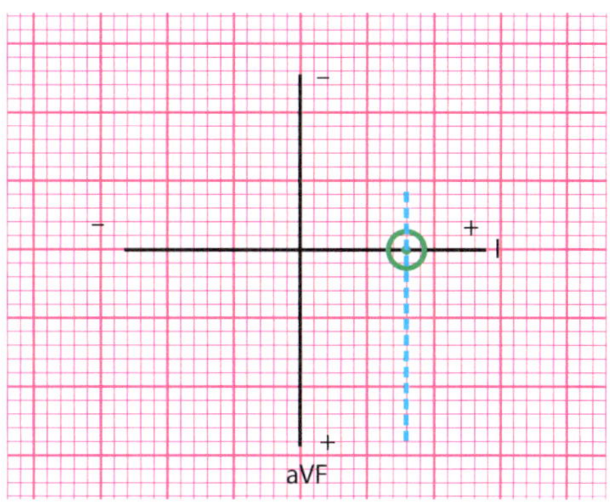

**Step V**

Next draw a perpendicular through the plotted point on lead aVF axis and prolong it to meet the perpendicular drawn on lead I axis (Fig. 7.14).

**Step VI**

Next draw a line joining the point of the intersection of axis of lead I and lead aVF and the point of intersection of the two perpendicular lines. The QRS axis is +51° (Figs. 7.15 and 7.16). This is normal QRS axis.

**Fig. 7.13** Plotting of +10 on axis of lead aVF

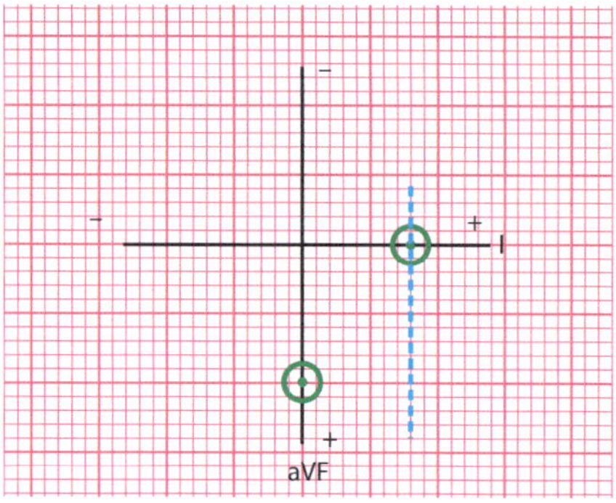


**Fig. 7.14** Perpendicular drawn on axis of lead aVF through +10

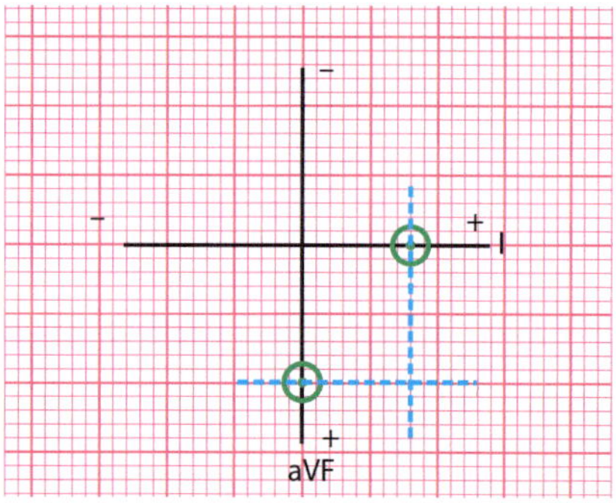


**Fig. 7.15** QRS axis is +51°

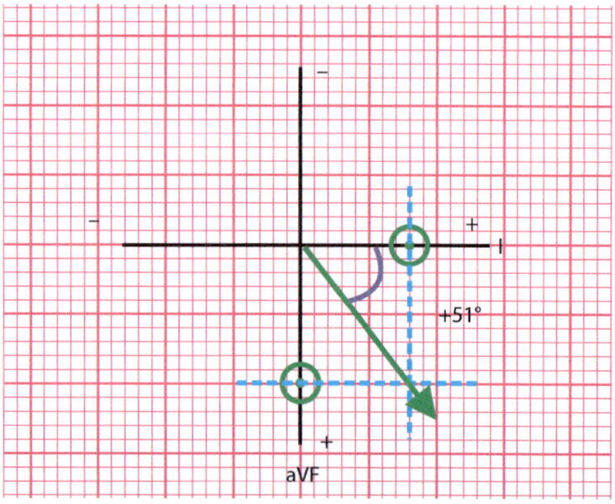

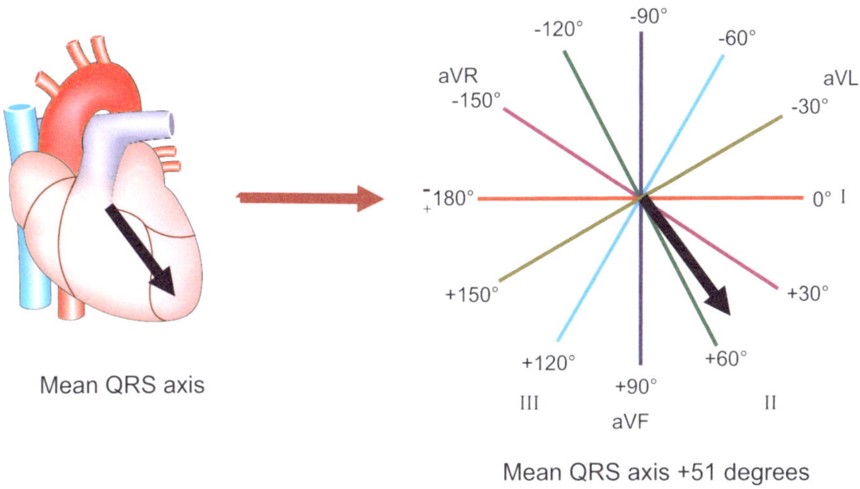


**Fig. 7.16** Mean QRS axis is +51°. This is normal QRS axis. The axis is directed towards the positive pole of lead II

**Tips and Tricks**

- Do not get confused. Axis determination is not very complicated.
- Only limb leads are studied to calculate the QRS axis.
- There is normal axis if lead I, II and III has R wave and the tallest R wave is present in lead II.
- Normal axis means there are dominant R waves in both leads I and aVF.
- Normal QRS axis lies between −30° and +90°.

**Self-Assessment Questions**

1. QRS axis is the mean direction of depolarization wavefront of the two ventricles. True or false?
2. The normal QRS axis lies between −60° and +90°. True or false?
3. In normal QRS axis, the R wave is taller in lead III than in lead II. True or false?
4. In normal QRS axis, R wave is seen in leads I, II and III. True or false?
5. In triaxial reference system each angle is separated by 30°. True or false?
6. **What is the normal range for the QRS axis on an ECG?**

   a. −30° to +90° b. −90° to +30° c. 0° to +180° d. −180° to 0°

7. **A QRS axis of −60° would be considered:**

   a. Normal b. Left axis deviation c. Right axis deviation d. Indeterminate axis

8. **A QRS axis of +120° would be considered:**

   a. Normal b. Left axis deviation c. Right axis deviation d. Indeterminate axis

9. **QRS axis of −20° would be considered:**

   a. Normal b. Left axis deviation c. Right axis deviation d. Indeterminate axis

**Case Studies**

1. Calculate the mean QRS axis, based on the six limb leads given below (Fig. 7.17).
2. Calculate the mean QRS axis based on lead I and lead aVF as shown in Fig. 7.18.

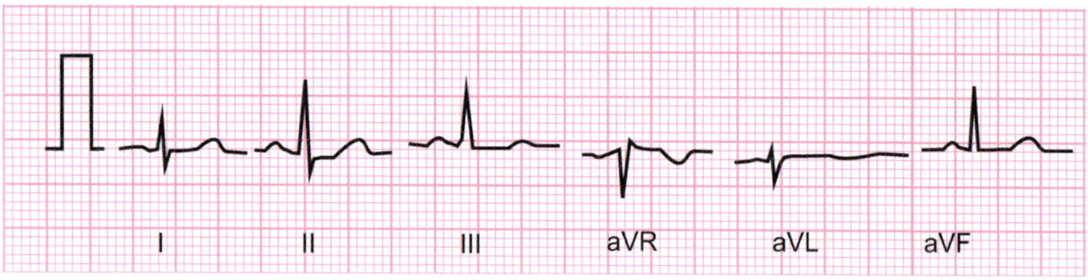


**Fig. 7.17** Calculate the mean QRS axis

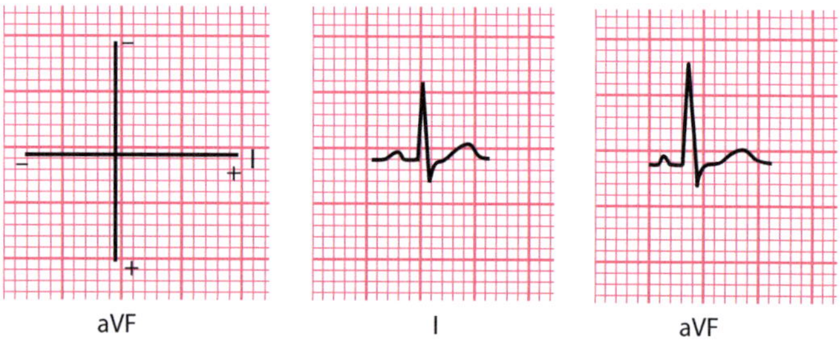


**Fig. 7.18** Calculate the mean QRS axis

**Answers**

1. True 2. False 3. False 4. True 5. False 6. a 7. b 8. c 9. a

**Case Studies**

1. Let us use method 1and method 3 to calculate the mean QRS axis.

   **Method 1:** There is predominantly positive wave in lead I and completely positive wave in lead aVF. Hence, the mean QRS axis is normal.

   **Method 2:** By using method 2, it can be seen that the algebraic sum of the deflections in lead I is +2 (+5 + [−3] = +2). Similarly, the resultant of the deflections in lead aVF is +10 (+10 + 0 = +10). Hence, by plotting the resultant on the ECG grid, the mean QRS axis calculated is +78° (Fig. 7.19).

2. The following steps are to be followed to calculate the QRS axis of the ECG (lead I and lead aVF shown) in Fig. 7.18.

   Step I

   Plot the lead axis of lead I and lead aVF (Fig. 7.20).

   Step II

   Calculate the total positive and total negative deflection of the QRS complex in lead I. For example, it is +7 (R wave) and −2 (S wave) in the given ECG. So the net resultant is +5 (+7 + [−2] = +5).

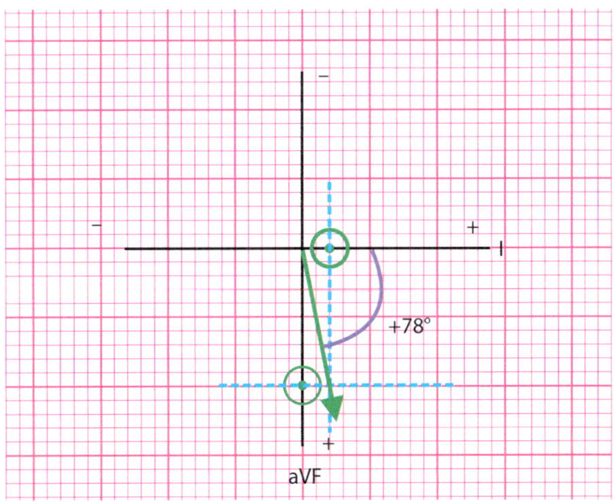


**Fig. 7.19** Mean QRS axis is +78°. This is normal QRS axis

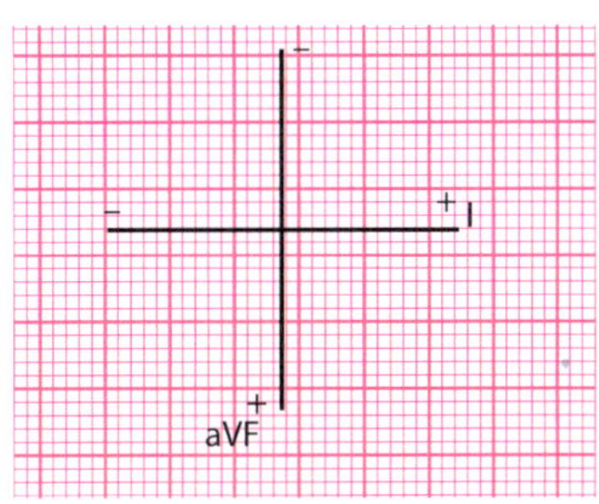


**Fig. 7.20** Lead axis of lead I and lead aVF

Now plot +5 in the lead axis of lead I (Fig. 7.21).

Step III

Draw a perpendicular through the plotted point on lead I axis (Fig. 7.22).

Step IV

Now similarly calculate the net resultant in lead aVF. In the given ECG, the net resultant is +7 (+9 + [−2] = +7). Now plot +7 in the lead axis of lead aVF (Fig. 7.23).

Step V

Draw a perpendicular through the plotted point on lead aVF axis and prolong it to meet the perpendicular drawn on lead I axis (Fig. 7.24).

Step VI

Draw a line joining the point of the intersection of axis of lead I and aVF and the point of intersection of the two perpendicular lines. The QRS axis is +55° (Fig. 7.25). So, it is normal QRS axis.

**Fig. 7.21** Plotting of +5 on axis of lead I

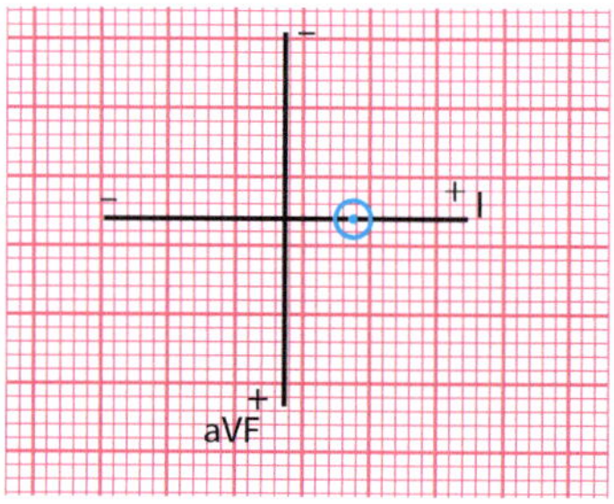


**Fig. 7.22** Perpendicular drawn on lead I axis through +5

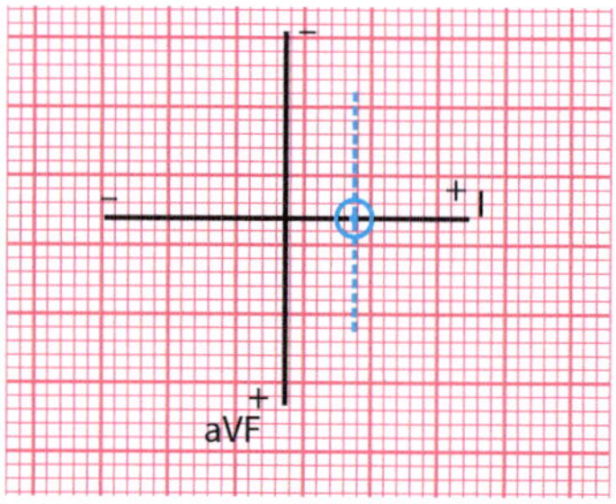


**Fig. 7.23** Plotting of +7 on axis of lead aVF

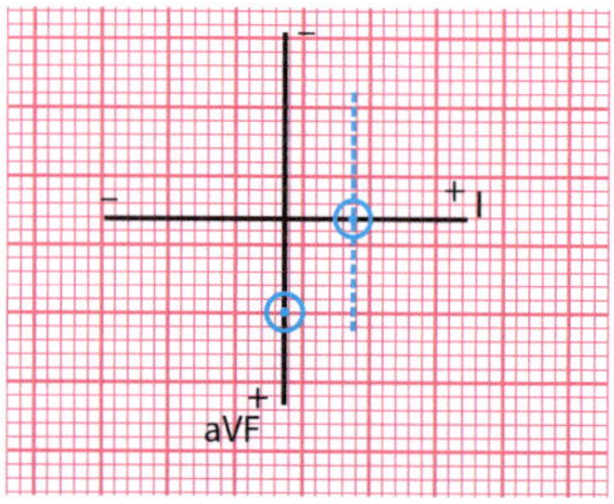

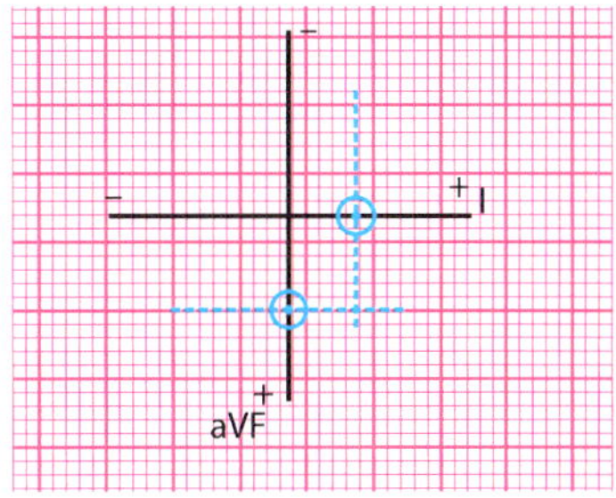


**Fig. 7.24** Perpendicular drawn on axis of lead aVF through +7

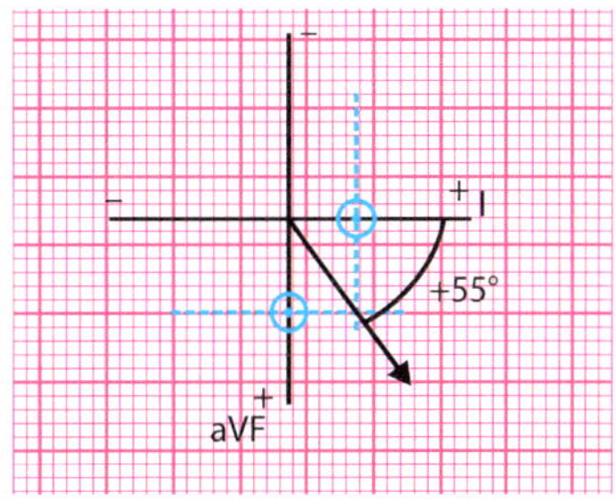


**Fig. 7.25** QRS axis is +55°

# Chapter 8
# Left Axis Deviation

**Learning Objectives**
After studying this chapter, the reader will learn about:

- Left axis deviation
- Calculation of left axis deviation
- Causes of left axis deviation

In left axis deviation (LAD), the QRS axis lies between −30° and −90°. QRS axis between −90° and −180° is very rare. To calculate QRS axis, let us consider the QRS tracing of Fig. 8.1. At first glance, it may be possible to say that there is a left axis deviation by using the first method as there is dominant R wave in lead I and dominant S wave in lead aVF. However, to calculate the exact QRS axis, the second method has to be followed.

**Step I**
At first, plot the lead axis of lead I and lead aVF.

**Step II**
Next calculate the total positive and total negative deflection of the QRS complex in lead I. For example, it is +4 (r wave) and −1 (s wave) in the given ECG. So, the net resultant is +3 (+4 + [−1] = +3).

Now, plot +3 in the lead axis of lead I (Fig. 8.2).

**Step III**
Now draw a perpendicular through the plotted point on lead I (Fig. 8.3).

**Step IV**
Similarly, calculate the net resultant in lead aVF. In the given ECG, the net resultant is −8 (−12 + [+4] = −8). Plot −8 in the lead axis of lead aVF (Fig. 8.4).



T. K. Koley, *Rapid Review of ECG*,
https://doi.org/10.1007/978-981-99-9116-7_8

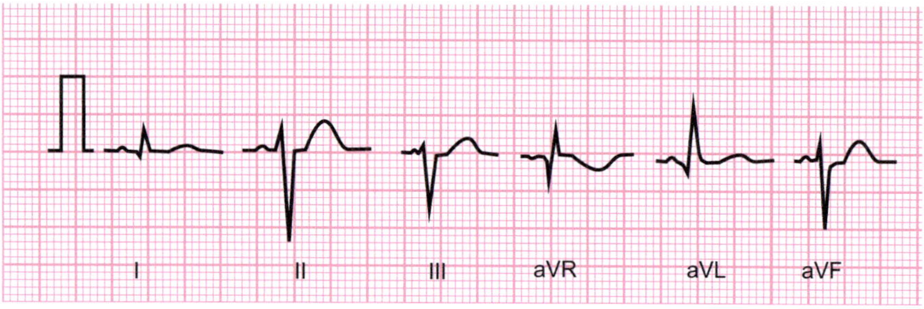


**Fig. 8.1** ECG tracing of standard leads

**Fig. 8.2** Plotting of +3 on axis of lead I

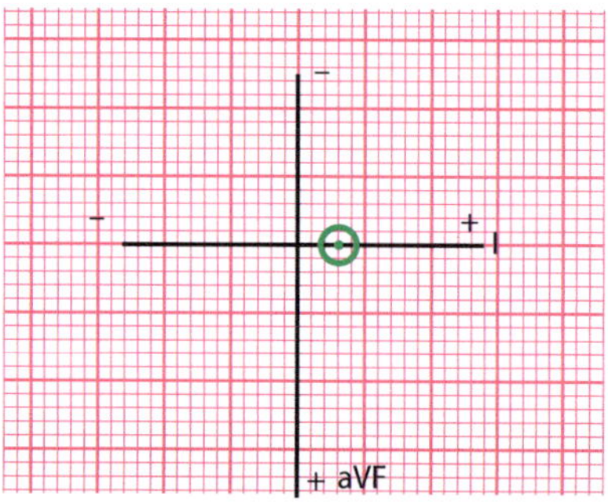


**Fig. 8.3** Perpendicular drawn on lead I axis through +3

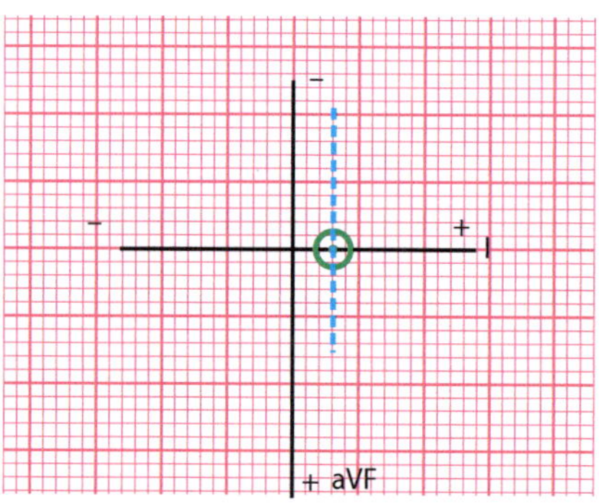


**Fig. 8.4** Plotting of −8 on axis of lead aVF

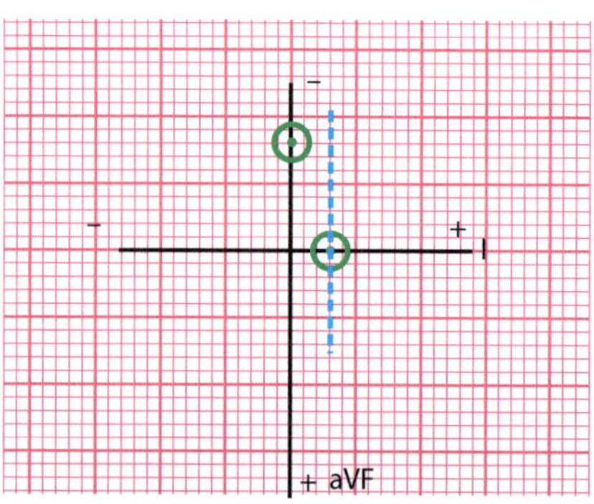

**Step V**

Next draw a perpendicular through the plotted point on lead aVF axis and prolong it to meet the perpendicular drawn on lead I axis (Fig. 8.5).

**Step VI**

In the last step, draw a line joining the point of the intersection of axis of lead I and aVF and the point of intersection of the two perpendicular lines. The QRS axis is −70° (Figs. 8.6 and 8.7).

The various causes of left axis deviation are enumerated in Box 8.1.

**Box 8.1 Causes of Left Axis Deviation**

Left anterior hemiblock
Left bundle branch block
Left ventricular hypertrophy
Inferior wall myocardial infarction
WPW syndrome
Ostium primum atrial septal defect
Hyperkalaemia
Emphysema
Mechanical shift: ascites and pregnancy
Normal variant or physiologic

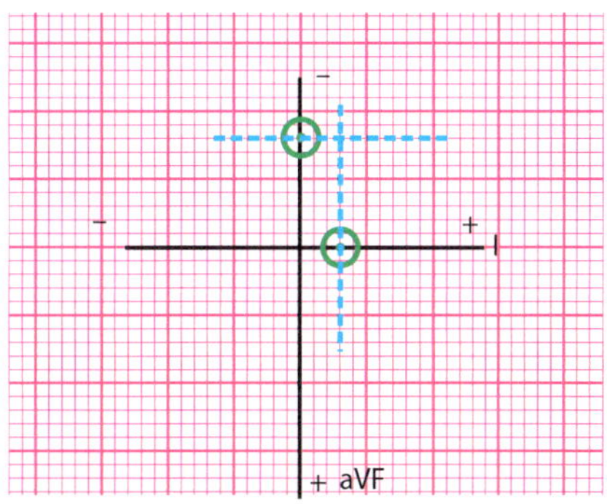


**Fig. 8.5** Perpendicular drawn on axis of lead aVF through −8

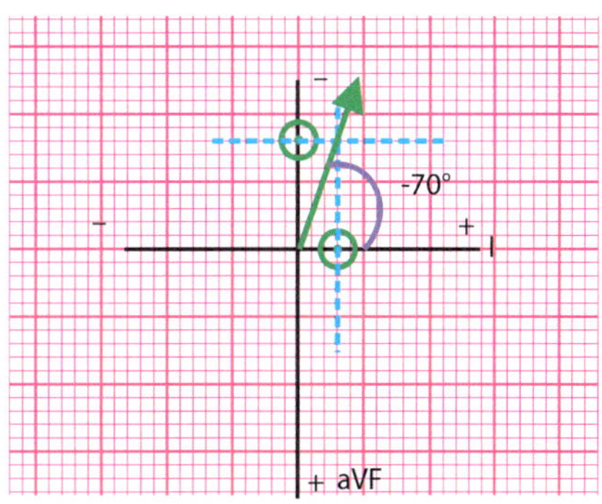


**Fig. 8.6** QRS axis is −70°. This is left axis deviation

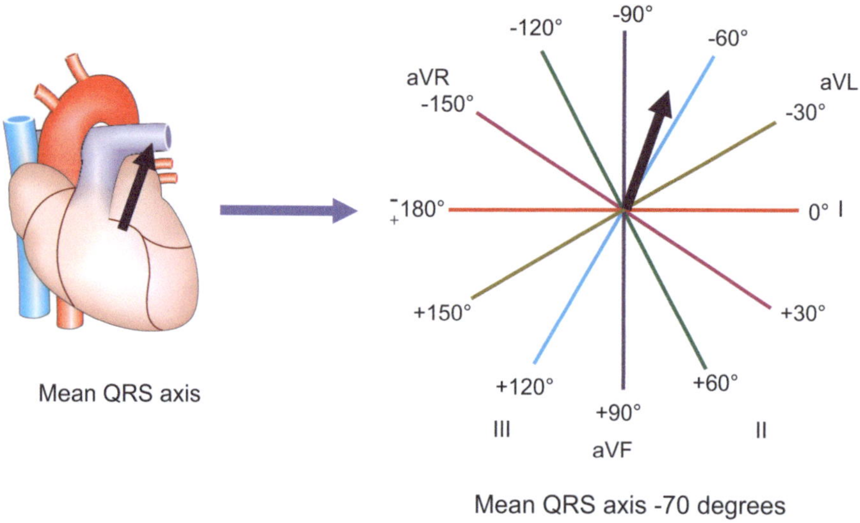


**Fig. 8.7** Left axis deviation (QRS axis −70°). The axis is directed towards the negative pole of lead III

**Tips and Tricks**

- In left axis deviation, QRS axis lies between −30° and −90°.
- Check the dominant waves in lead I and lead aVF.
- If lead I has dominant R wave and lead aVF has dominant S wave, it is left axis deviation.
- Any doubt, use method 2.
- In the presence of left axis deviation, always rule out LVH and LAHB. Rule out hypertension in these patients.
- Asymptomatic patients with left axis deviation do not require any treatment.

**Self-Assessment Questions**

1. Left axis deviation on an ECG may be a normal finding. True or false?
2. Left axis deviation is seen in ostium secundum ASD. True or false?
3. Left axis deviation is typically caused by a blockage in the right bundle branch of the heart. True or false?
4. Left axis deviation is observed in individuals with long standing uncontrolled hypertension. True or false?
5. In left axis deviation, the QRS vector is directed upward and to the left. True or false?

**Case Study**

1. Based on the six limb leads shown below (Fig. 8.8), calculate the mean QRS axis. If you can detect any axis deviation, name one condition where you will get such axis deviation.

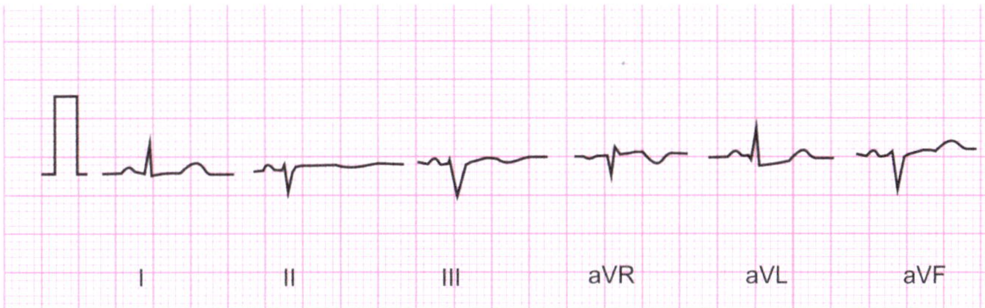


**Fig. 8.8** Calculate the mean QRS axis

**Answers**

1. True 2. False 3. False 4. True 5. True

**Case Study**

1. To calculate the mean QRS axis, let us use method 1 and method 2.

   **Method 1:** There is positive deflection in lead I and negative deflection in lead aVF. Hence, there is left axis deviation.

   **Method 2:** By using method 2, it can be seen that the algebraic sum of the deflections in lead I is +5 (+5 + 0 = +5). Similarly, the resultant of the deflections in lead aVF is −4 (−5 + 1 = −4). Hence, by plotting the resultant on the ECG grid, the mean QRS axis calculated is −41° (Fig. 8.9). Thus, the ECG shows left axis deviation. Because of left axis deviation, there is tall R wave in lead I (mean depolarization wavefront moving towards the positive pole of lead I), deep S wave in lead III (mean depolarization wavefront moving away from the positive pole of lead III, Fig. 8.10) and rS complex in lead II (mean depolarization wavefront moving slightly towards, but mainly away from the positive pole of lead II), where the depth of S wave is more than the height of r wave.

   In left anterior hemiblock, there is left axis deviation. Besides this, there is deep S waves in both lead II and lead III, and the depth of S wave in lead III is more than that of S wave in lead II. This is an important feature of left anterior hemiblock, about which you will read in details in subsequent chapter.

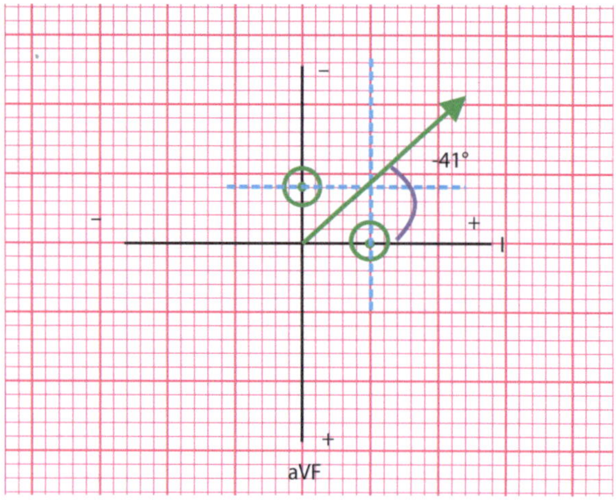


**Fig. 8.9** Mean QRS axis is −41°. There is left axis deviation

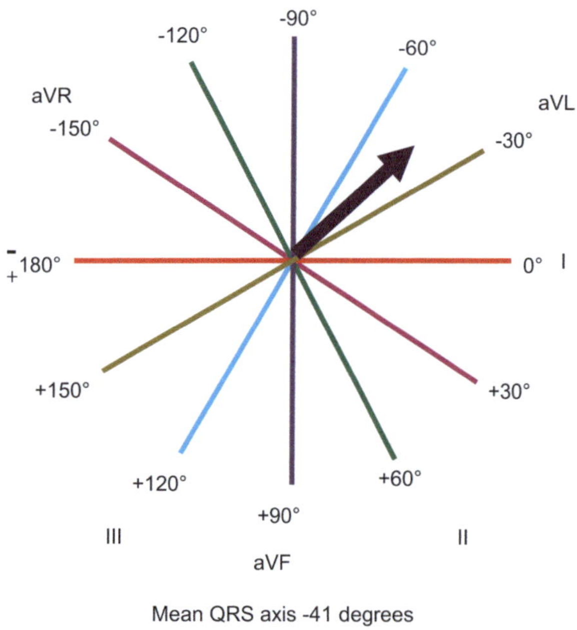


**Fig. 8.10** Mean QRS axis is directed towards the negative pole of axis of lead III

# Chapter 9
# Right Axis Deviation

**Learning Objectives**
After studying this chapter, the reader will learn about:

- Right axis deviation
- Calculation of right axis deviation
- Causes of right axis deviation

In right axis deviation (RAD), the axis is between +90° and +180° (Fig. 9.1). The QRS vector would be directed downward and to the right. Right axis deviation occurs in various conditions including right bundle branch block, left posterior hemiblock, right ventricular hypertrophy, etc.

To calculate axis, let us consider the QRS tracing in lead I and lead aVF of Fig. 9.2. There is a positive deflection in lead aVF and a negative deflection in lead

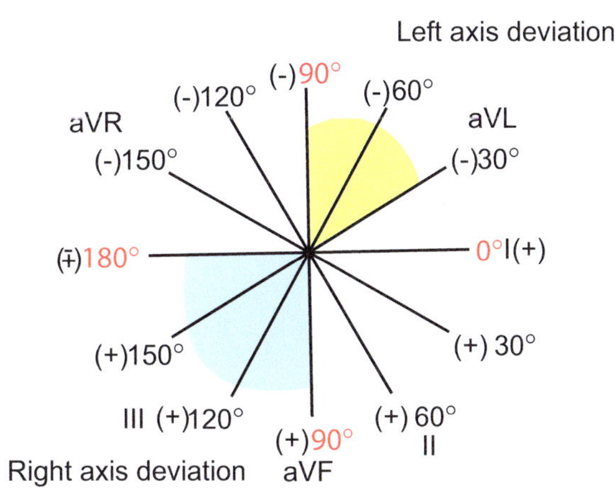


**Fig. 9.1** Orientation of the cardiac axis. The area shaded light blue is right axis deviation, and thc arca shaded yellow is left axis deviation



T. K. Koley, *Rapid Review of ECG*,
https://doi.org/10.1007/978-981-99-9116-7_9

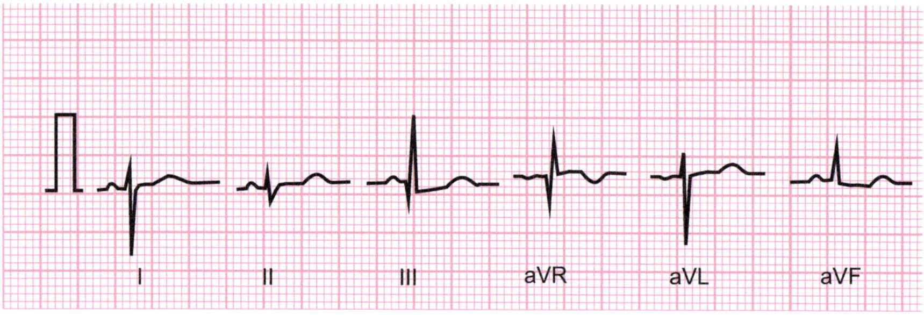


**Fig. 9.2** ECG tracing of standard leads

**Fig. 9.3** Plotting of −-5 on axis of lead I

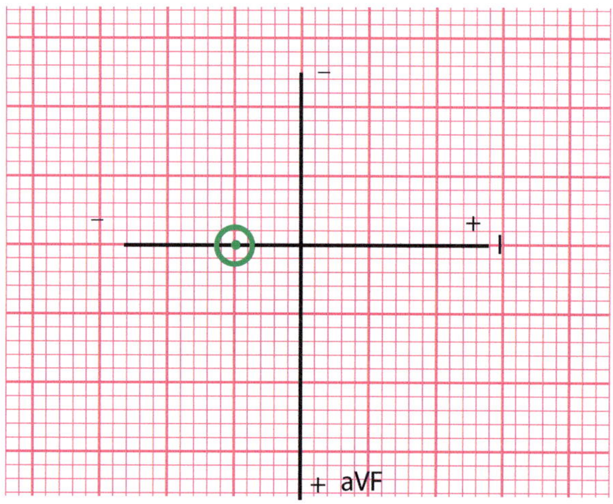


I. If we use the first method to calculate the QRS axis, we can say that there is a right axis deviation but a more accurate axis can be determined by this method. Let us calculate the axis by the second method and follow the steps as mentioned below.

### Step I

At first, plot the lead axis of lead I and lead aVF.

### Step II

Next calculate the total positive and total negative deflection of the QRS complex in lead I. For example, it is +4 (r wave) and −9 (S wave) in the given ECG. So, the net resultant is −5 (+4 + [−9] = −5).

Now, plot −5 in the lead axis of lead I (Fig. 9.3).

**Step III**

Now draw a perpendicular through the plotted point on lead I (Fig. 9.4).

**Step IV**

Similarly, calculate the net resultant in lead aVF. In the given ECG, the net resultant is +6 (+6 + 0) = +6). Now, plot +6 in the lead axis of lead aVF (Fig. 9.5).

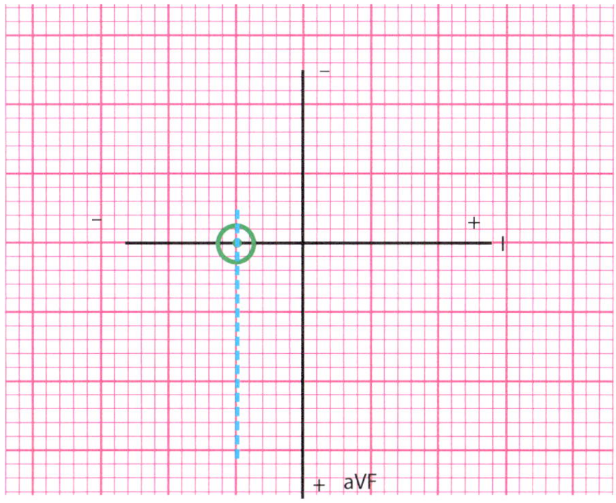


**Fig. 9.4** Perpendicular drawn on lead I axis through −5

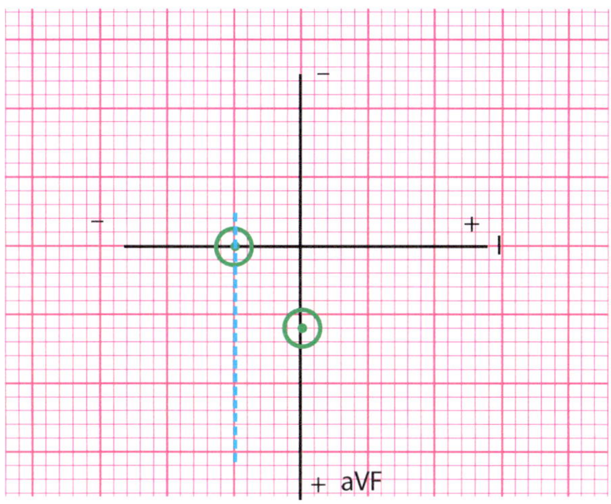


**Fig. 9.5** Plotting of +6 on axis of lead aVF

**Step V**

Next draw a perpendicular through the plotted point on lead aVF axis and prolong it to meet the perpendicular drawn on lead I axis (Fig. 9.6).

**Step VI**

In the last step, draw a line joining the point of the intersection of axis of lead I and aVF and the point of intersection of the two perpendicular lines. The QRS axis is +130° (Figs. 9.7 and 9.8).

The various causes of right axis deviation are enumerated in Box 9.1.

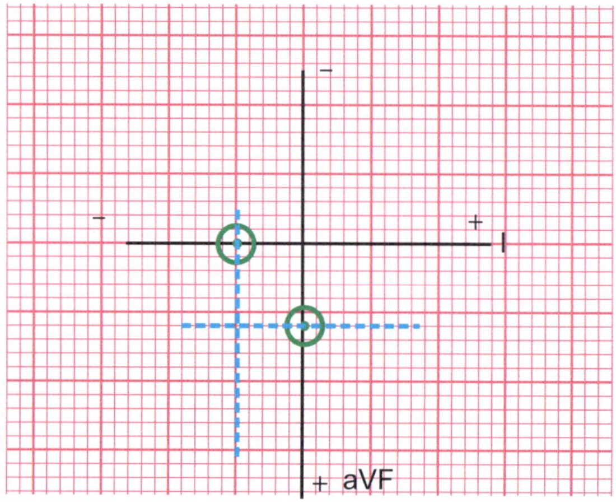


**Fig. 9.6** Perpendicular drawn on axis of lead aVF through +6

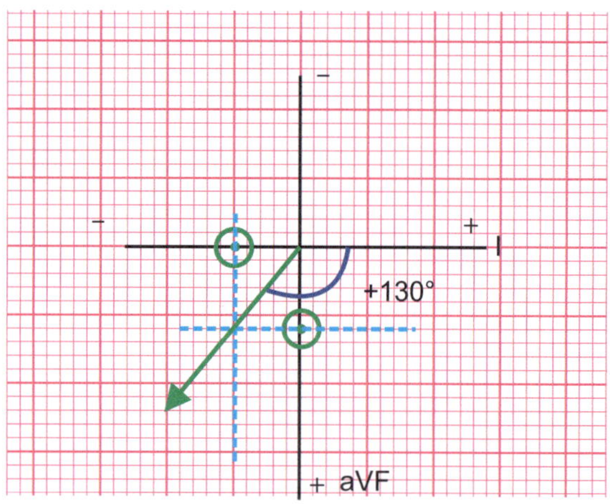


**Fig. 9.7** QRS axis is +130°. There is right axis deviation

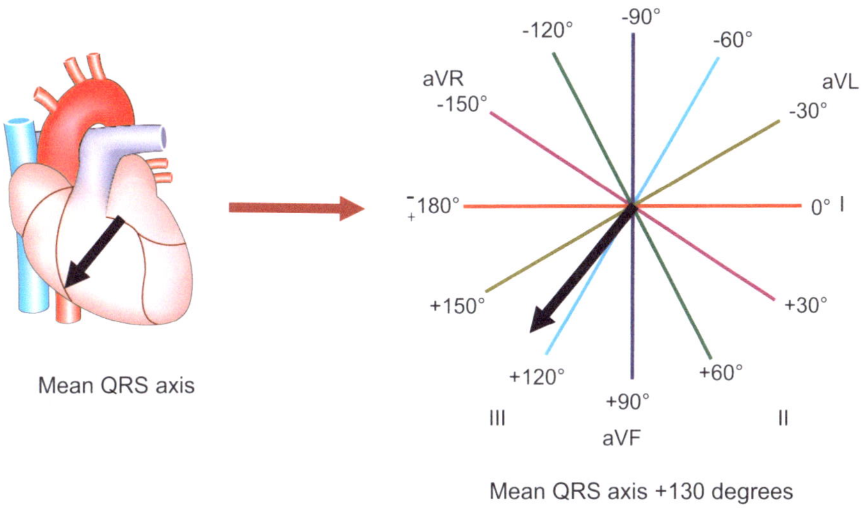


**Fig. 9.8** Right axis deviation (QRS axis + 130°). The axis is directed to the positive pole of lead III

**Box 9.1 Causes of Right Axis Deviation**

Right ventricular hypertrophy
COPD
RBBB
Left posterior hemiblock
Limb lead reversal
Lateral wall myocardial infarction
Ostium secundum ASD
Pulmonary embolism
Dextrocardia
Anterolateral myocardial infarction
WPW syndrome
Normal variant
Left pneumothorax

**Tips and Tricks**

- In right axis deviation, QRS axis lies between +90° and +180°.
- Check the dominant waves in lead I and lead aVF.
- If lead I has dominant S wave and lead aVF has dominant R wave, it is right axis deviation.
- Any doubt, use method 2.

**Self-Assessment Questions**

1. **Which of the following is the range for the QRS axis in RAD?**

   a. −30° to +90° b. +90° to +180° c. 0° to +180° d. −180° to 0°

2. **Which of the following is associated with RAD on an ECG?**

   a. LVH b. Sinus arrhythmia c. Atrial fibrillation d. RVH

3. **Which of the following conditions is not typically associated with RAD on an ECG?**

   a. Acute myocardial infarction b. Chronic obstructive pulmonary disease c. Pulmonary embolism d. Pulmonary hypertension

4. **Which of the following statements about RAD is true?**

   a. It always indicates some cardiac disease b. It is always a normal finding c. It can be either a pathologic or a normal finding, depending on the underlying cause d. It is always seen in athletes

5. **Positive deflection is seen in lead aVF and negative deflection is seen in lead I. The QRS axis is:**

   a. LAD b. RAD c. Normal QRS axis d. Northwest axis

**Case Study**

1. Calculate the mean QRS axis from the six limb leads shown below (Fig. 9.9). If you can detect any axis deviation, name one condition where you will get such axis deviation.

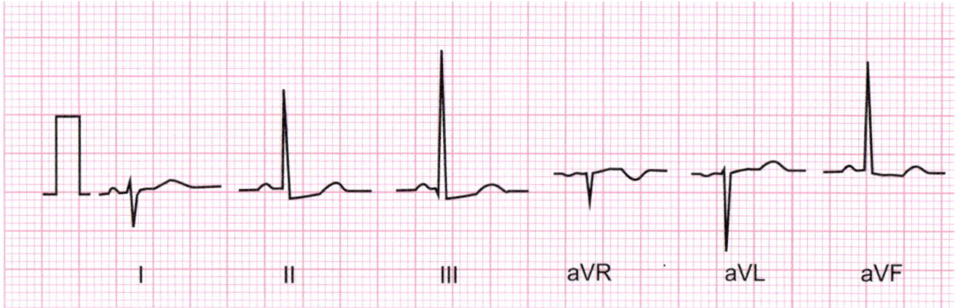


**Fig. 9.9** Calculate the mean QRS axis

### Answers

1. b 2. d 3. a 4. c 5. b

### Case Study

1. For calculating the mean QRS axis, method 1 and 2 will be used.

**Method 1:** There is negative deflection in lead I and positive deflection in lead aVF. Hence, there is right axis deviation.

**Method 2:** The algebraic sum of the deflections in lead I is −4 (+2 + [−6] = −4). Similarly, the resultant of the deflections in lead aVF is +14 (+14 + 0 = +14). Hence, by plotting the resultant on the ECG grid, the mean QRS axis calculated is +105° (Fig. 9.10). Thus, the ECG shows right axis deviation.

Because of right axis deviation, there is tall R wave in lead III and lead aVF (mean depolarization wavefront moving towards the positive pole of lead III and lead aVF) (Fig. 9.11), and the height of R wave is more in lead III as compared to the height of R wave in lead II (mean depolarization wavefront is moving more towards the positive pole of lead III as compared to the positive pole of lead II). Right axis deviation is seen in right ventricular hypertrophy, about which you will read in subsequent chapters.

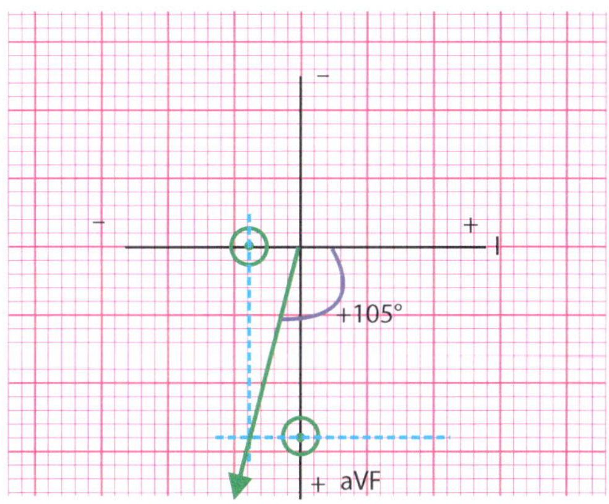


**Fig. 9.10** Mean calculated QRS axis is +105°. There is right axis deviation

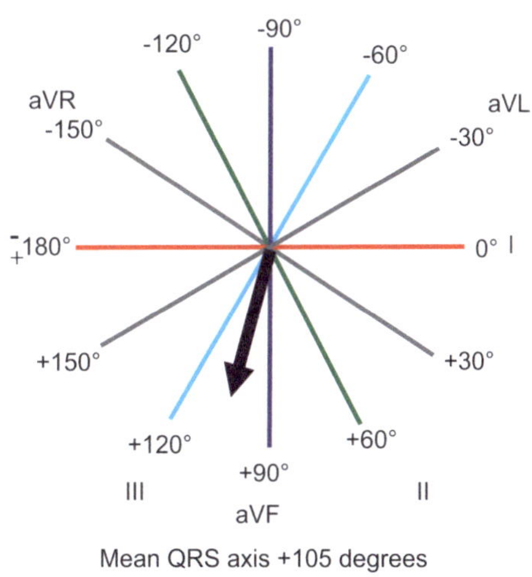


**Fig. 9.11** The axis is directed between the positive poles of lead III and lead aVF

# Chapter 10
# Normal ECG and Its Variants

**Learning Objectives**
After studying this chapter, the reader will learn about:

- Normal ECG
- Early repolarization syndrome
- Persistent juvenile pattern
- Nonspecific T wave changes
- Method of interpretation of ECG

## 10.1 Normal ECG

For a beginner, one of the most complex part of learning ECG is to remember the normal morphology of P, QRS and T waves in all the 12 leads. If one can confidently interpret a normal ECG, he may consider himself to have crossed one of the major hurdles in the process of learning of ECG. However, one must remember, it comes only by constant practice. Before proceeding further, let us recapitulate what we have learnt about normal ECG.

- In frontal plane leads, the P wave is positive in lead II and negative in lead aVR. This simple observation tells us that impulse has originated from SA node.
- In rest of the limb leads, the P wave is generally positive.
- The QRS complex and T wave morphology are also similar to the P wave morphology in limb leads. However, there are lots of normal variants, which are discussed later in this chapter.
- In lead aVR, all the waves are negative.
- The T wave generally follows the main deflection of the QRS complex in any lead.



T. K. Koley, *Rapid Review of ECG*,
https://doi.org/10.1007/978-981-99-9116-7_10

- In chest leads, P wave may be positive, negative or biphasic in lead V1. In rest of the leads, the P wave is positive.
- In lead V1, rS complex is recorded, and in lead V6, qRs complex is recorded. There is progression of R wave amplitude, and the transition zone is recorded in lead V3 or lead V4.
- In electrically vertical heart, QRS complex in lead aVF and lead V6 is similar.
- In electrically horizontal heart, QRS complex in lead aVL and lead V6 is similar.
- S-T segment is isoelectric.
- The normal P-R interval is 0.12–0.20 s.
- The normal QRS interval is less than 0.12 s.
- The normal range of Q-Tc is 0.35–0.44 s (men) or 0.45 s (women).
- Heart rate = 1500/R-R interval. Normal heart rate is between 60 and 100 bpm.

A normal ECG is shown in Fig. 10.1. The P, QRS and T waves in all the 12 leads are normal. All the waves are inverted in lead aVR. Transition zone is recorded in lead V3. QRS axis is normal. The different time intervals are also within normal limit. In infants, the ECG will simulate that of right ventricular hypertrophy in adults. Tall R waves are present in right precordial leads. There is right axis deviation. There is no initial q wave in lead V1, and the VAT is not prolonged. The T waves are normally inverted in leads V1–V4. The tall R waves in right precordial leads usually disappear after the age of 5 years. But the inverted T waves may persist even up to the second decade. The QRS axis gradually shifts to left.

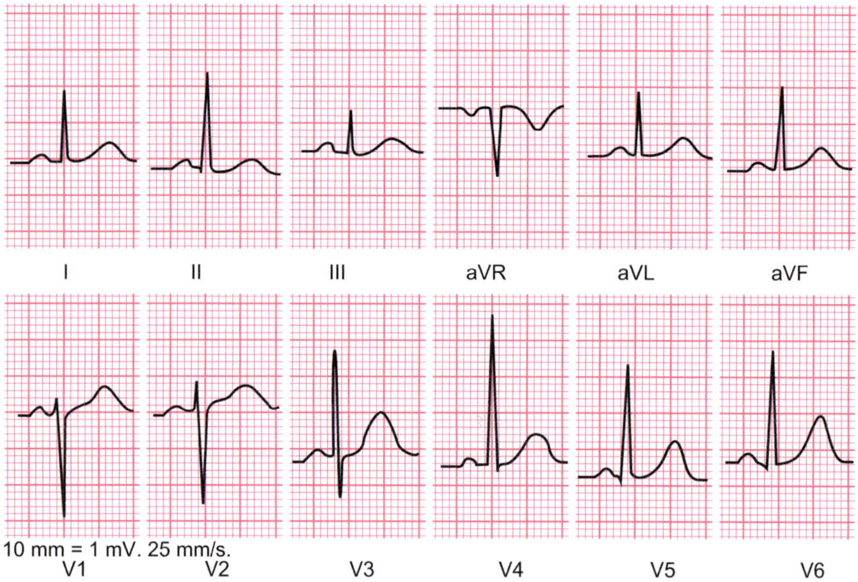


**Fig. 10.1** Normal ECG. P wave is rounded and upright in lead II. Lead aVR reflects completely negative complex. P-R interval and QRS duration are normal. rS complex is recorded in lead V1 and qR complex is recorded in lead V6. Transition zone is recorded in lead V3. QRS axis is normal

Another normal ECG is shown in Fig. 10.2. The QRS axis is normal. All the complexes in lead aVR are inverted. P-R interval and QRS duration are normal. The transition zone is located in lead V3. rS complex is recorded in lead V1, and Rs complex is recorded in lead V6. All the complexes in respective leads are normal in configuration.

**Tips and Tricks**

- Never look at the computerized interpretation of ECG.
- If any doubt, repeat the ECG after a few minutes.

## 10.2 Normal ECG Variants

Variants of normal ECG can be defined as ECG readings which seem abnormal but are found in ordinary healthy people. ECG readings are based on a range of factors including age, sex, body mass index, heart position, race, food consumption and exercise. It is easy to recognize some of the normal variants that have been identified and given names such as persisting juvenile pattern, early repolarization syndrome. It is important to recognize the normal variants to avoid confusion with cardiac anomalies. However, the ECG should always be interpreted in context of the clinical features of the patient. Some of the important normal variants are enumerated in Box 10.1.

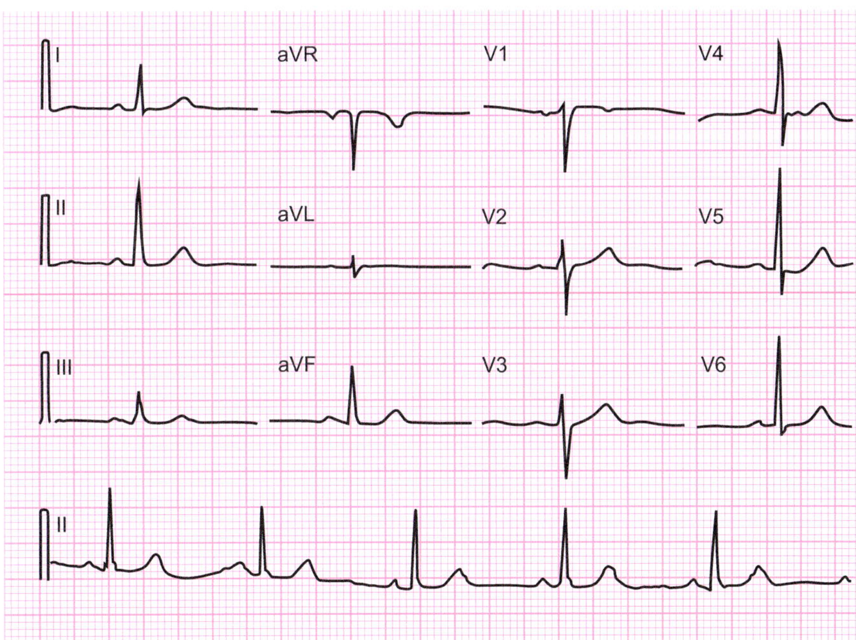


**Fig. 10.2** Normal ECG from a 35-year-old gentleman

**Box 10.1 Normal ECG Variants**

Variations of P wave: Notching or peaking of P waves with normal duration.

A short P-R interval may be normal in young adults or healthy children.

Variation of Q wave: Prominent Q waves of normal duration may appear in normal persons depending upon the heart position and body built.

Variation of T waves: Abnormally tall T waves may appear without any other abnormality. Besides this non-specific T wave inversion is also common in normal healthy people.

Variation of QRS complex: High amplitude of R and S waves may appear in precordial leads in thin persons. Low amplitude of R and S waves may be seen in obese persons.

Abnormal looking Q wave and T wave inversion in lead III which disappear on taking a deep breath. The T wave becomes upright.

Non-specific widening of QRS complex, which does not fulfil the criteria of any bundle branch block pattern. Incomplete right bundle branch block is commonly seen in young people.

S-T segment may be elevated by 1 mm or more in lead V2 and less in lead V3.

Early repolarization syndrome.

Persistent juvenile pattern.

## *10.2.1 Well-Recognized Variants of Normal ECG*

### 10.2.1.1 Early Repolarization Syndrome

Early repolarization syndrome is a common variant and is often confused with myocardial infarction and pericarditis. The main ECG feature is elevation of J point and S-T segment. The J point elevation often creates a distinct notch or hook in the distal or descending limb of the QRS complex, called J wave.

The S-T segment elevation is usually about 2–3 mm but may be up to 5 mm in some cases. The S-T segment is concave upwards (in contrast to myocardial infarction) and it is more prominent in leads V4–V6 (Fig. 10.3). Serial ECG recordings, however, do not show any evolutionary changes, as observed in myocardial infarction. The S-T segment elevation frequently returns to baseline with exercise. The ECG manifestations are the following:

- Concave upwards S-T segment elevation
- J point elevation
- Prominent J waves
- Tall R waves in leads V4–V6
- Tall and symmetrical T waves
- Narrow q waves in leads V4–V6
- Sinus bradycardia

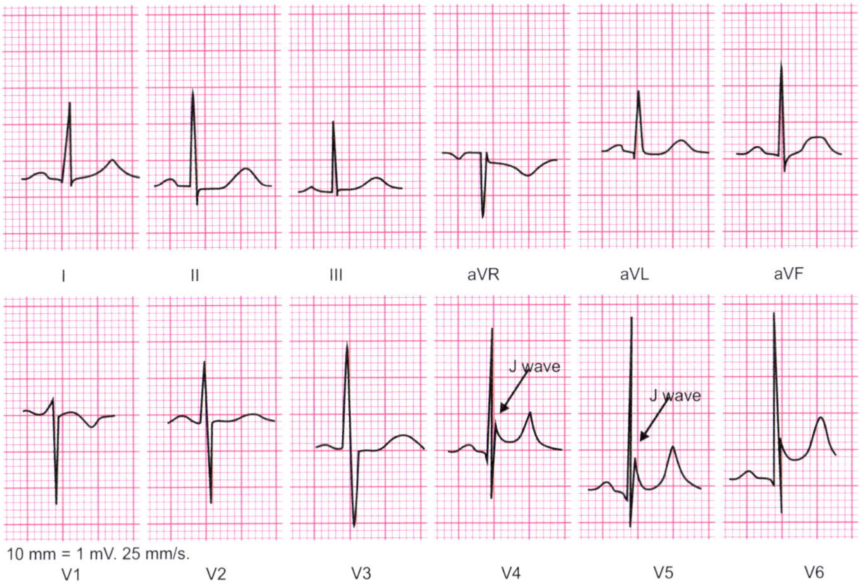


**Fig. 10.3** Early repolarization syndrome. This ECG is taken from a 30-year-old gentleman who presented with chest pain. Note the concave upwards S-T segment elevation in leads V4, V5 and V6. Note also the prominent J waves in leads V4 and V5. This type of ECG is often confused with S-T segment elevation of myocardial infarction

#### 10.2.1.2 Persistent Juvenile Pattern

The T wave is normally inverted in leads V1–V4 in infancy and childhood, and if these changes persist in adulthood, it is known as persistent juvenile pattern (Fig. 10.4). It is more common in females and is frequently associated with other normal variants. The main ECG feature is T wave inversion which is not symmetric or deep. It should be differentiated from other conditions, which may produce T wave inversion in chest leads, including anterior wall myocardial ischaemia, myocarditis and pulmonary embolism.

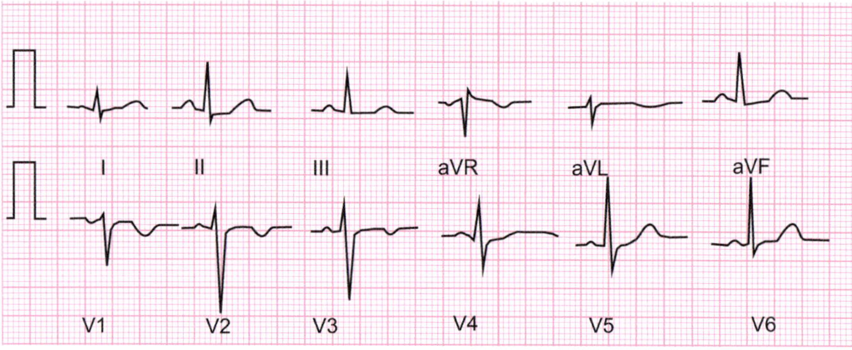


**Fig. 10.4** Persistent juvenile pattern. Note the inversion of T waves in lead V1 to lead V3. Rest of the ECG is normal

#### 10.2.1.3 Non-specific T Wave Changes

Often we come across normal persons in whom the T waves are inverted, and detailed examination and investigation do not reveal any anatomical or pathological changes in the heart. T waves may be inverted in athletes in leads V4–V6. The T waves may be inverted in the following conditions also:

- After hyperventilation
- Anxiety and fear
- After heavy meal

**Tips and Tricks**
- The ECG of early repolarization syndrome, persistent juvenile pattern and non-specific T wave changes is often confused with myocardial infarction due to S-T segment elevation and T wave changes.
- You may repeat the ECG after deep inspiration if there is T wave inversion.
- If there is confusion, repeat the ECG and look for any serial change.
- In myocardial infarction, the ECG findings change with time, whereas in early repolarisation syndrome, the ECG findings are fixed.
- If doubt persists, take help of other investigations like Trop I estimation and echocardiography.

## 10.3 Method of Interpretation of ECG

The interpretation of ECG starts with the history and clinical examination of the patient. This is often the most neglected step. ECG should always be interpreted in light of the clinical findings. This gives us the clue based on which it becomes easier to read ECG. This step is very important for the beginners, as it enhances the accuracy of interpretation of ECG. Clinical diagnosis and ECG are complimentary to each other. The study of an ECG should be systematic; otherwise, important findings will be missed and the diagnosis will become difficult. The following points should be considered while studying an ECG to arrive at a diagnosis:

### 10.3.1 Rate

The rate should be calculated to rule out bradycardia or tachycardia.

### 10.3.2 Rhythm

The rhythm should be checked in the beginning. It is important to observe if the rhythm is regular or irregular. If regular, it should be checked whether the complexes are originating from SA node (sinus rhythm) or from any supraventricular or ventricular focus. If irregular, it is important to rule out sinus arrhythmia in the beginning, i.e. before considering any supraventricular or ventricular arrhythmia. The relation between P wave and QRS complex should be noted. If there are abnormalities, then they should be written down and correlated with the clinical findings. In normal ECG, every P wave should be followed by a QRS complex. Rhythm should always be examined in lead II or lead V1 in a rhythm strip.

### 10.3.3 P-R Interval

The P-R interval should be checked in the leads where the P waves are seen very clearly, e.g. lead II. Prolongation of P-R interval indicates first-degree heart block. Short P-R interval with delta wave indicates WPW syndrome.

### 10.3.4 P Waves

It is important to rule out any right or left atrial enlargement by examination of P waves in all the 12 leads but especially in lead II and lead V1. The P wave is always inverted in lead aVR and it may be biphasic in lead V1. If P wave is upright in lead aVR, then there may be dextrocardia. Inverted P waves in leads II, III and aVF indicate nodal/junctional rhythm.

### 10.3.5 QRS Complexes

The QRS complexes should be studied in all the 12 leads and it should be checked if they are of normal configuration and correspond to the normal complexes in all the 12 leads. The following points should be studied in the QRS complexes:

(a) Duration
(b) VAT
(c) Presence of normal or pathological Q waves
(d) Amplitude of R and S waves
(e) QRS axis: To rule out left or right axis deviation

### *10.3.6 T Waves*

It should be checked whether the T waves are upright or inverted. The T wave is normally inverted in lead aVR. Deep and symmetric T wave inversion is a sign of myocardial ischaemia. Asymmetric inversion is a feature of strain pattern associated with left or right ventricular hypertrophy.

### *10.3.7 U Waves*

It should be checked whether the U waves are present or absent. If present, they may be normal or may be a feature of hypokalaemia.

### *10.3.8 S-T Segment*

S-T segment should be carefully examined to rule out any elevation or depression. S-T segment elevation indicates myocardial infarction or pericarditis or ventricular aneurysm. S-T segment depression indicates myocardial ischaemia. S-T segment depression with a reverse check sign or scooped S-T segment depression is a feature of digitalis effect.

### *10.3.9 Left or Right Ventricular Hypertrophy*

The presence of left or right ventricular hypertrophy should be checked. For LVH one must look for the sum of amplitude of S wave in lead V1 and amplitude of R wave in lead V5 or lead V6. If it is more than 35 mm, then one should look for rest of the features as described in Chapter 12. For RVH, one should look for the R:S ratio in lead V1. If it is more than 1, then one must look for the other features of RVH. You will read in details about ECG features of right and left ventricular hypertrophy in Chapter 12.

### *10.3.10 Conduction Disturbance*

Conduction disturbances like first, second and third degree heart block should be checked. Left or right bundle branch block should be excluded. If rSR' pattern is seen in lead V1, then look for other features of RBBB and if rSR' pattern is seen in lead V6, then look for other features of LBBB. You will read in details about conduction disturbances in Chapter 13.

**Reporting of ECG**

ECG reporting should be done in details and the diagnosis should be mentioned clearly. ECG should be reported in the following format.

Name:________ Age:__________ Sex:_____ Drugs: ___________

Date & Time: ________

Rate: _________ Rhythm: _______ P wave: _______ P-R interval: _______

Q-T interval: _________

QRS complex:

a) Configuration________________

b) Duration____________________

c) QRS axis____________________

d) VAT________________________

S-T segment:__________________

T wave: ________________

U wave: _________________

Diagnosis: ________________

**Tips and Tricks**

- It is always preferable to look at any previous ECG for comparison before reporting an ECG.

**Self-Assessment Questions**

1. J point is elevated in early repolarization syndrome. True or false?
2. Biphasic P wave is seen in normal persons not suffering from any cardiac disease. True or false?
3. In early repolarization syndrome, there is S-T segment depression in leads V4–V6. True or false?
4. In young people, T wave inversion is often seen normally in leads V1–V3. True or false?
5. T wave inversion in lead III only indicates inferior wall ischaemia? True or false?
6. **The normal rhythm in ECG is:**

   a. Sinus rhythm b. Atrial fibrillation c. Ventricular fibrillation d. Asystole
7. **The normal upper limit of the P-R interval in ECG is:**

   a. 0.10 s b. 0.20 s c. 0.30 s d. 0.40 s
8. **Prolonged Q-T interval is seen in:**

   a. Hypocalcaemia b. Hyponatraemia c. Hypercalcaemia d. Hypernatraemia
9. **The normal S-T segment is:**

   a. Isoelectric b. Elevated with concavity upwards c. Depressed below the isoelectric line d. Elevated with convexity upwards
10. **Wide QRS complex is seen in:**

    a. Left bundle branch block b. Inferior wall MI c. Pericarditis d. Atrial flutter

11. **P wave is always inverted in lead:**

    a. aVL b. aVR c. aVF d. V1

12. **U wave is usually in the same direction as that of:**

    a. S wave b. S-T segment c. Tp wave d. T wave

13. **Hyperventilation can lead to inversion of:**

    a. P wave b. R wave c. R' wave d) T wave

14. **The normal upper limit of QRS interval is:**

    a. 0.10 s b. 0.12 s c. 0.15 s d. 0.20 s

15. **The QRS axis in ECG with R waves in Leads I, II and III with the tallest R wave in lead II is:**

    a. Left axis deviation b. Right axis deviation c. Northwest axis d. Normal axis

**Case Studies**

1. A 32-year-old gentleman had an electrocardiogram as part of a medical check-up. Examine his 12-lead ECG given in Fig. 10.5 and answer the following questions:

   a. What is the heart rate?
   b. Calculate the P-R interval.
   c. Calculate the QRS duration.
   d. Is normal sinus rhythm present?
   e. What is your final interpretation?

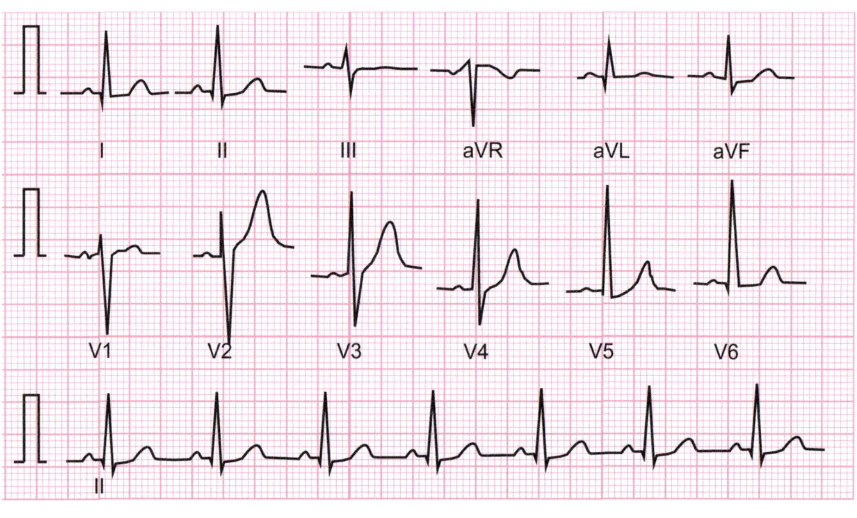


**Fig. 10.5** Calculate the P-R interval and QRS duration and interpret it

2. A 28-year-old gentleman got his ECG done during renewal of medical insurance policy. He has no chest pain, palpitation or dyspnoea. He does not smoke or drink alcohol. He is not suffering from hypertension or diabetes. His lipid profile is normal. Examine his 12-lead ECG given in Fig. 10.6 and answer the following questions.

   a. Calculate the P-R interval.
   b. Calculate the QRS duration.
   c. Is normal sinus rhythm present?
   d. What is the shape of the S-T segment?
   e. Can you identify any special wave in leads V3 and V4.
   f. What is your final interpretation?

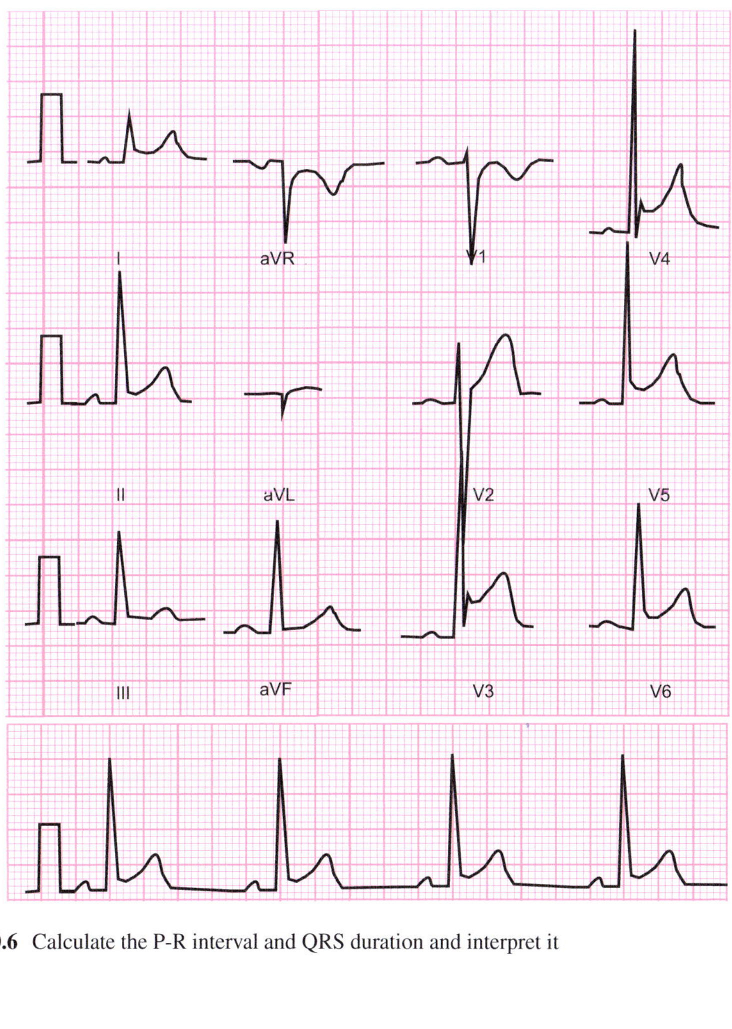


**Fig. 10.6** Calculate the P-R interval and QRS duration and interpret it

3. 12-lead ECG of a 25-year-old lady is given in Fig. 10.7. Examine it carefully and answer the following questions.

   a. Calculate the P-R interval.
   b. Calculate the QRS duration.
   c. Is normal sinus rhythm present?
   d. Identify the transition zone.
   e. What is your final interpretation?

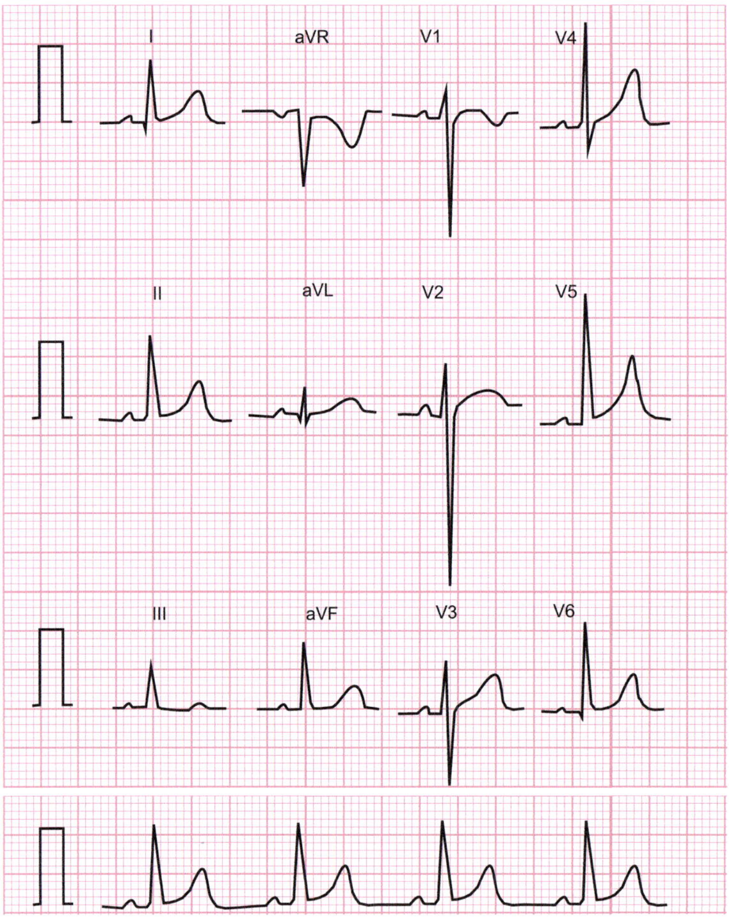


**Fig. 10.7** Calculate the P-R interval and QRS duration and interpret it

4. A 29-year-old gentleman's 12-lead ECG is given in Fig. 10.8. He is asymptomatic. Examine his ECG and answer the following questions.

   a. Calculate the P-R interval.
   b. Calculate the QRS duration.
   c. Is normal sinus rhythm present?
   d. Can you identify any abnormality of T waves.
   e. What is your final interpretation?

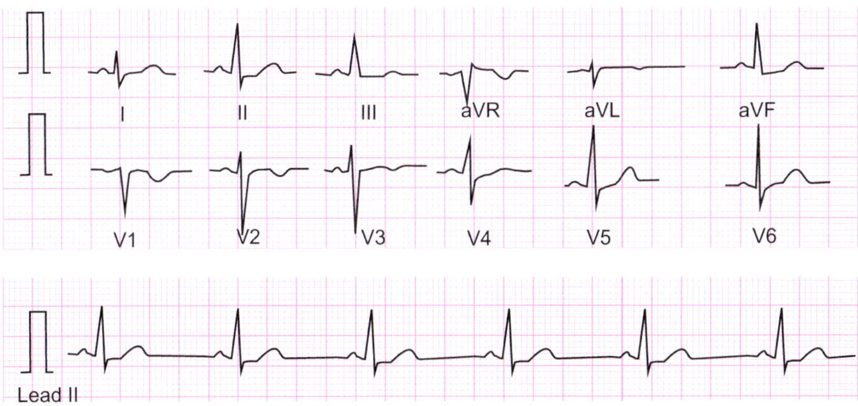


**Fig. 10.8** Calculate the P-R interval and QRS duration and interpret it

**Answers**

1. True 2. True 3. False 4. True 5. False 6. a 7. b 8. a 9. a 10. a 11. b 12. d 13. d 14. b 15. d

**Case Studies**

1. a. The heart rate is 1500 ÷ 17 = 88.23 bpm. It may be considered as 88 bpm.
   b. The P-R interval is 3 × 0.04 s = 0.12 s.
   c. The QRS duration is 2 × 0.04 s = 0.08 s.
   d. Normal sinus rhythm is present as evident by presence of smooth, round and upright P waves in leads II, III and aVF.
   e. For interpretation of a 12-lead ECG, the following aspects should be checked carefully—rate, rhythm (whether sinus or not, and whether regular or irregular), P wave (morphology of P wave and whether every P wave is followed by QRS complex or not), P-R interval, QRS duration, S-T segment, T wave, Q-T interval, QRS axis and special features. Complete analysis of ECG (Fig. 10.5):

   - Rate: 88 bpm.
   - Rhythm: Sinus rhythm, regular.
   - P wave: Smooth, round, upright and every P wave is followed by QRS complex.
   - P-R interval: 0.12 s.
   - QRS duration: 0.08 s.
   - S-T segment: Isoelectric.
   - T wave: Normal.
   - Q-T interval: 9 × 0.04 s = 0.36 s.
   - QRS axis: Normal.
   - Special feature: Nil.

   Every P wave is followed by a QRS complex. The QRS complexes are normal in all the 12 leads. P-R interval, QRS duration and heart rate are normal. The rhythm is regular. There is normal progression of R wave amplitude in chest leads. The transition zone is situated in lead V3. Hence, it is a normal electrocardiogram.
2. a. The P-R interval is 5 × 0.04 s = 0.20 s.
   b. The QRS duration is 2 × 0.04 s = 0.08 s.
   c. Every QRS complex is preceded by P wave. The P wave is smooth, round and upright in leads II, III and aVF. Hence, normal sinus rhythm is present.
   d. The S-T segment is elevated with concavity upwards in leads I, II, V3, V4, V5 and V6. J wave is present in leads V3 and V4.
   e. Complete analysis of ECG (Fig. 10.6):

   - Rate: 1500 ÷ 25 or 300 ÷ 5 = 60 bpm.
   - Rhythm: Sinus rhythm, regular.

- P wave: Smooth, round, upright and every P wave is followed by QRS complex.
- P-R interval: 0.20 s.
- QRS duration: 0.08 s.
- S-T segment: The S-T segment is elevated with concavity upwards in leads I, II, V3, V4, V5 and V6.
- T wave: Normal.
- Q-T interval: 9 × 0.04 s = 0.36 s.
- QRS axis: Normal.
- Special feature: J wave is present in leads V3 and V4; tall R waves in lead V3 and V4.

The ECG belongs to a young man. He is asymptomatic and has no risk factors for coronary artery disease. There are tall R waves in precordial leads with concave upwards elevated S-T segment and J waves in leads V3 and V4. These features point towards the diagnosis of early repolarization syndrome. This type of ECG is often confused with ECG of myocardial infarction.

3. a. The P-R interval is 3 × 0.04 s = 0.12 s.
   b. The QRS duration is 2 × 0.04 s = 0.08 s.
   c. Every QRS complex is preceded by P wave. The P wave is smooth, round and upright in leads II, III and aVF. Hence, the normal sinus rhythm is present.
   d. The transition zone is situated in lead V3.
   e. Complete analysis of ECG (Fig. 10.7):

- Rate: 1500 ÷ 19 = 78.94 bpm. This may be considered as 79 bpm.
- Rhythm: Sinus rhythm, regular.
- P wave: Smooth, round, upright and every P wave is followed by QRS complex.
- P-R interval: 0.12 s.
- QRS duration: 0.08 s.
- S-T segment: Isoelectric.
- T wave: Normal.
- Q-T interval: 9 × 0.04 s = 0.36 s.
- QRS axis: Normal.
- Special feature: Nil.

The QRS complexes are normal in all the 12 leads. P-R interval and QRS duration are normal. There is normal progression of R wave amplitude in chest leads. The transition zone is situated in lead V3. Hence, it is a normal electrocardiogram.

4. a. The P-R interval is $3 \times 0.04$ s = 0.12 s.
   b. The QRS duration is $2 \times 0.04$ s = 0.08 s.
   c. Every QRS complex is preceded by P wave. The P wave is smooth, round and upright in leads II, III and aVF. Hence, the normal sinus rhythm is present.
   d. The T waves are inverted in leads V1–V3.
   e. Complete analysis of ECG (Fig. 10.8):

- Rate: $1500 \div 23 = 65.21$ bpm. This may be considered as 65 bpm.
- Rhythm: Sinus rhythm, regular.
- P wave: Smooth, round, upright and every P wave is followed by QRS complex.
- P-R interval: 0.12 s.
- QRS duration: 0.08 s.
- S-T segment: Isoelectric.
- T wave: Inverted in leads V1–V3 and lead aVL.
- Q-T interval: $9 \times 0.04$ s = 0.36 s.
- QRS axis: Normal.
- Special feature: Inversion of T wave in leads V1–V3.

The ECG belongs to a young asymptomatic man. Except for T wave inversion in leads V1–V3, rest of the ECG is normal. Hence, the final interpretation is persistent juvenile pattern, which is a variant of normal ECG.

# Part II
# ECG Patterns in Chamber Enlargement

# Chapter 11
# Atrial Enlargement

**Learning Objectives**
After studying this chapter, the reader will learn about:

- Right atrial enlargement
- Left atrial enlargement
- Combined right and left atrial enlargement

In the previous chapters, the basic aspects of normal ECG were described. Now, the abnormal ECG patterns seen in various diseases will be described. This chapter will focus on the abnormal ECG patterns seen in atrial enlargement.

There may be hypertrophy or enlargement of atria, ventricles or both. The term enlargement implies the presence of dilatation or hypertrophy or both. Dilatation is an increase in internal diameter of a chamber of heart caused by volume overload. Hypertrophy is thickening of muscular wall of a chamber of heart due to pressure overload. The term enlargement is usually used for atria and hypertrophy is used for ventricles.

**Tips and Tricks**
- In atrial enlargement, the changes are mainly seen in P waves, whereas in ventricular hypertrophy, the changes are mainly seen in QRS complexes.

Atrial enlargement is common ECG change encountered in day-to-day clinical practice. The enlargement of the atria occurs in various conditions, for example, chronic obstructive pulmonary disease, rheumatic heart disease and congenital heart disease with pulmonary hypertension. In atrial enlargement, the changes are primarily seen in the P waves. Lead II and lead V1 are the two most important leads that reflect the changes of P wave in atrial enlargement.



T. K. Koley, *Rapid Review of ECG*,
https://doi.org/10.1007/978-981-99-9116-7_11

## 11.1 Right Atrial Enlargement

Enlargement or hypertrophy of right atrium is commonly seen in various conditions including mitral stenosis, cor pulmonale, ASD, tricuspid stenosis, pulmonary stenosis and tricuspid regurgitation. Prolonged increase in right atrial pressure leads to right atrial enlargement. In right atrial enlargement, there is increase in the amplitude of the P wave, without any increase in duration. In this condition, the electrical vector generated in right atrium is strong due to the enlarged right atrium. This electrical vector is oriented mainly in the direction of lead II, but also towards lead aVF and lead III. In all these leads an unusually large (i.e. > 0.25 mV or 2.5 mm) P wave is seen. The ECG features of right atrial enlargement are:

- P pulmonale
- P pulmonale is diagnosed by presence of tall and peaked P waves in lead II, III and aVF (Figs. 11.1 and 11.2). The amplitude is more than 2.5 mm. It is called p pulmonale because it is frequently seen in diseases involving the lungs causing pulmonary hypertension.
- P wave may be normal or biphasic with a slight increase in amplitude (> 1.5 mm) of the initial component in lead V1.
- The axis of the P wave is deviated to right (between +80° and +90°). The normal P wave axis is around +60°. The enlargement of right atrium may result in right atrial electrical dominance over the left atrium. This results in rightward swing of the vector of atrial depolarization, leading to a rightward deviation of P wave axis.

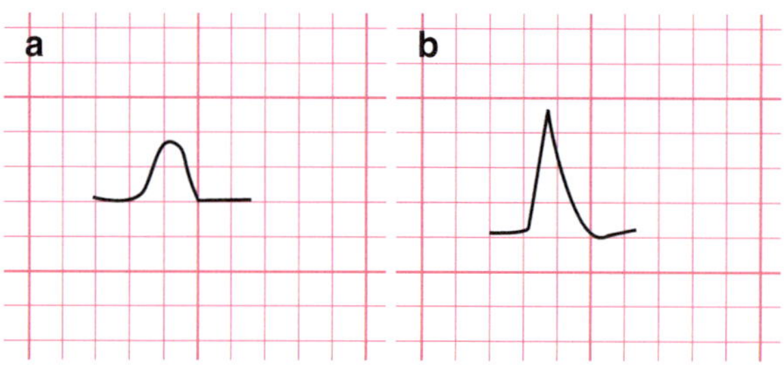


**Fig. 11.1** Diagram of normal P wave and tall P wave of right atrial enlargement. Note the round contour of normal P wave (**a**) and the tall and peaked contour of P wave of right atrial enlargement (**b**). The height of P wave of right atrial enlargement is more than 2.5 mm

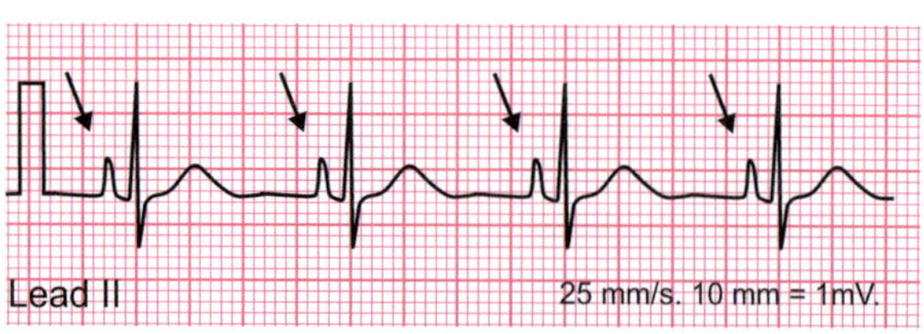


**Fig. 11.2** P pulmonale. This ECG is recorded from a 42-year-old lady suffering from pulmonary hypertension. Note the tall and peaked P waves (arrow)

- Two features of QRS complex suggest right atrial enlargement. There is a high incidence of RVH in presence of right atrial enlargement. Besides this, right ventricle is also displaced by an enlarged right atrium. These two features are:
  (a) qR complex in lead V1
  (b) Decrease in size of QRS complex in lead V1 with a marked increase in QRS amplitude in lead V2

## 11.2 Left Atrial Enlargement

Enlargement of left atrium is often seen secondary to left ventricular hypertrophy in various conditions including hypertensive heart disease, cardiomyopathy, aortic stenosis, mitral regurgitation and VSD. The enlargement is an anatomical change due to prolonged increased left atrial pressure. As mentioned earlier, the left atrial depolarization results in second half of the P wave. The first half of P wave is due to right atrial depolarization. Hence, the ECG changes of left atrial enlargement are mainly due to abnormalities in the second half of the P wave. In left atrial enlargement, the electrical vector generated in enlarged left atrium is strong and is directed towards positive pole of lead I and away from the positive pole of lead V1. The longer lasting depolarization of enlarged left atrium results in prolongation and often bifidity of the P wave. This is known as P mitrale (commonly seen in mitral stenosis, hence the term). The specific diagnostic criterion for left atrial enlargement is the terminal portion of the P wave in lead V1, having duration ≥ 0.04 s and negative amplitude ≥ 0.1 mV (more than 1 × 1 small squares). This results in a biphasic P wave with a prominent negative component in lead V1. The ECG features of left atrial enlargement are:

- P mitrale
  P mitrale is diagnosed by presence of a wide, double peaked, prolonged P wave. The P wave duration is more than 0.11 s. The duration between the two peaks of P wave is greater than 0.04 s (Figs. 11.3 and 11.4). This is best seen in lead II.
- P wave is biphasic with a deep and wide terminal negative component in lead V1 (Fig. 11.5). P terminal force also known as Morris Index is calculated by multiplying the depth of the negative component (in mm) by the duration of the nega-

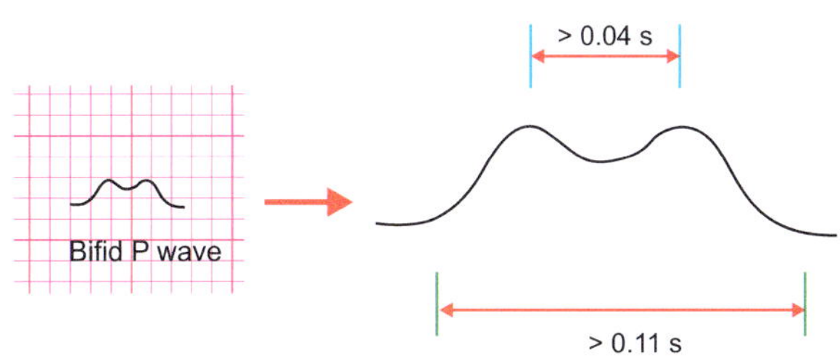


**Fig. 11.3** Diagram of P mitrale. The total duration of P wave is more than 0.11 s and the interval between the two peaks of P wave is more than 0.04 s

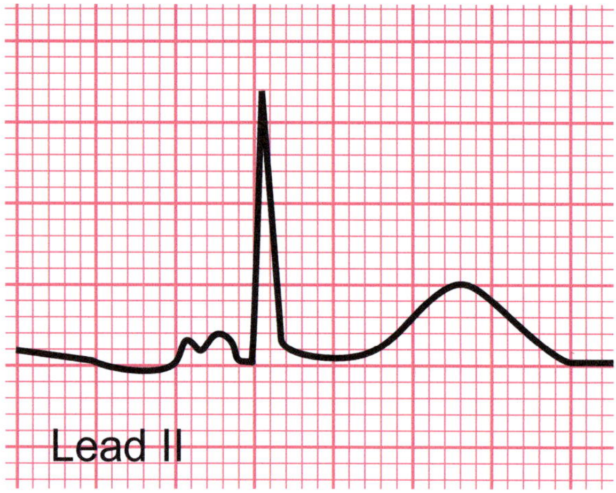


**Fig. 11.4** P mitrale. Note the bifid P wave

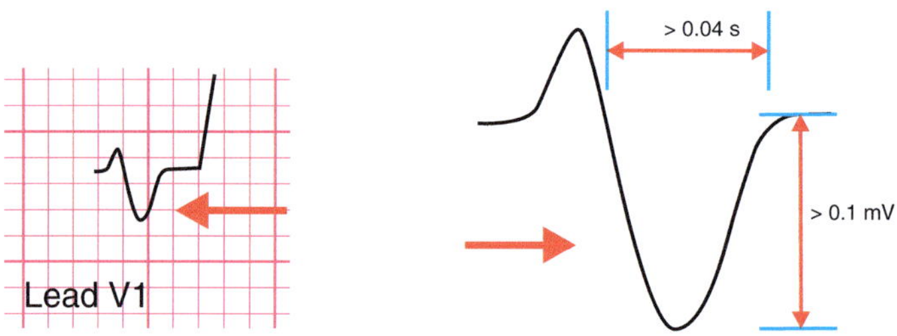


**Fig. 11.5** Diagram of P wave of left atrial enlargement in lead V1. Note the deep and wide negative component of the biphasic P wave (arrow)

tive component (in second). It is expressed in millimetre-second. Normally it is less than 0.03 mm-s. P terminal force more than 0.03 mm-s represents left atrial enlargement.

- Left axis deviation of P wave

## 11.3 Combined Left and Right Atrial Enlargement

In biatrial enlargement, there is combination of ECG features of left and right atrial enlargement. The ECG features are the following:

- The P wave is wide and notched with increased amplitude. When this type of P wave is associated with an initial component that is taller than the terminal component, it is known as p tricuspidale. It is commonly seen in diseases affecting the tricuspid valve.

- In lead V1, there will be a large biphasic P wave. The initial component of this P wave is tall and peaked (more than 1.5 mm), and the terminal component is wide, deep and delayed (1 mm in amplitude and more than 0.04 s in duration). The initial component is due to right atrial enlargement and the terminal component is due to the left atrial enlargement.
- Tall and peaked P wave (more than 1.5 mm) in right sided chest leads and wide, notched P wave in left sided chest leads and limb leads (Fig. 11.6).
- Various conditions associated with biatrial enlargement are enumerated in Box 11.1.

**Box 11.1 Conditions Associated with Biatrial Enlargement**
Mitral stenosis with severe pulmonary hypertension
Mitral stenosis with tricuspid stenosis
ASD
Mitral stenosis with tricuspid regurgitation
Lutembacher's syndrome, i.e. ASD with acquired rheumatic mitral stenosis

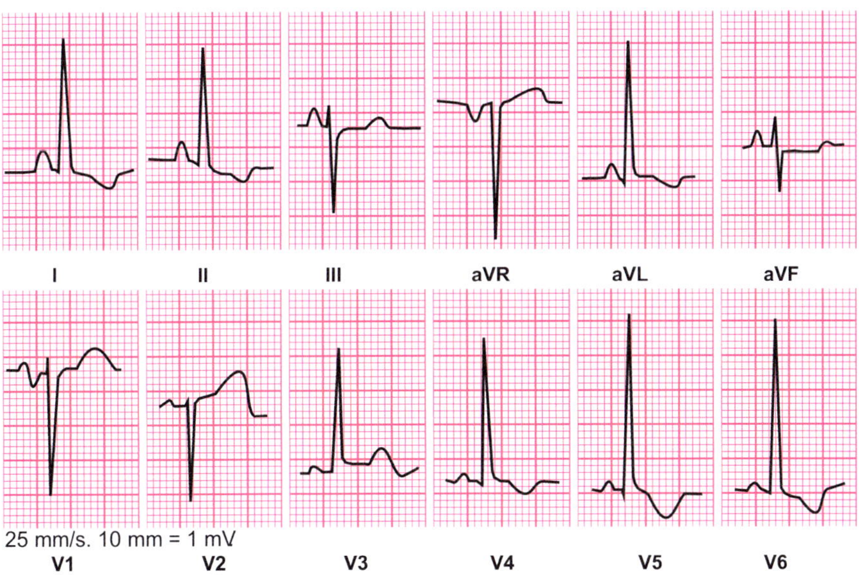


**Fig. 11.6** Biatrial enlargement. Note the tall P waves in limb leads and a broad biphasic P wave in lead V1

**Tips and Tricks**

- To diagnose right atrial enlargement, look at the height of P wave (more than 2.5 mm).
- To diagnose left atrial enlargement, look at the width of P wave (more than 0.11 s).
- If P pulmonale is present, diagnosis is right atrial enlargement.
- If P mitrale is present, diagnosis is left atrial enlargement.
- If P tricuspidale is present, diagnosis is biatrial enlargement.

**Self-Assessment Questions**

1. Pressure overload leads to hypertrophy of muscular wall of cardiac chamber. True or false?
2. Biatrial enlargement is seen in Lutembacher's syndrome. True or false?
3. The height of P wave is more than 2.5 mm in P pulmonale. True or false?
4. To diagnose atrial enlargement, focus should be on QRS complex. True or false?
5. Biatrial enlargement is diagnosed by P mitrale. True or false?
6. **Right atrial enlargement is characterized by:**

   a. Increased amplitude of the P wave in lead II b. Prolonged P-R interval c. Widened QRS complex d. Tall and peaked T waves

7. **In biatrial enlargement, the P wave in lead V1 may be:**

   a. Large and biphasic b. Negative, with an inverted shape c. Positive, with a tall and peaked appearance d. Absent

8. **Right atrial enlargement may be caused by:**

   a. Pulmonary hypertension b. Left ventricular hypertrophy c. Aortic stenosis d. Mitral regurgitation

9. **Left atrial enlargement is characterized by:**

   a. Increased amplitude of the P wave in lead II b. Prolonged P-R interval c. Bifid P wave d. Tall and peaked T waves

10. **To diagnose left atrial enlargement, P wave should be examined in:**

    a. Lead V5 and V6 b. Lead aVR and aVL c. Lead I and aVL d. Lead II and V1

**Case Studies**

1. A 23-year-old young lady suffering from breathlessness arrived at the emergency. She had mid-diastolic murmur, opening snap and a loud S1. Her ECG (lead II) is given below (Fig. 11.7). Can you identify the abnormality?
2. Lead V1 of a 12-lead ECG is shown in Fig. 11.8. Identify the abnormality and name two conditions in which you will find this abnormality.
3. A 50-year-old gentleman came to emergency department with severe breathlessness. He has similar attacks in the past for which he ignored treatment. He is a chronic smoker. His chest X-ray revealed increased bilateral bronchovascular marking, hyperinflated lungs with flattened hemidiaphragms. Lead II of a 12-lead ECG is shown in Fig. 11.9. Identify the abnormality and name two conditions in which you will find this abnormality.

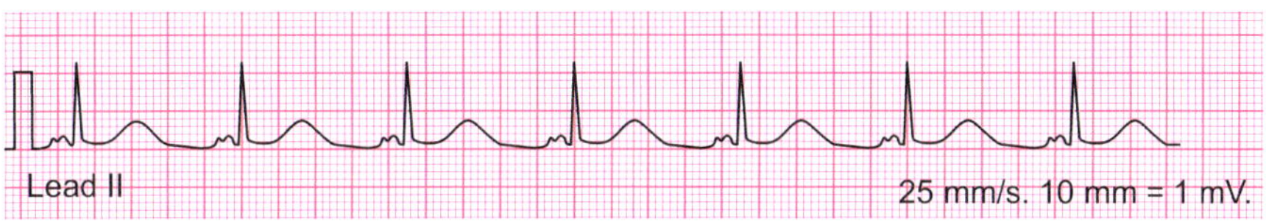


**Fig. 11.7** Identify the ECG abnormality

**Fig. 11.8** Identify the ECG abnormality

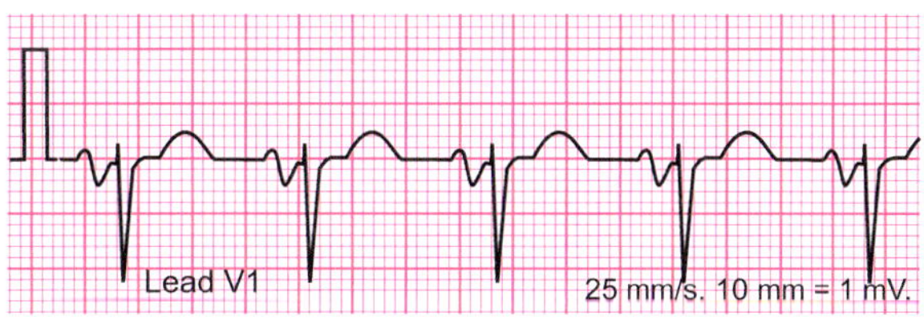


**Fig. 11.9** Identify the ECG abnormality

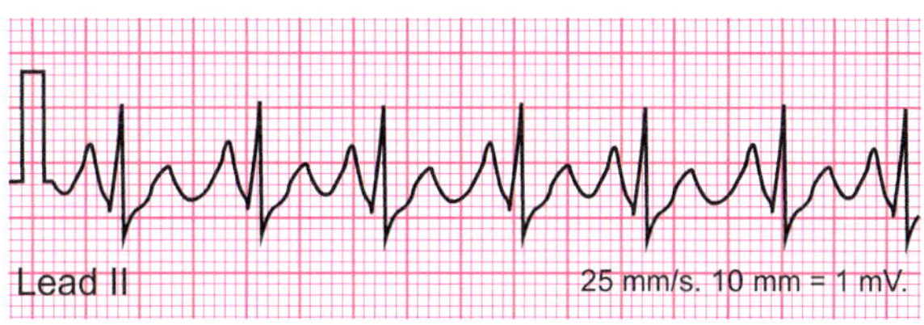

**Answers**

1. True 2. True 3. True 4. False 5. False 6. a 7. a 8. a 9. c 10. d

**Case Studies**

1. There are bifid P waves. The P wave has two peaks and the two peaks are more than 0.04 s apart. This is P mitrale. It is suggestive of left atrial enlargement. Mid-diastolic murmur with opening snap and loud S1 indicates mitral stenosis. So it is a case of mitral stenosis. However, this patient should be further investigated and echocardiography should be done to treat her properly. She may need a mitral valve replacement.
2. There is a biphasic P wave in lead V1 with deep and wide terminal negative component. The negative component is more than 0.04 s in duration and more than 1 mm (0.1 mV) in depth. This indicates left atrial enlargement. It is observed in mitral stenosis and mitral regurgitation.
3. There are tall and peaked P waves. These are called P pulmonale which indicates right atrial enlargement. History of similar past attacks in presence of smoking indicates chronic obstructive pulmonary disease. Chest X-ray further confirms the diagnosis. P pulmonale is also seen in pulmonary hypertension and tricuspid regurgitation.

# Chapter 12
# Ventricular Hypertrophy

**Learning Objectives**
After studying this chapter, the reader will learn about:

- Left ventricular hypertrophy
- Right ventricular hypertrophy
- Biventricular hypertrophy

Ventricular hypertrophy is caused by pressure or volume overload of ventricles. Concentric hypertrophy is caused by pressure overload, and eccentric hypertrophy is caused by volume overload. Changes in the amplitude of the R and S waves are reflected in ECG.

## 12.1 Pressure (Systolic) Overload

Pressure overload occurs when the heart pumps against an increased resistance, as in systemic hypertension. Chronic increase in resistance results in concentric hypertrophy, in which the ventricular wall thickens as compared to the ventricular cavity. In hypertrophy, the cardiac muscle fibres increase in size. In ECG, the main changes are increased voltage of QRS complex, depression of S-T segment and asymmetric inversion of T wave in the chest leads.



T. K. Koley, *Rapid Review of ECG*,
https://doi.org/10.1007/978-981-99-9116-7_12

## 12.2 Volume (Diastolic) Overload

Persistent increased volume, as seen in valvular regurgitation, results in stretching or dilatation of the ventricular chamber. This is known as eccentric hypertrophy in which the ventricular wall thickness remains normal relative to the increase in the radius of the ventricle. Volume and pressure overload often occur together.

## 12.3 Left Ventricular Hypertrophy

Prolonged raised pressure in left ventricle leads to anatomical changes of left ventricle hypertrophy (LVH). The various causes of LVH are enumerated in Box 12.1. Diagnosis of LVH (Fig. 12.1) is important because it indicates the future possibility of major cardiovascular complications. The ECG criteria for diagnosis of LVH are quite specific. However, one must always remember that similar ECG changes may be seen in young persons and athletes as well. Besides this, the ECG criteria are not

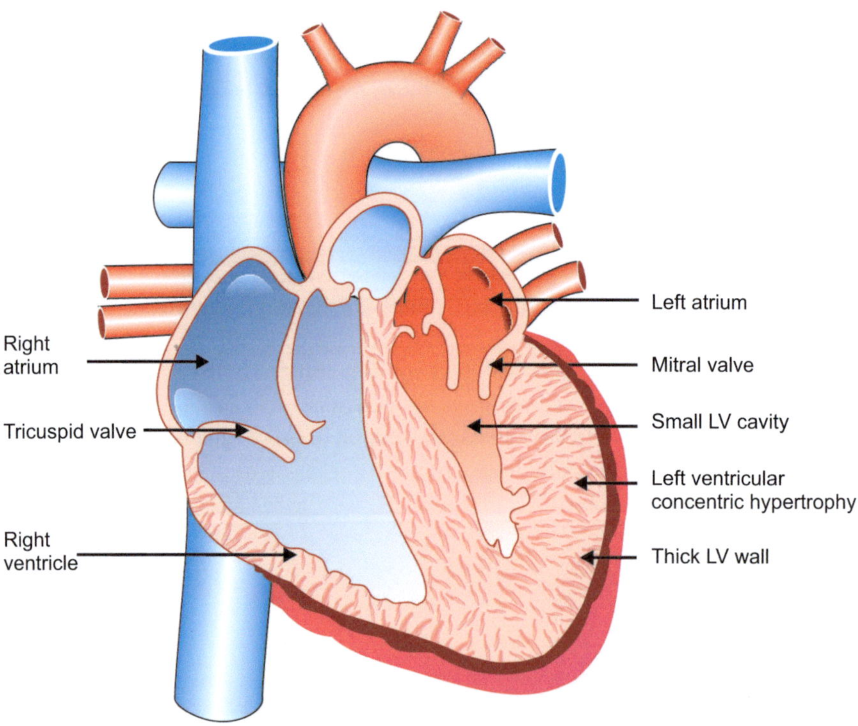


**Fig. 12.1** Left ventricular hypertrophy. Note the wall thickness of left ventricle and the small left ventricular cavity

always reliable in presence of bundle branch block, WPW syndrome and previous myocardial infarction. Hence, all ECG changes should be interpreted in light of the clinical findings.

**Box 12.1 Some Important Causes of LVH**
Aortic stenosis
Aortic regurgitation
Mitral regurgitation
Hypertensive heart disease
Congenital heart disease like PDA, coarctation of aorta and tricuspid atresia
Hypertrophic cardiomyopathy

After the neonatal period, the left ventricle becomes hypertrophied as compared to right ventricle. The left ventricular electrical dominance is reflected in ECG by tall R waves in left-sided chest leads and deep S waves in right sided chest leads. In presence of LVH, there is further dominance of the electrical forces generated in the left ventricle. This is reflected in ECG by increase in the height of R waves in left-sided chest leads and depth of S waves in right sided chest leads.

The following are the ECG changes of left ventricular hypertrophy:

- Abnormalities of QRS complex
- Abnormalities of S-T segment and T wave
- Abnormalities of QRS axis
- Inversion of U wave
- Left atrial enlargement

## *12.3.1 Abnormalities of QRS Complex*

### 12.3.1.1 Increased Amplitude of QRS Complex

The amplitude of the QRS complex is increased in LVH due to increase in left ventricular mass. Since ventricular activation occurs from endocardium to epicardium, the amplitude of the R and S waves indicates the thickness of the ventricular wall. The amplitude of the QRS complex is increased in LVH. There is deep S wave in lead V1 and tall R wave in leads V5 and V6 (Fig. 12.2). In an adult above 35 years of age if the sum of R wave in lead V5 and the depth of S wave in lead V1 exceed 35 mm, it indicates LVH. Sokolow-Lyon voltage criteria are used for diagnosis of LVH (Box 12.2) in adults over 35 years of age.

**Box 12.2 Sokolow-Lyon Voltage Criteria for LVH**
RI + SIII ≥ 2.5 mv (25 mm)
R in aVL > 1.2 mv (12 mm)
R in aVF > 2.0 mv (20 mm)
S in VI ≥ 2.4 mv (24 mm)
R in V5 or V6 > 2.6 mv (26 mm)
R in V5 or V6 + S in VI > 3.5 mv (35 mm)

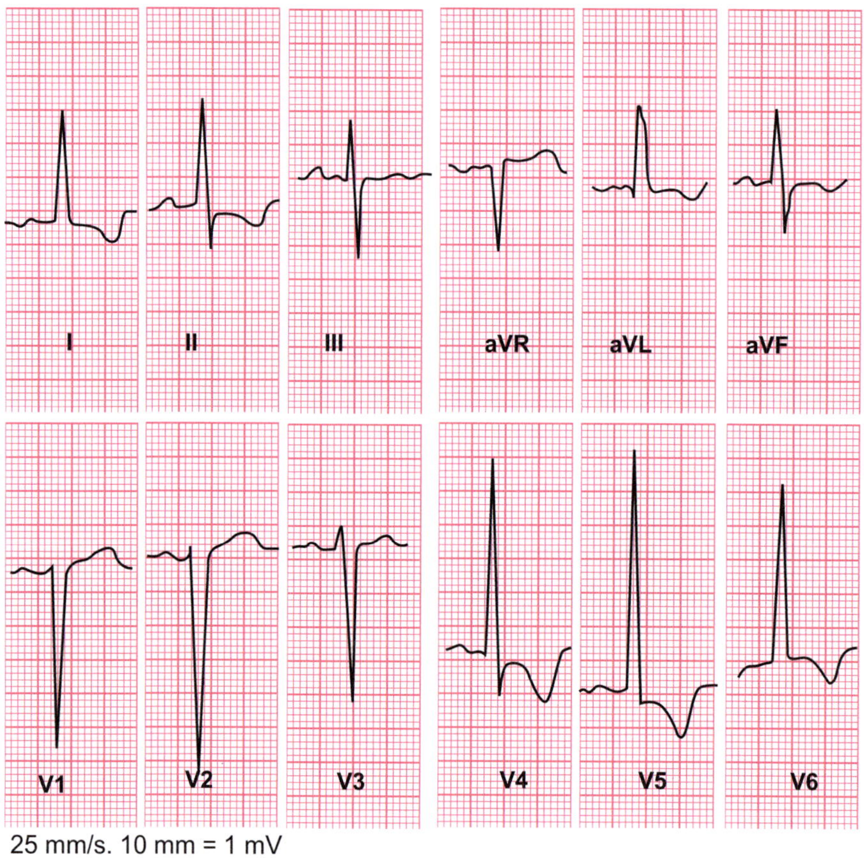


**Fig. 12.2** Left ventricular hypertrophy. This ECG is recorded from a 64-year-old gentleman suffering from hypertension for last 20 years. Note the S-T segment, T wave change in leads V4, V5 and V6. SV1 + RV5 is 61 mm

### 12.3.1.2 Increase in Ventricular Activation Time

Ventricular activation time is increased in LVH to more than 0.05 s in lead V5 or lead V6 due to increase in wall thickness.

#### 12.3.1.3 Counterclockwise Electric Rotation

The counterclockwise electric rotation of heart leads to shifting of transition zone to lead V3 or even lead V2.

### *12.3.2 Abnormalities of S-T Segment and T Wave*

The left ventricle is under strain in LVH and it is manifested by S-T segment depression and T wave inversion in leads V5, V6, aVL and lead I. This is termed left ventricular strain (Fig. 12.3).

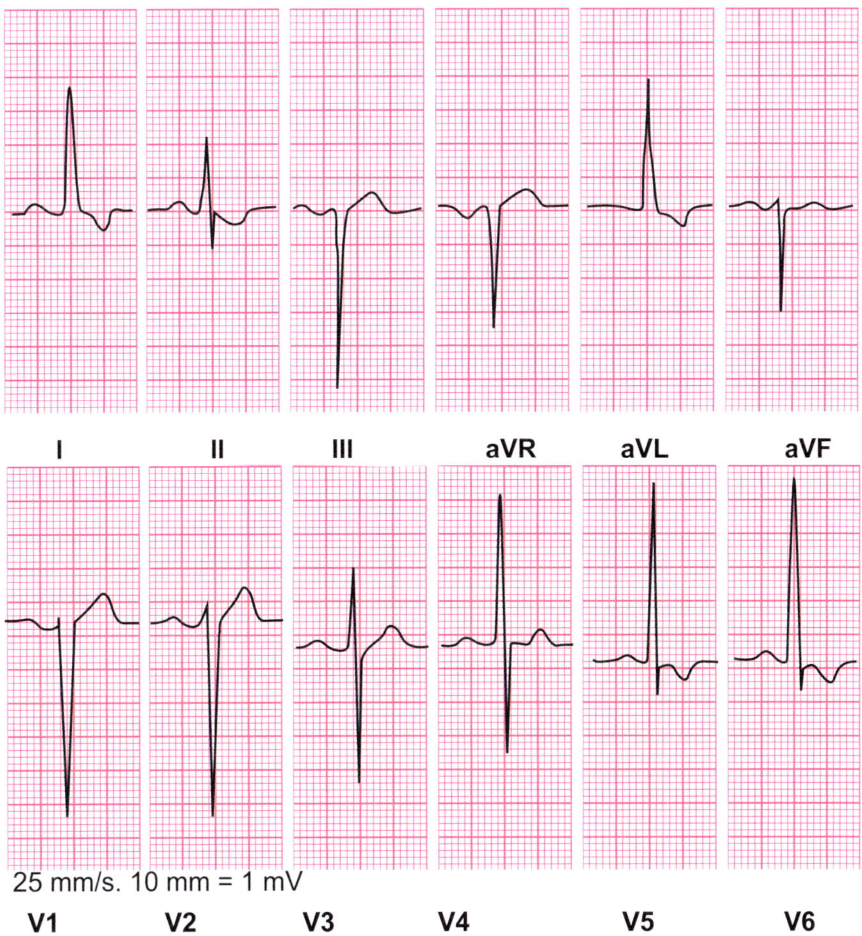


**Fig. 12.3** Left ventricular hypertrophy. SV1 + RV5 is more than 35 mm. There is tall R wave in lead aVL and left axis deviation. There are S-T segment, T wave changes in leads V5 and V6

### 12.3.3 Abnormalities of QRS Axis

Normal QRS axis is seen in early and uncomplicated LVH. However, in long standing LVH, especially that associated with hypertension leads to fibrosis, which affects the left anterior fascicle resulting in left anterior hemiblock. This results in left axis deviation.

### 12.3.4 Inversion of U Wave

There is inversion of U wave in left-sided chest leads.

### 12.3.5 Left Atrial Enlargement

Left atrial enlargement provides contributory evidence of left ventricular hypertrophy. It helps in diagnosis of LVH in presence of left bundle branch block. There may be wide and notched P wave in lead II and there may be biphasic P wave in lead V1 with a deep negative component.

Romhilt and Estes point score system combines several of the above mentioned criteria. A score of 4 indicates probable LVH and a score of 5 indicates LVH. All the diagnostic criteria of Romhilt and Estes point score system are enumerated in Box 12.3. The important diagnostic criteria of LVH are enumerated in Box 12.4.

**Box 12.3 Romhilt and Estes Point Score**

1. Voltage criteria (any of the following):
   - Largest R or S wave in limb leads ≥ 20 mm 3 Points
   - S wave in V1 or V2 ≥ 30 mm
   - R wave in V5 or V6 ≥ 30 mm
2. ST-T abnormalities (left ventricular strain pattern):
   - ST-T vector opposite to QRS without digitalis 3 Points
   - ST-T vector opposite to QRS with digitalis 1 Point
3. (Left atrial abnormality)
   - P terminal force in V1 is 1 mm or more in depth with a duration ≥ 0.04 s 3 Points
4. Left axis deviation (QRS axis of −30° or more) 2 points
5. QRS duration ≥ 0.09 s 1 Point
6. Intrinsicoid deflection in V5 or V6 (> 0.05 s) 1 Point

LVH due to diastolic overload (excess blood flow in left ventricle) as happens in aortic incompetence or mitral incompetence has the following features:

Like in systolic overload, there are tall R waves in leads V5 and V6. They may be even taller than what is seen in systolic overload.

There are narrow and deep Q waves in leads V5 and V6. These do not indicate any old myocardial infarction.

The T waves in leads V5 and V6 are taller than the normal T waves in those leads. Often they are pointed with arrowhead appearance.

The S-T segment in leads V5 and V6 are slightly elevated with concavity upwards (Fig. 12.4).

**Box 12.4 Diagnostic Criteria of LVH**
Increased amplitude of QRS complex
Increase in VAT in lead V5 or V6
Counterclockwise rotation of heart
S-T, T strain pattern in lead V5 or V6
Left axis deviation
Inversion of U wave
Left atrial enlargement
Romhilt and Estes point of 5 or more

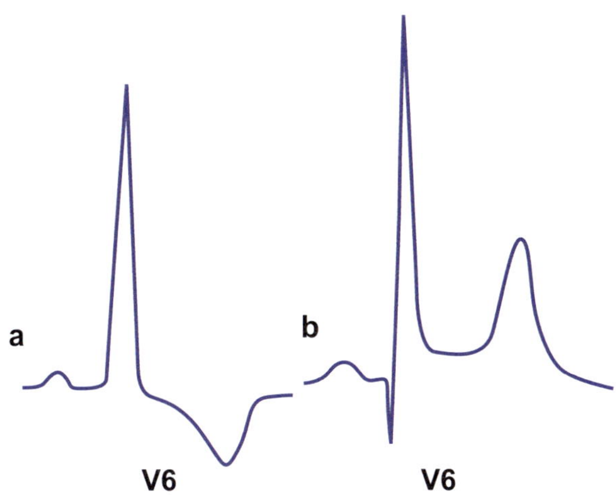


**Fig. 12.4** Diagram showing QRS complex in lead V6 in LVH: systolic (**a**) and diastolic (**b**) overload. In systolic overload, the initial q wave often disappears, whereas in diastolic overload, the initial q wave becomes prominent. The amplitude of R wave is increased in both. The T wave is inverted with S-T segment depression in systolic overload but in diastolic overload the S-T segment may be minimally elevated with upward concavity

**Tips and Tricks**

- If you come across an ECG with big QRS amplitudes in chest leads, think of LVH. However, it can be seen in healthy persons also.
- To diagnose LVH calculate SV1 + RV5. If it is more than 35, think about the possibility of LVH.

## 12.4 Right Ventricular Hypertrophy

The ECG features for diagnosis of right ventricular hypertrophy (RVH) are specific but lack sensitivity. Conditions like hyperinflated lungs, young age, bundle branch block and body build often make the diagnosis of RVH difficult. The diagnosis is further difficult in young children, as there are prominent R waves in right-sided chest leads due to physiological dominance of right ventricle over the left.

Right ventricular hypertrophy (RVH) is seen in various conditions including pulmonary stenosis, tetralogy of Fallot, cor pulmonale, mitral stenosis, tricuspid incompetence and idiopathic pulmonary hypertension. Prolonged raised pressure in right ventricle leads to anatomical changes of right ventricular hypertrophy (Fig. 12.5). Because of strong vectors generated in the dominant left ventricle, severe RVH must be present to dominate and manifest on the ECG. As a result, it is difficult to diagnose minor degrees of right ventricular hypertrophy.

The lead V1 is close to the right ventricular mass, hence, it is the most sensitive lead to record the changes of RVH. In normal condition, prominent S wave and a small r wave are recorded in lead V1. The dominant left ventricular vector neutralizes the right ventricular vector. As it is directed away from the positive pole of lead V1, a prominent S wave is recorded. In RVH, the right ventricular vector becomes strong and it neutralizes the left ventricular vector. It is directed towards the positive pole of lead V1, hence, a tall R wave is recorded instead of a deep S wave. Therefore, a tall R wave, a small s wave or a change in R:S ratio are seen in lead V1.

RVH should not be diagnosed only on the basis of ECG changes seen in lead V1. It is important to look for as many features as possible in ECG to arrive at a correct diagnosis. The ECG features should always be interpreted in light of the clinical features. More the ECG features, better is the chance of correct diagnosis. Right ventricular hypertrophy is characterized by the following ECG abnormalities:

- Abnormalities of QRS complex
- Abnormalities of S-T segment and T wave
- Abnormality of QRS axis
- Right atrial enlargement

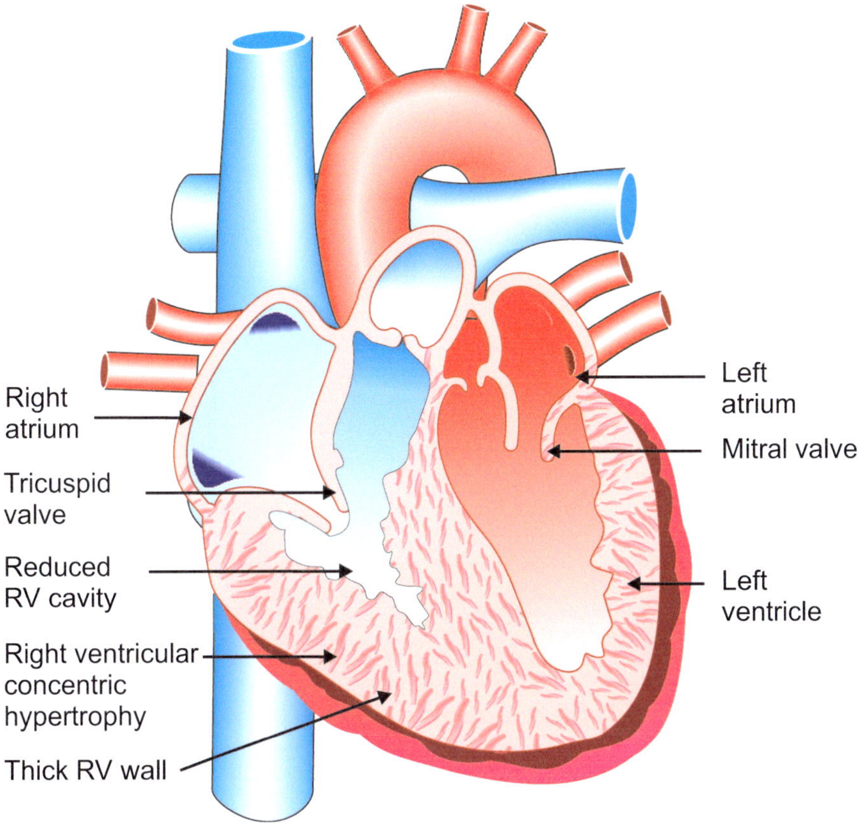


**Fig. 12.5** Right ventricular hypertrophy. Note the thickness of right ventricular wall and decrease in cavity size. This is concentric hypertrophy

## *12.4.1 Abnormalities of QRS Complex*

### 12.4.1.1 Dominance of R Wave in Right-Sided Chest Leads

The R wave in lead V1 becomes prominent in comparison to S wave in RVH. There is gradual, progressive increase in height of R wave and diminution of S wave, which is expressed as R:S ratio (Fig. 12.6). If the ratio exceeds 1, then RVH is diagnosed. The amplitude of R wave is more than 5 mm in lead V1. The S waves are prominent in V5 and V6. It is important to remember that there are several other causes of tall R wave in lead V1 including posterior wall myocardial infarction, persistent juvenile pattern, RBBB, dextrocardia and WPW syndrome.

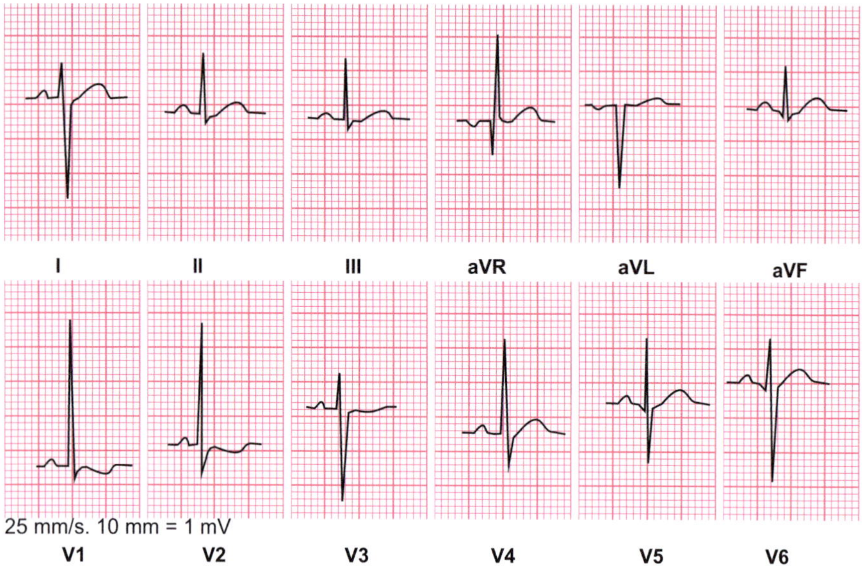


**Fig. 12.6** Right ventricular hypertrophy. R:S ratio is more than 1 in lead V1. There is right axis deviation with clockwise rotation

#### 12.4.1.2 In Lead V1 There Is Increase in VAT (> 0.02 s)

#### 12.4.1.3 Clockwise Electric Rotation

Clockwise rotation is reflected by the shifting of transition zone to lead V5 or V6. All the chest leads may show prominent R waves only.

#### 12.4.1.4 Right Bundle Branch Block

Complete or incomplete RBBB is often associated with RVH.

### *12.4.2 Abnormalities of S-T Segment and T Wave*

Strain pattern in right-sided chest leads is often seen in RVH. The S-T segment is slightly depressed with inversion of T waves in lead V1–V4.

### *12.4.3 Abnormalities of QRS Axis*

QRS axis is deviated to right in RVH. The QRS axis lies between +110° and +180°. Sometimes it is the only feature of RVH.

### *12.4.4 Right Atrial Enlargement*

ECG features of right atrial enlargement are often associated with RVH. The P waves become tall and pointed in lead II. The diagnostic criteria of RVH are enumerated in Box 12.5.

**Box 12.5 Diagnostic criteria of RVH**
R:S ratio greater than 1 in lead V1
Increase in VAT in lead V1 or V2
Clockwise rotation of heart
Right axis deviation
S-T, T strain pattern in leads V1–V4
Right atrial enlargement

**Tips and Tricks**

- To diagnose RVH, look at lead V1 and calculate the R:S ratio. If it is more than 1 and the height of R wave is more than 5 mm, think about the possibility of RVH.

## 12.5 Biventricular Hypertrophy

Hypertrophy of both the ventricles is not an uncommon condition. It is frequently observed in Eisenmenger's syndrome. The various other conditions are enumerated in Box 12.6.

**Box 12.6 Causes of Biventricular Hypertrophy**
Dilated cardiomyopathy
Congenital heart disease: Eisenmenger's syndrome
Multiple valvular lesions

It is not always easy to diagnose biventricular hypertrophy in ECG. The ECG features of LVH may be masked by the development of RVH. The ECG may actually become normal. However, one must look for the following features diagnostic of biventricular hypertrophy:

- Right axis deviation with ECG features of LVH
- Clockwise rotation, i.e. transition zone in lead V5 or V6 with ECG features of LVH
- ECG features of LVH along with tall R wave in lead V1 especially if R:S ratio is greater than 1 indicate biventricular hypertrophy
- Katz-Wachtel phenomenon: Large biphasic complexes in lead V2 or V3
- P mitrale with R:S ratio greater than 1 in lead V1 or right QRS axis deviation
- Tall R waves in left-sided chest leads with disproportionately small S waves in lead V1 or inverted T wave in right precordial leads

**Self-Assessment Questions**

1. Left ventricular hypertrophy is seen in mitral stenosis. True or false?
2. Romhilt Estes point score is used for diagnosis of LVH. True or false?
3. VAT is increased in RVH in lead V1 or V2. True or false?
4. Katz-Wachtel phenomenon is seen in biventricular hypertrophy. True or false?
5. Clockwise electric rotation is seen in LVH. True or false?
6. **Features of RVH are all except:**

   a. Right axis deviation (> 90°) b. Tall R waves in left-sided chest leads; deep S waves in right-sided chest leads c. RV strain pattern d. May see incomplete RBBB pattern or qR pattern in V1

7. **All of the following are features of LVH except:**

   a. Increased QRS amplitude b. Delayed intrinsicoid deflection in lead V1 c. Left ventricular strain pattern d. Biphasic P wave in lead V1 with prominent negative component

8. **ECG features of LVH with right axis deviation indicate:**

   a. Biventricular hypertrophy b. LVH c. RVH d. Biatrial hypertrophy

9. **A 25-year-old lady is suffering from mitral stenosis for last 10 years. She has not taken any treatment for mitral stenosis. What is not expected in her ECG?**

   a. P pulmonale b. P mitrale c. SV1 + RV5 more than 35 mm d. Tall R waves in lead V1.

10. **Which ECG lead is most commonly used to assess right ventricular hypertrophy (RVH)?**

    a. Lead I b. Lead aVR c. Lead V1 d. Lead V6

**Case Studies**

1. Examine the 12-lead ECG (Fig. 12.7) and answer the following questions:

   a. What is your diagnosis?
   b. Name three important points in favour of your diagnosis.
   c. Name two conditions where you will get such an abnormality.

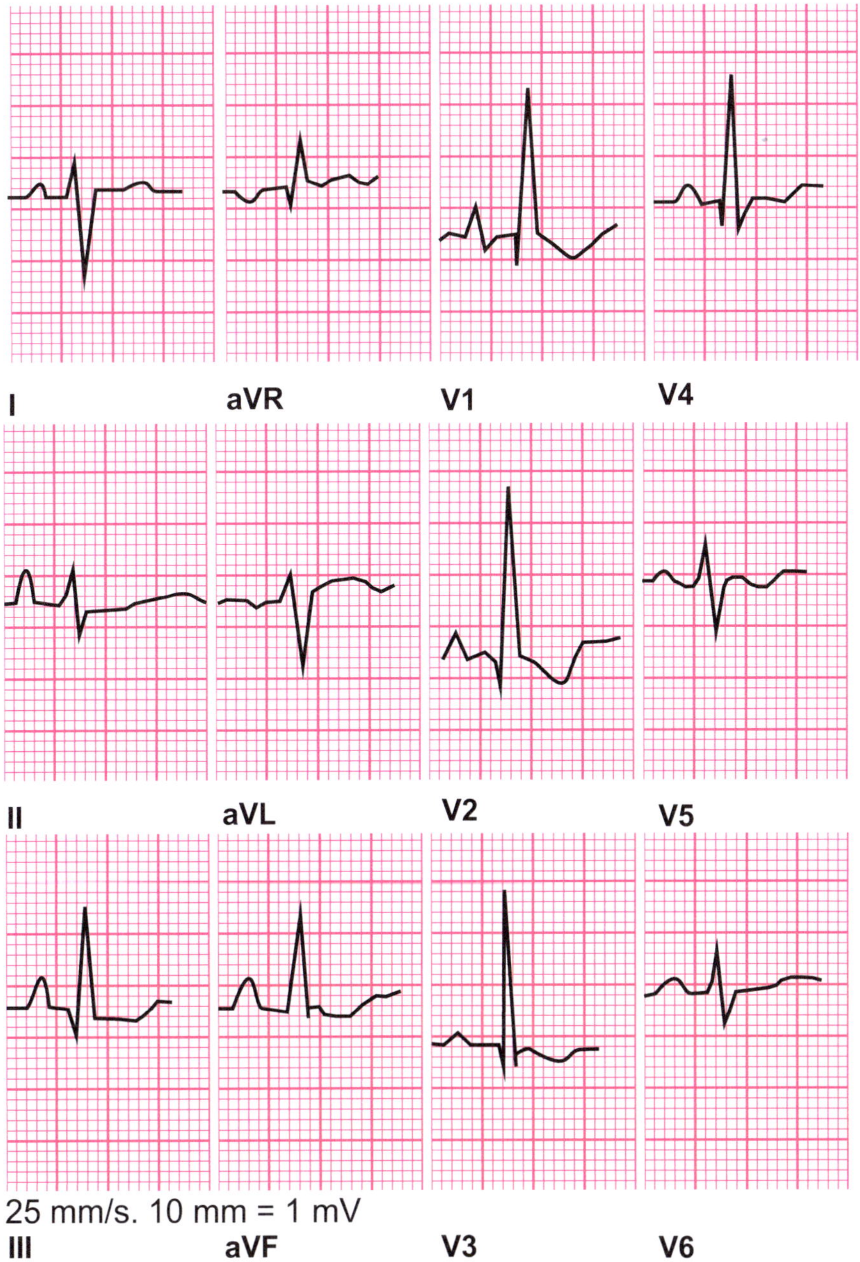


**Fig. 12.7** Identify the ECG

2. A 75-year-old gentleman presented with history of breathlessness and dizziness. On examination, an ejection systolic murmur was audible in aortic area. Examine the 12-lead ECG (Fig. 12.8) and answer the following questions:

   a. What is your diagnosis?
   b. Name two important points in favour of your diagnosis.
   c. Name one condition where you will get such an abnormality.

3. Examine the 12-lead ECG (Fig. 12.9) and answer the following questions:

   a. What is your diagnosis?
   b. Name two important points in favour of your diagnosis.

4. A patient suffering from pulmonary stenosis came to the OPD. His ECG was mixed up with that of another patient. Do you think the given ECG (Fig. 12.10) belongs to this patient? If yes, give two points in favour of your conclusion.

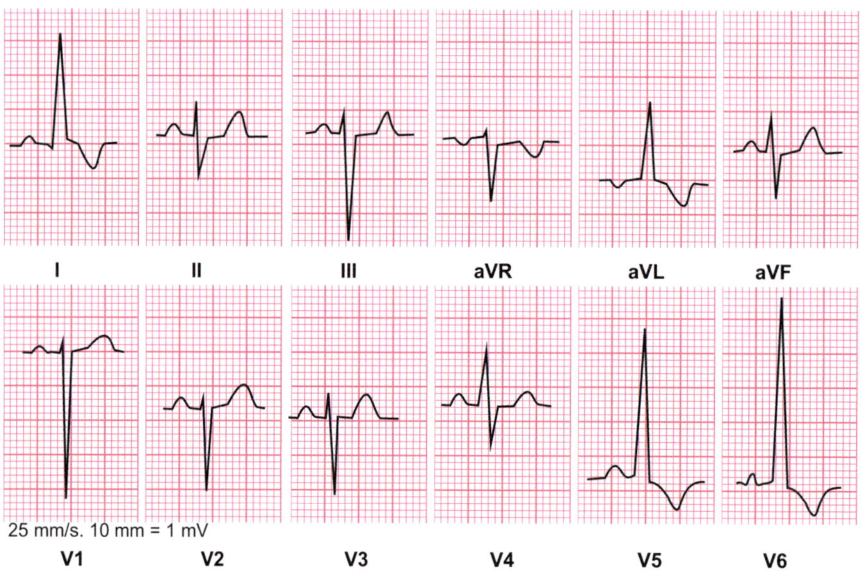


**Fig. 12.8** Identify the ECG

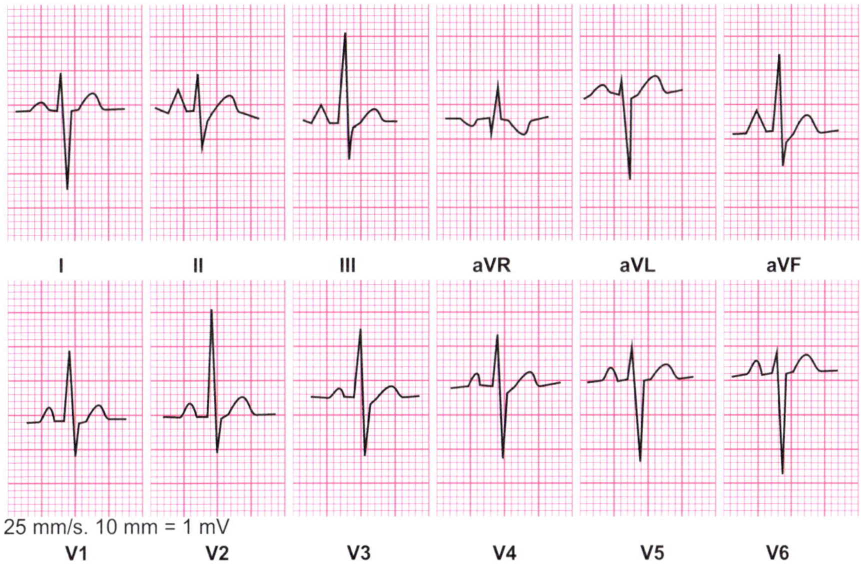


**Fig. 12.9** Identify the ECG

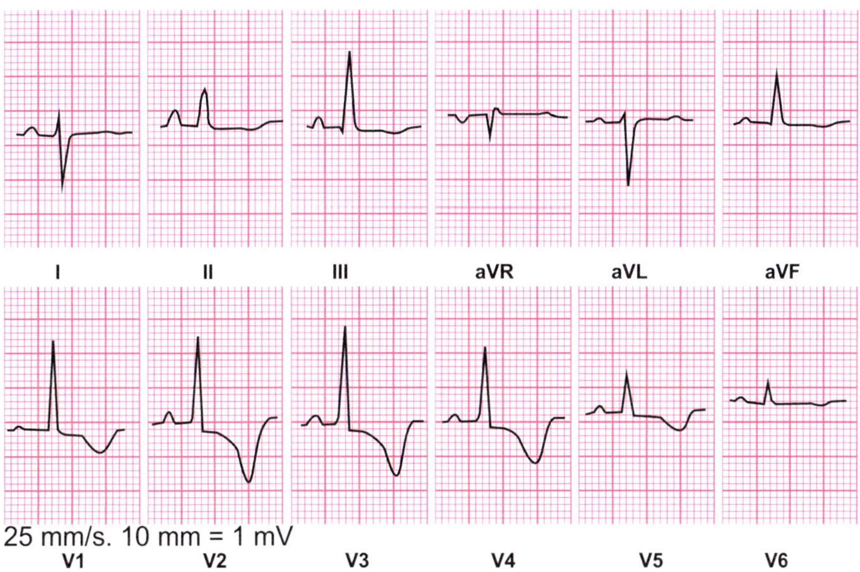


**Fig. 12.10** Identify the ECG

5. A 50-year-old patient was suffering from hypertension for 12 years. He used to take his medicines irregularly. Examine his 12-lead ECG (Fig. 12.11) and make your diagnosis. Give three points in favour of your diagnosis.
6. A 65-year-old lady suffering from off and on breathlessness presents for evaluation. She had mild dyspnoea. There was no cyanosis. There was bilateral wheeze and a loud second heart sound in pulmonary area. Examine the 12-lead ECG (Fig. 12.12). Make your diagnosis. Give three points in favour of your diagnosis and name two conditions where you get similar changes in ECG.

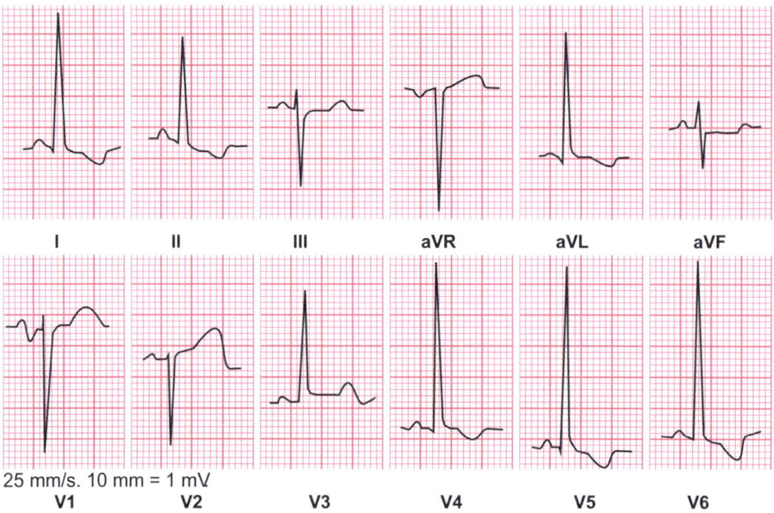


**Fig. 12.11** Identify the ECG

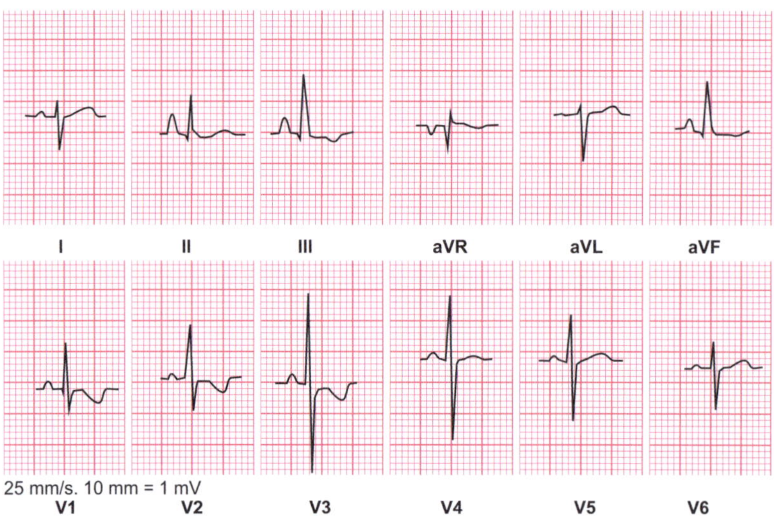


**Fig. 12.12** Identify the ECG

**Answers**

1. False 2. True 3. True 4. True 5. False 6. b 7. b 8. a 9. c 10. c

**Case Studies**

1. a. The diagnosis is RVH.
   b. Three diagnostic points are:
      i. P pulmonale
      ii. qR pattern in lead V1.
      iii. S-T, T changes (strain pattern) in lead V1–V5, which is more prominent in leads V1 and V2.
   c. Mitral stenosis and tetralogy of Fallot.
2. a. The diagnosis is LVH.
   b. Two diagnostic points are:
      i. SV1 + RV5 is more than 35 mm.
      ii. Strain pattern in lead V5 and lead V6.
   c. The patient is most likely suffering from aortic stenosis. Ejection systolic murmur with LVH in ECG points towards aortic stenosis. History of dizziness and breathlessness indicate severe obstruction and may lead to sudden cardiac death. He needs urgent further investigation and management. Similar ECG changes can also be observed in patients suffering from hypertensive heart disease.
3. a. The diagnosis is RVH.
   b. The two diagnostic points are:
      i. Tall R wave in lead V1 with R:S ratio more than 1.
      ii. P pulmonale (lead II) indicates right atrial enlargement.
4. This ECG most likely belongs to the patient suffering from pulmonary stenosis. In pulmonary stenosis, right atrial and right ventricular hypertrophy are observed. The two points in favour of diagnosis are:
   a. Tall R wave in lead V1 with S-T, T changes indicate RVH.
   b. P pulmonale in lead II indicates right atrial enlargement.
5. The diagnosis is LVH. Three diagnostic points are:
   i. SV1 + RV5 is more than 35 mm.
   ii. Strain pattern in lead V5 and lead V6.
   iii. Biphasic P wave in lead V1 with wide (> 0.04 s) and deep (> 1 mm) terminal negative component.
6. The diagnosis is RVH. The points in favour of diagnosis are:
   i. Tall R wave in lead V1 with R:S ratio more than 1.
   ii. Strain pattern in leads V1 to V3.
   iii. P pulmonale (lead II).

   Bilateral wheeze with loud second heart sound indicates obstructive airway disease with pulmonary hypertension. ECG features of RVH are seen in COPD with cor pulmonale and idiopathic pulmonary hypertension.

# Part III
# Conduction Disturbance

# Chapter 13
# Sinoatrial and Atrioventricular Block

**Learning Objectives**
After studying this chapter, the reader will learn about:

- Sinoatrial block
- Atrioventricular block
  - First degree block
  - Second degree block
  - Third degree (complete) block

Conduction disturbance is an abnormality in the transmission of an electrical impulse through the normal conducting system of the heart. Conduction disturbance may range from delay in conduction to complete interruption in transmission of electrical impulse. It can be divided broadly into three categories:

1. Sinoatrial block (conduction disturbance at the sinoatrial junctional tissue)
2. Atrioventricular block (conduction disturbance at the AV node, AV junctional tissue, His bundle)
3. Intraventricular block (conduction disturbance in the bundle branches)

**Tips and Tricks**
- Abnormal conduction in SA node or atrial myocardium will affect the P waves.
- Abnormal conduction through the AV node will affect the P-R interval and the relationship between P wave and QRS complex.
- Conduction abnormality beyond the AV node affects the simultaneous depolarization of the ventricles resulting in widening of QRS complex.

In this chapter, sinoatrial and atrioventricular block will be discussed.



T. K. Koley, *Rapid Review of ECG*,
https://doi.org/10.1007/978-981-99-9116-7_13

## 13.1 Sinoatrial Block

Sinoatrial block (SA block) is characterized by blocking of the electrical impulse at the junction of SA node and atrial myocardium. As a result, atrial and ventricular activation does not occur and an entire PQRST complex is not recorded (Fig. 13.1). There is a 'pause' in the ECG or a prolonged isoelectric line that indicates a complete temporary absence of electrical activity.

SA block is commonly a manifestation of increased vagal tone. It may be seen in normal persons also. The various causes of SA block are enumerated in Box 13.1.

**Box 13.1 Causes of SA Block**
Digitalis toxicity
Rheumatic fever
Sick Sinus Syndrome
Hypokalaemia
Acute myocardial infarction
Myocarditis
Young athletes
Uraemia
Carotid sinus sensitivity

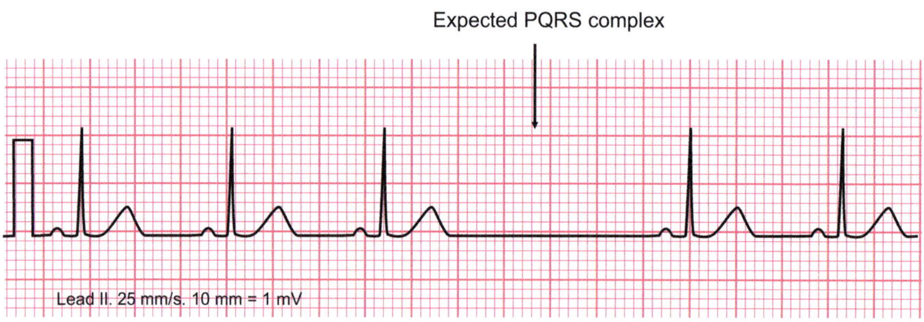


**Fig. 13.1** Sinoatrial block. Note that after three normal complexes, there is a drop of entire PQRS complex followed by normal rhythm

## 13.2 Atrioventricular Block

Atrioventricular block (AV block) is characterized by disturbance in conduction of atrial impulse through the atrioventricular conducting system, i.e. the AV node, the bundle of His or His-Purkinje system. AV block leads to prolonged atrioventricular conduction time or complete failure of conduction of one or more impulses due to prolonged refractory period of the AV junctional tissue. It can result from either a functional or pathologic defect in the AV node, bundle of His or bundle branches. The functional block may result from increased vagal tone.

A variety of factors may lead to AV block. Myocardial ischaemia or infarction is a common cause. The block may be temporary or permanent in presence of myocardial infarction. Drug toxicity, electrolyte imbalance, cardiac surgery, radiofrequency ablation may lead to development of AV block. The clinical significance of AV block depends upon the number of blocked impulses and the resulting ventricular rate. A slow ventricular rate can decrease the cardiac output.

In general, there are three degrees of AV block:

1. First degree of AV block: Delay in conduction
2. Second degree of AV block: Intermittent interruption in conduction
3. Third degree or complete AV block: Complete interruption in conduction

### 13.2.1 *First Degree AV Block*

In first degree AV block, there is delay in conduction of every electrical impulse through the AV conducting system (Fig. 13.2). Hence, there is prolongation of P-R interval above 0.20 s in every PQRS complex (Fig. 13.3). The rhythm is regular without any dropped beat. All the beats are conducted to the ventricles and the ventricles are activated, meaning every P wave is followed by a QRS complex. The duration and morphology of QRS complex are normal. The T wave, Q-T interval

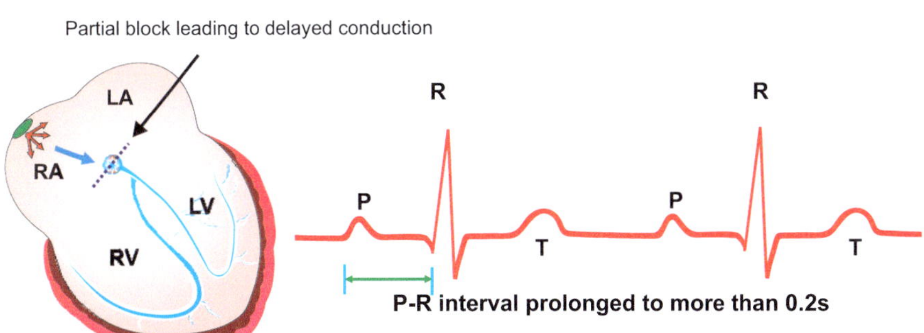


**Fig. 13.2** First degree AV block

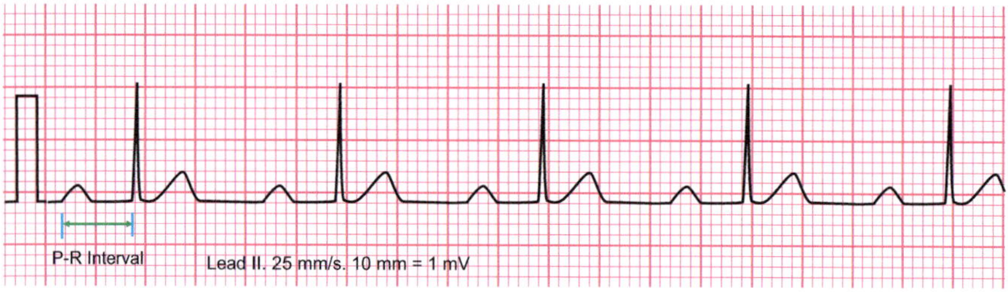


**Fig. 13.3** First degree AV block. In this ECG, the P-R interval is 0.28 s (0.04 s × 7 boxes). This patient was taking atenolol (beta-blocker) for hypertension. In his case, the P-R interval became normal after stopping atenolol

and the S-T segments are also normal. The various causes of first degree AV block are enumerated in Box 13.2. It must be kept in mind that prolonged P-R interval may be normal in some persons.

**Box 13.2 Causes of First Degree AV Block**
Increased vagal tone
Coronary artery disease
Rheumatic fever
Drugs—Beta-blocker, Quinidine
Digitalis toxicity
Hyperkalaemia
ASD
Ebstein's anomaly
Idiopathic

**Tips and Tricks**
- First degree AV block is often seen in normal healthy persons.
- Think of the possibility of acute rheumatic fever and acute myocardial infarction as the most likely cause.

## *13.2.2 Second Degree AV Block*

In second degree AV block, there is intermittent interruption of AV conduction. Some of the impulses are conducted to the ventricles while others are blocked. As a result the P wave is not followed by the QRS complex as the ventricles are not depolarised. The second degree AV block may be constant or variable.

There may be physiologic AV block. During atrial flutter, the atrial rate may be 300 bpm, whereas the ventricular rate may be 150 bpm. This does not mean that a true AV block persists; rather it is a physiologic protective AV block. It will be a 2:1 conduction rather than block.

Second degree AV block is usually due to organic heart disease. The various causes of second degree AV block are enumerated in Box 13.3.

**Box 13.3 Causes of Second Degree AV Block**
Coronary artery disease
Beta-blocker and verapamil toxicity
Digitalis toxicity
Rheumatic carditis
Hyperkalaemia
Increased vagal tone
In presence of atrial fibrillation and flutter (physiological)
Diphtheria myocarditis

There are two types of second degree AV block: Mobitz type I and Mobitz type II.

#### 13.2.2.1 Mobitz Type I AV Block

In Mobitz type I AV block (Wenckebach phenomenon), the conduction of impulse through the AV conducting system becomes increasingly difficult and ultimately an impulse fails to conduct to the ventricles. This results in an initial PQRST complex with normal P-R interval followed by gradual prolongation of P-R interval in successive beats followed by dropping of a QRS complex (P wave without a following QRS complex). After this, the AV conduction system recovers and the sequence is repeated (Figs. 13.4 and 13.5). Usual site of block is below the AV node. The P-R interval after the nonconducted beat is shorter than the P-R interval preceding the nonconducted beat.

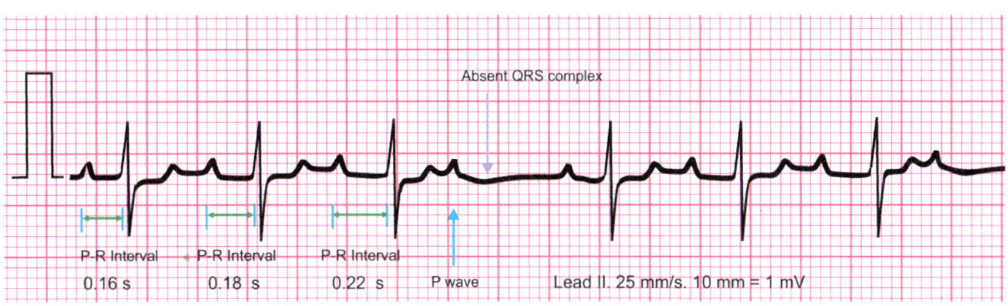


**Fig. 13.4** Wenckebach phenomenon. This ECG was recorded from a 14-year-old patient suffering from acute rheumatic carditis. This conduction disturbance became normal with treatment of rheumatic fever. Note the gradual prolongation of P-R interval in the first three QRS complexes, which are followed by a P wave with loss of QRS complex. After this, there is a recovery of conduction and there is a normal P-R interval followed by gradual prolongation of the P-R interval

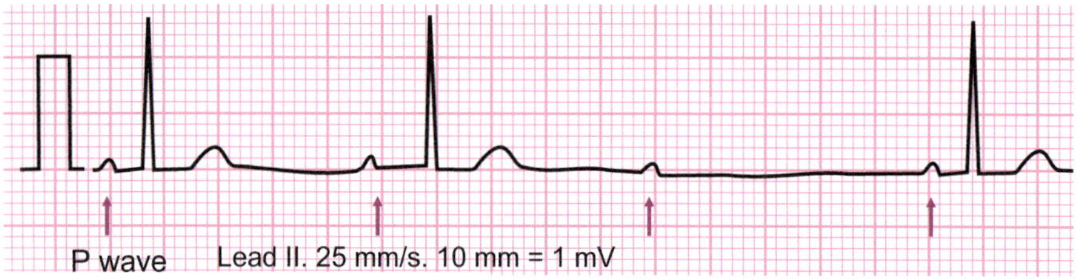


**Fig. 13.5** Wenckebach phenomenon (Mobitz type I block)

The various causes of Mobitz type I second degree AV block are drugs (beta-blockers, calcium channel blockers, digoxin), myocardial ischaemia, inferior wall myocardial infarction, physiologic increase in vagal tone and rheumatic fever. Clinically, the patients are without any symptoms unless the ventricular rate is very slow.

**Tips and Tricks**

- If there is clustering of QRS complexes separated by a pause, suspect Wenckebach phenomenon.
- Next look for progressive lengthening of P-R interval to diagnose Wenckebach phenomenon.
- Sometimes it may be seen in athletes.

#### 13.2.2.2 Mobitz Type II AV Block

Mobitz type II second degree AV block is more serious but less common than type I second degree AV block. There is regular or irregular interruption of conduction of electrical impulse through AV conducting system (Fig. 13.6). For a specified number of P waves, the number of QRS complexes are less, for example, if the number of P waves are 2 and the number of QRS complexes are 1, then the block will be 2:1 AV block (Fig. 13.7).

In Mobitz type II AV block, there is no gradual prolongation of P-R interval. Usual site of block is in His Purkinje system. Atrial rhythm is regular. Ventricular rhythm is irregular (regular in 2:1 AV block). P waves are normal in shape and size. P-R interval is within normal limits. QRS complex duration is usually 0.10 s or greater but they are periodically absent after the P waves.

It can be seen in anterior wall MI, where it carries a much more grave prognosis in contrast to type I block (Fig. 13.8). These patients may progress to complete AV block. Degenerative changes in conducting system may also lead to this type of AV block.

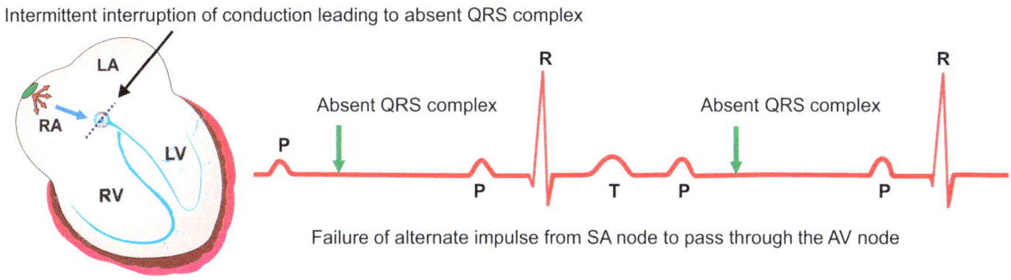


**Fig. 13.6** Diagrammatic representation of Mobitz type II AV block

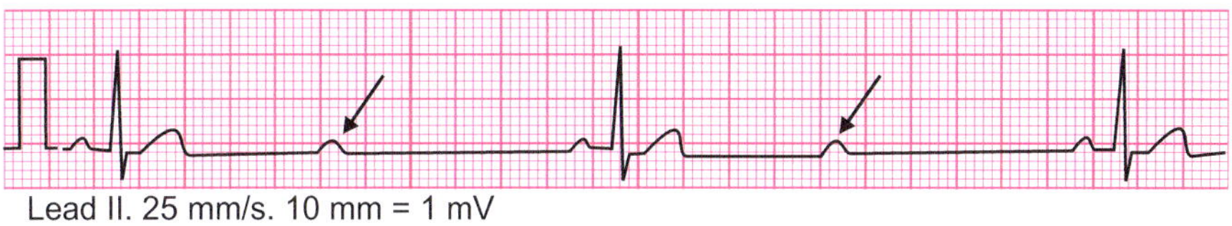


**Fig. 13.7** 2:1 AV block. Note that after every normal PQRTS complex there is a P wave, which is not followed by a QRS complex (arrows). So there are two P waves and one QRS complex and thus the block is 2:1 AV block

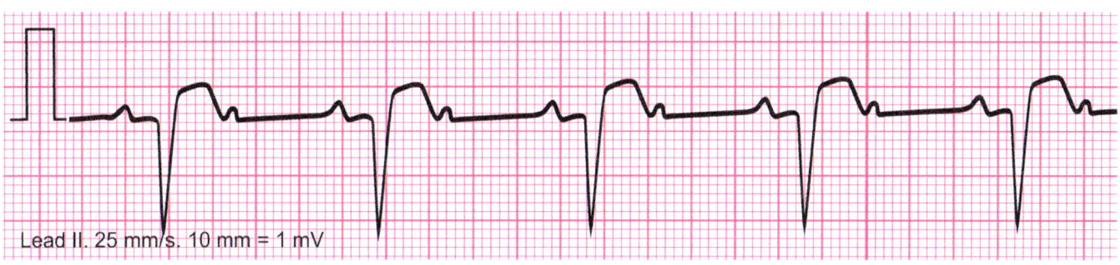


**Fig. 13.8** Mobitz type II second degree AV block in presence of myocardial infarction

As long as cardiac output is maintained, majority of the patients remain asymptomatic. As the number of dropped beats increase, patient may suffer from fatigue, dyspnoea, light headedness and syncope. Hypotension, regular or irregular pulse rate with bradycardia are observed in these patients.

### Tips and Tricks

- Second degree AV block usually indicates heart disease.
- It is often seen after acute myocardial infarction.
- In haemodynamically unstable patients, pacemaker may be required.

### 13.2.3 Third Degree AV Block

Third degree AV block also known as complete heart block (CHB) is characterized by complete and permanent failure of conduction through AV conducting system (Fig. 13.9). The block may occur at the AV node, bundle of His or bundle branches. The ventricles are activated by an ectopic pacemaker situated either in AV node junction below the block or in the ventricles. This is a type of escape mechanism whereby the ventricles take over the task of generating an impulse of its own in absence of any electrical current coming to it via the normal conducting system. Thus, the atria and the ventricles are activated by two different pacemakers and the two rhythms are asynchronous. Hence, there is atrioventricular dissociation (Figs. 13.10, 13.11 and 13.12). The EGG manifestations are the following:

1. AV dissociation: There is no relation between the P waves and QRS complexes.
2. Slow ventricular rate: The ventricles beat at a slower rate, usually in the range of 30–35 bpm. The atrial rate is more than the ventricular rate and the atrial and ventricular rhythms are regular.
3. QRS configuration: The QRS configuration depends on the location of the ectopic pacemaker. If the pacemaker is situated in the Purkinje fibres or in myocardium, the QRS complexes become broad, slanted, bizarre in shape. However, if the pacemaker is situated in AV junction or in the bundle of His proximal to the bundle branches, then the QRS configuration is normal or near normal.

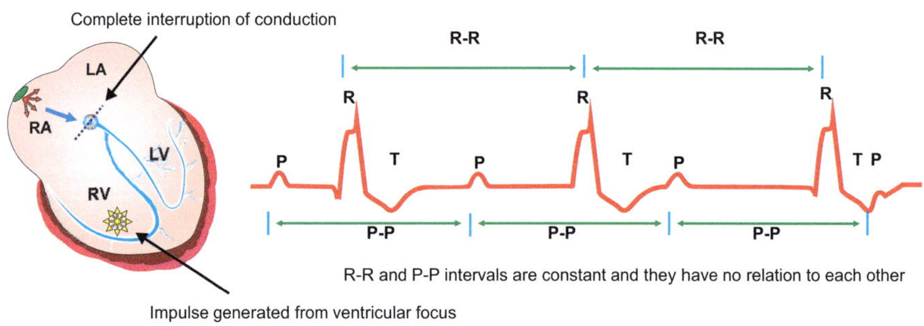


**Fig. 13.9** Complete AV block

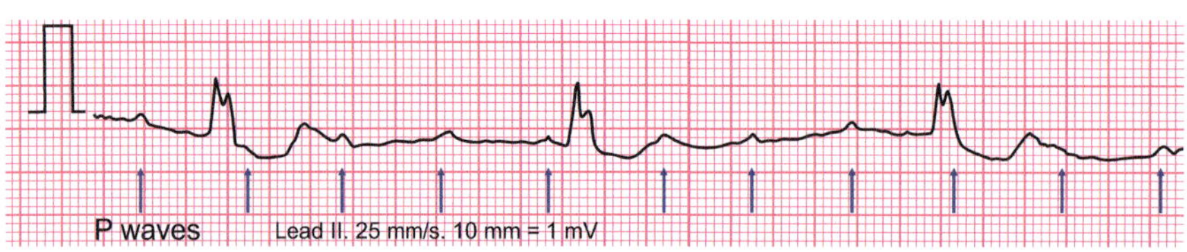


**Fig. 13.10** Complete heart block. The P waves are shown with arrows. Note the wide QRS complexes with left bundle branch block configuration. The ventricular rate is about 35 bpm

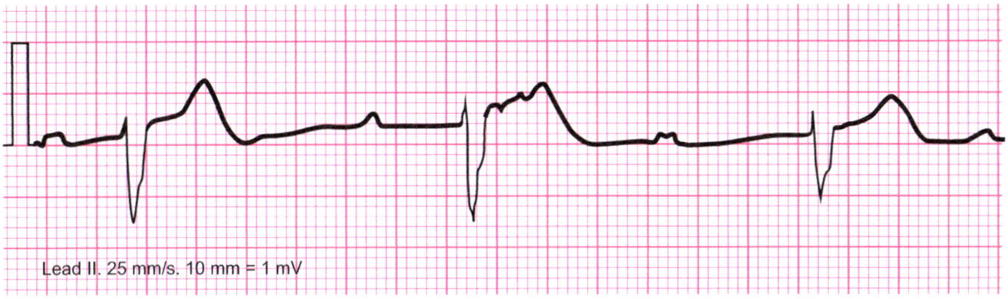


**Fig. 13.11** Complete heart block

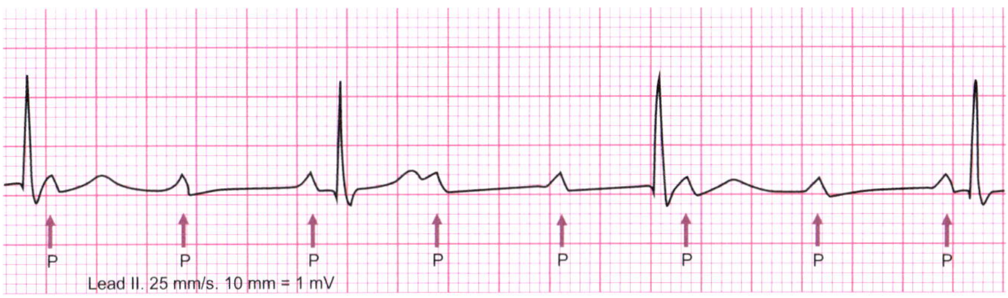


**Fig. 13.12** Complete heart block

Digitalis intoxication, degenerative changes of the conducting system, myocardial infarction and bacterial endocarditis may cause complete AV block. Anterior wall myocardial infarction complicated by a complete heart block is a very dangerous condition which requires prompt pacemaker insertion. Clinically, complete AV block with wide QRS complexes tends to be less stable as compared to complete AV block with narrow QRS complexes. The various causes of complete AV block are enumerated in Box 13.4.

**Box 13.4 Causes of Complete AV Block**

Coronary artery disease
Congenital complete AV block
Drugs: Digitalis, quinidine
Myocarditis and endocarditis
Intracardiac surgery
Congenital heart disease: Corrected transposition of the great vessels, VSD, ostium primum type of ASD
Acute rheumatic carditis
Lenegre's disease, Lev's disease
Amyloid heart disease
Miscellaneous: Chaga's disease, intracardiac tubercle, gumma, granuloma, tumour

**Tips and Tricks**

- First degree AV block rarely requires any treatment.
- To study SA block and AV block, rhythm strip needs to be studied. Chest leads are usually not required.
- Focus should be on grouping of QRS complexes, P-R interval, missing of P wave and/or QRS complex and the relation between P wave and QRS complex.
- If P-R interval is fixed in all the complexes in the rhythm strip, it is either first degree AV block or Mobitz type II second degree AV block.
- To differentiate between them, calculate the P-R interval correctly. If it is prolonged (more than 0.2 s) in all the leads, it is first degree AV block.
- If P-R interval is varying, then think about Mobitz type I second degree AV block and third degree AV block.
- If there is progressive increase in P-R interval, it is Mobitz type I second degree AV block.
- Look for AV dissociation to diagnose complete heart block.
- Complete heart block always indicates some heart disease.
- Temporary or permanent pacemaker is required in complete heart block.

**Self-Assessment Questions**

1. SA block may be due to digitalis toxicity. True or false?
2. In SA block, an entire PQRS complex is not recorded. True or false?
3. AV dissociation is a feature of SA block. True or false?
4. First degree AV block is always pathological. True or false?
5. Wenckebach block is more serious than Mobitz type II second degree AV block. True or false?
6. **Spot the wrong statement about complete AV block.**

   a. The ventricles and atria beat independently of each other b. Both P waves and QRS complexes are present c. P waves bear no relation to the QRS complexes d. Ventricles beat faster than atria.

7. **Which of the following is seen in Mobitz type I AV block?**

   a. Progressive prolongation of P-R interval followed by a dropped QRS complex b. Progressive shortening of Q-T interval c. Progressive decrease in P-R interval d. Longest P-R interval is less than twice the shortest P-R interval

8. **Which of the following ECG findings is characteristic of a second-degree atrioventricular block (AV block) type II?**

   a. Progressive prolongation of P-R interval until a dropped beat occurs b. Constant P-R interval with intermittent dropped beats c. Absence of P waves d. Narrow QRS complex

9. **In a third-degree atrioventricular block (AV block), what is the relationship between the atrial and ventricular rhythms on the ECG?**

   a. Atrial and ventricular rhythms are regular and independent of each other b. Atrial rhythm is regular, but ventricular rhythm is irregular c. Atrial rhythm is irregular, but ventricular rhythm is regular d. Atrial and ventricular rhythms are both irregular

10. **Which ECG lead is commonly used to assess the type of atrioventricular block (AV block)?**

    a. Lead I b. Lead II c. Lead V1 d. Lead aVR

11. **Which of the following ECG findings is characteristic of a third-degree atrioventricular block (AV block)?**

    a. Normal P-R interval b. Regular P-P intervals c. Normal QRS duration d. Absence of AV conduction

**Case Studies**

1. A 30-year-old gentleman wants to get your advice before joining an exercise program. He has history of smoking and positive family history of coronary artery disease. He has a sedentary lifestyle. He has no complaints. On examination, his blood pressure is 140/90 mmHg. His ECG is given in Fig. 13.13. Can you identify any abnormality?
2. A 62-year-old lady was admitted with history of syncope. As a part of her workup, an ECG was obtained (Fig. 13.14). Can you identify the conduction disturbance? Mark the points where the absent P waves are expected.
3. A 55-year-old gentleman came to the medicine outdoor for routine medical checkup. He has no symptoms. No family history of CAD, hypertension and diabetes. Clinical examination revealed irregular pulse rate. His ECG (Fig. 13.15) is given below. Identify the abnormality and mark all the P waves.

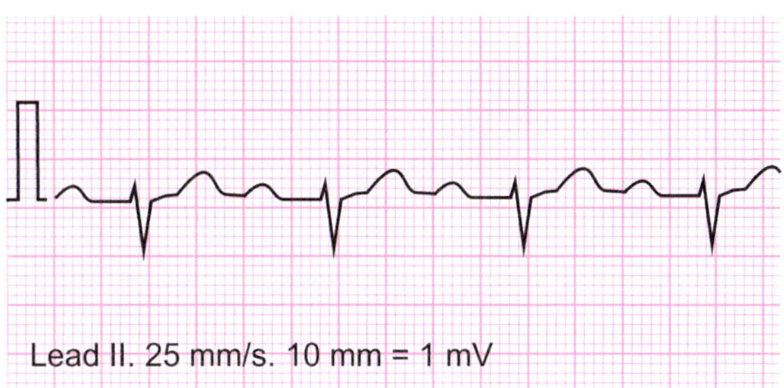


**Fig. 13.13** Identify the ECG abnormality

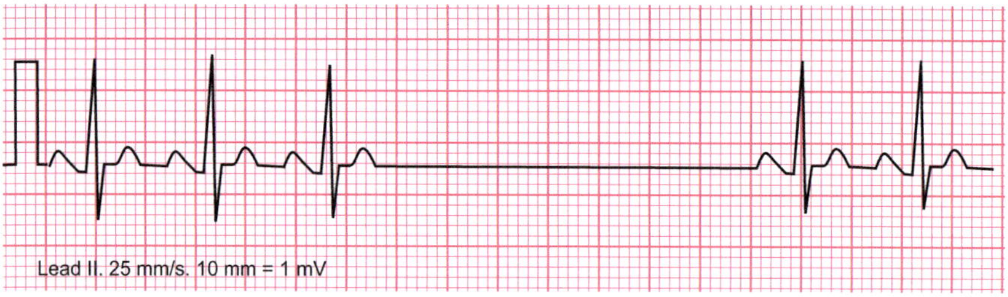


**Fig. 13.14** Identify the conduction disturbance

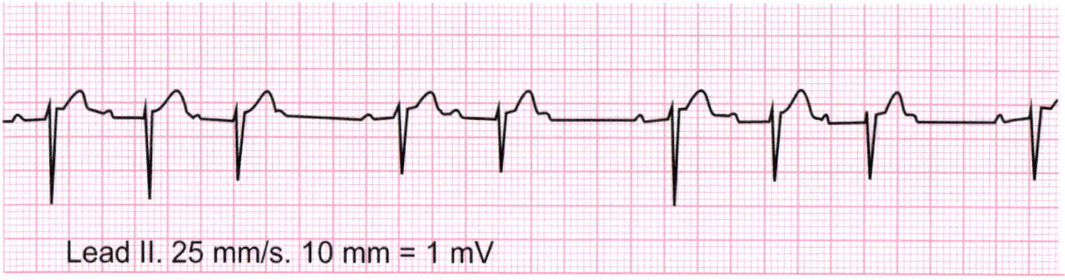


**Fig. 13.15** Identify the abnormality in the ECG and mark the P waves

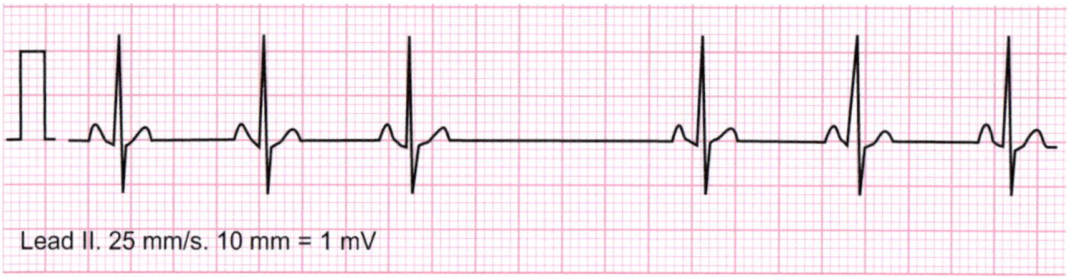


**Fig. 13.16** Identify the ECG abnormality

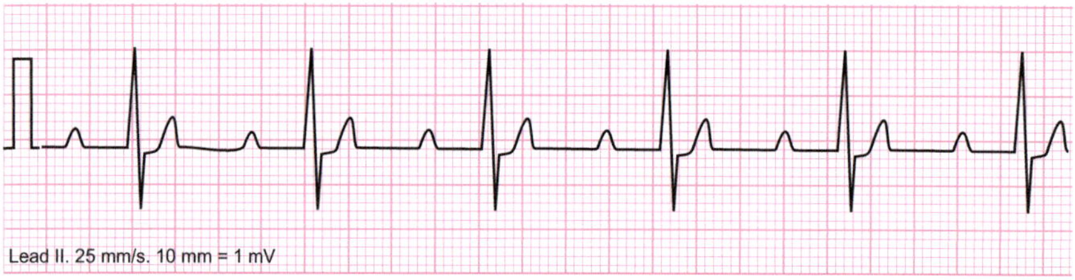


**Fig. 13.17** Identify the ECG abnormality

4. A 76-year-old gentleman is admitted with history of syncope. His ECG is given below (Fig. 13.16). Can you identify the abnormality?
5. An asymptomatic 30-year-old gentleman was investigated during renewal of medical insurance. His ECG (Fig. 13.17) is given below. Identify the abnormality.

6. Identify the conduction disturbance in the given ECG (Fig. 13.18).
7. An 80-year-old gentleman comes to the emergency department with history of dizziness, fatigue and weakness. He has past history of hypertension, diabetes and CAD. Identify the conduction disturbance in the given ECG (Fig. 13.19) and mark all the P waves in the ECG.
8. A 57-year-old gentleman was admitted with history of fainting spells. He is breathless and complains of uneasy feeling. Blood pressure is 70/50 mmHg. Identify the conduction disturbance in the given ECG (Fig. 13.20) and mark all the P waves in the ECG. What is the treatment?
9. A 55-year-old woman was admitted with history of palpitation. Her ECG (Fig. 13.21) is given below. Identify the conduction disturbance and mark all the P waves in the ECG.

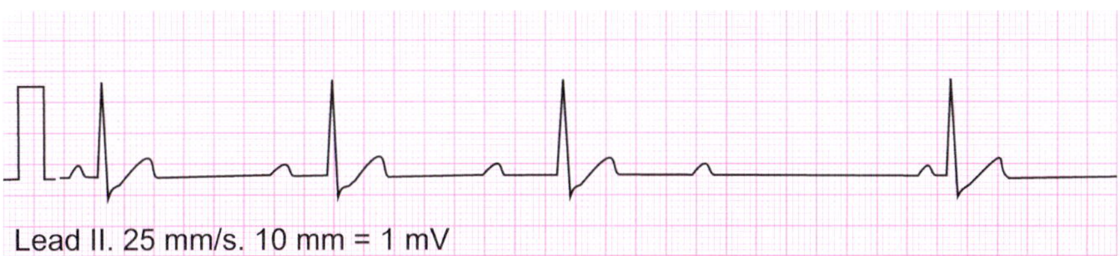


**Fig. 13.18** Identify the ECG abnormality

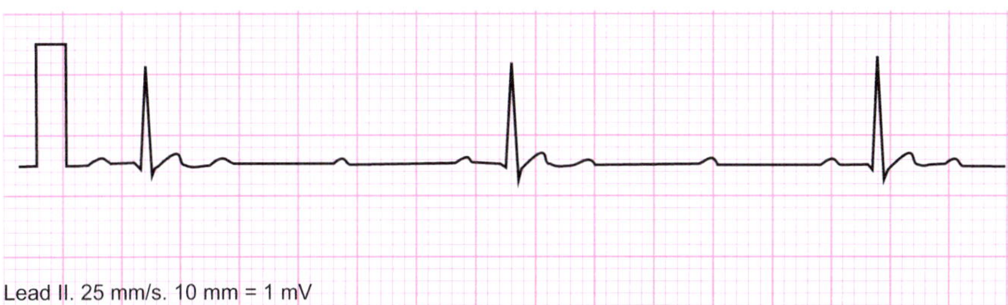


**Fig. 13.19** Identify the ECG abnormality and mark all the P waves

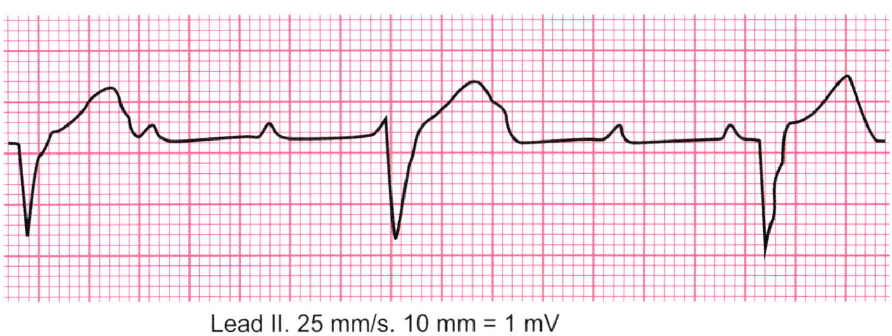


**Fig. 13.20** Identify the ECG abnormality and mark all the P waves

10. A 75-year-old gentleman was admitted with history of syncope and palpitation. His ECG (Fig. 13.22) is given below. Identify the conduction abnormality and mark all the P waves.
11. Given below is the ECG (Fig. 13.23) of an asymptomatic 34-year-old woman. Identify the conduction abnormality.
12. Identify the conduction disturbance in the given ECG (Fig. 13.24) and mark the position of all the P waves.

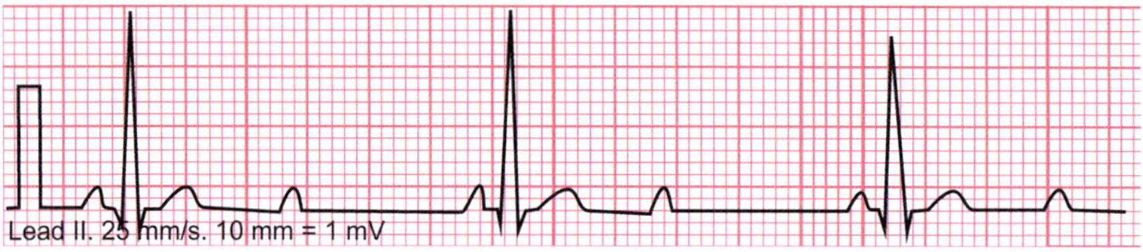


**Fig. 13.21** Identify the ECG abnormality and mark all the P waves

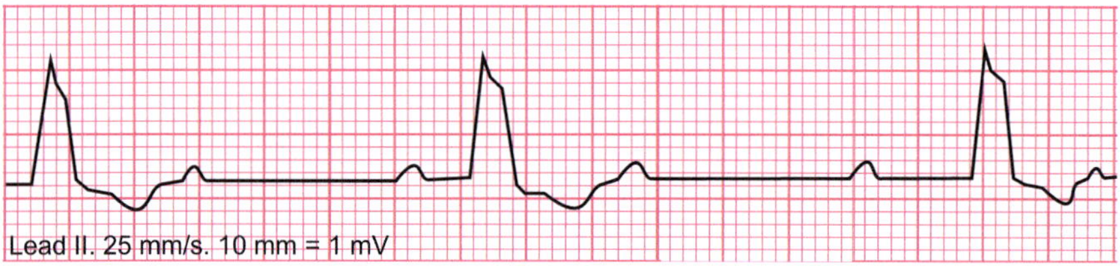


**Fig. 13.22** Identify the ECG abnormality and mark all the P waves

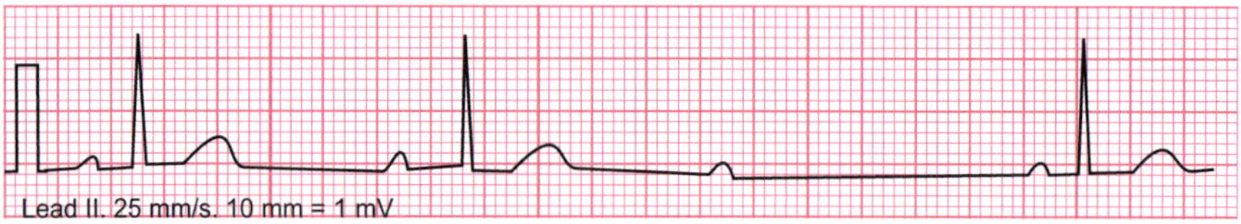


**Fig. 13.23** Identify the ECG abnormality

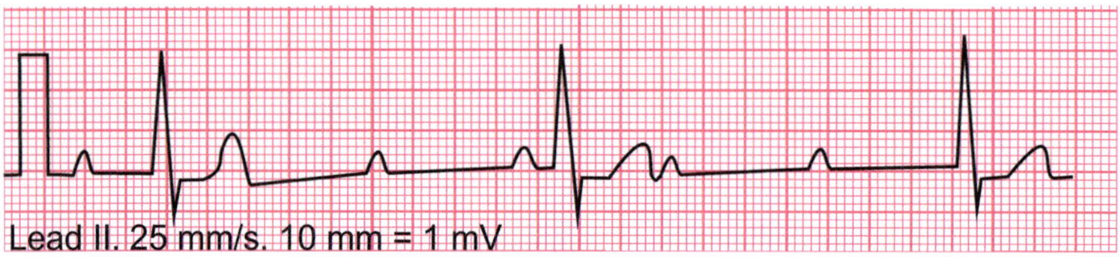


**Fig. 13.24** Identify the ECG abnormality and mark all the P waves

## Answers

1. True 2. True 3. False 4. False 5. False 6. d 7. a 8. b 9. a 10. b 11. d

## Case Studies

1. The conduction disturbance is first degree AV block. The P-R interval is prolonged (0.32 s) in all the complexes. Every P wave is followed by QRS complex. The morphology and duration of QRS complexes are normal.

   In this case, it must be remembered that often first degree heart block is seen in normal healthy persons and no active intervention is required.
2. The patient has developed SA block. There is a pause in the rhythm strip. Entire PQRS complexes are absent after the first three complexes. After the pause, the rhythm has recovered. The P-R intervals are normal and constant. The QRS complexes are of normal shape and duration. The absent P waves are marked in the ECG (Fig. 13.25).

   In this case, the patient has history of syncope which may be due to SA block. This patient should be subjected to proper investigation. Sinus node dysfunction at an advanced age with syncope is a serious condition and pacemaker should be implanted without delay.
3. The patient has developed Mobitz type I AV block (Wenckebach block). Note there is progressive increase in P-R interval of the first three complexes. This is followed by a P wave which is not followed by the QRS complex. The P-R interval of fifth PQRS complex is more than the P-R interval of fourth PQRS complex. This is again followed by a P wave which is not followed by the QRS complex. The same sequence is repeated in the sixth, seventh and eighth PQRS complexes. Note the P waves which are marked in Fig. 13.26.

   This patient is asymptomatic. Hence, pacemaker or any other active intervention is not required. However, he should be investigated to rule out the possibility of any further progression to higher degrees of AV block.
4. The patient is suffering from SA block. The main diagnostic feature is a pause after the first three complexes. The pause is because an entire PQRST complex is absent.

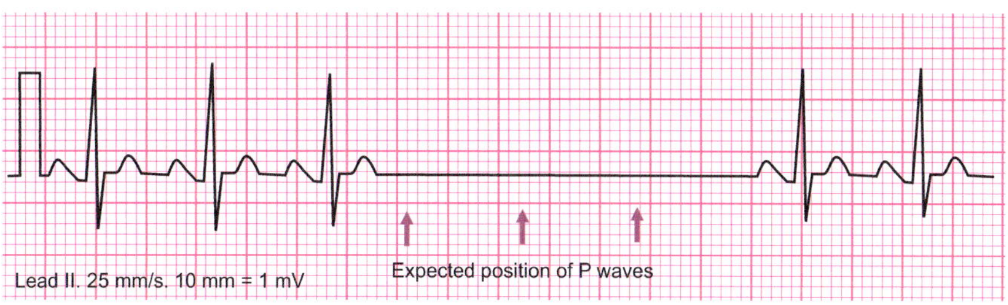


**Fig. 13.25** SA block

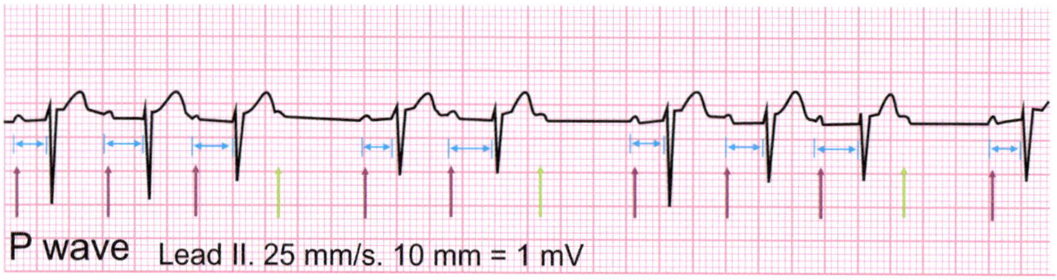


**Fig. 13.26** Mobitz type I AV block. The blocked P waves are represented by green arrows

5. The ECG shows first degree AV block. First degree AV block is diagnosed by prolonged P-R interval. In this case, the P-R interval is 0.28 s. The QRS complexes are normal in shape and duration. Every P wave is followed by QRS complex. Remember that first degree AV block is also seen in asymptomatic persons.
6. The conduction disturbance is Mobitz type I second degree AV block (Wenckebach). Note the progressive lengthening of P-R interval in the first three PQRS complexes. The first three P waves are followed by QRS complexes; however, after the fourth P wave, the QRS complex is absent. The P-R interval of first PQRS complex is 0.2 s. The P-R interval of second PQRS complex is 0.36 s. The P-R interval of third PQRS complex is 0.48 s. Hence, there is gradual prolongation of P-R interval. The P-R interval of the fourth PQRS complex is 0.2 s.
7. The conduction abnormality is Mobitz type II second degree AV block. The second, third, fifth, sixth and eighth P waves are not followed by QRS complexes. All the P waves are marked in Fig. 13.27.

   There is a high possibility that it may progress to complete heart block. Pacemaker is indicated in this patient. Symptomatic Mobitz type II second degree AV block is an indication for pacemaker implantation without any delay.
8. The patient is suffering from complete heart block. All the P waves are marked in Fig. 13.28. Note that there is no correlation between the P waves and QRS complexes. This means the atria and the ventricles are activated by two different pacemakers (atrioventricular dissociation). The wide and bizarre QRS complexes with slow ventricular rate suggest that the ventricular pacemaker is situated in the ventricular myocardium. If it was situated in the His bundle or in the bundle branches, then the QRS complexes would have been narrow with higher ventricular rate.

   Since the patient is feeling uneasy and suffering from hypotension, temporary pacemaker should be inserted as early as possible. Later on, permanent pacing will be required if the cause of complete heart block is irreversible.
9. The patient has developed Mobitz type II second degree AV block. The P waves are marked in Fig. 13.29.

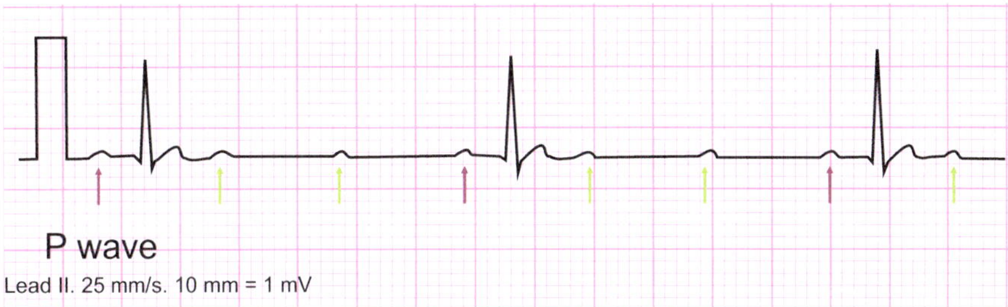


**Fig. 13.27** Mobitz type II second degree AV block. The blocked P waves are marked by green arrows

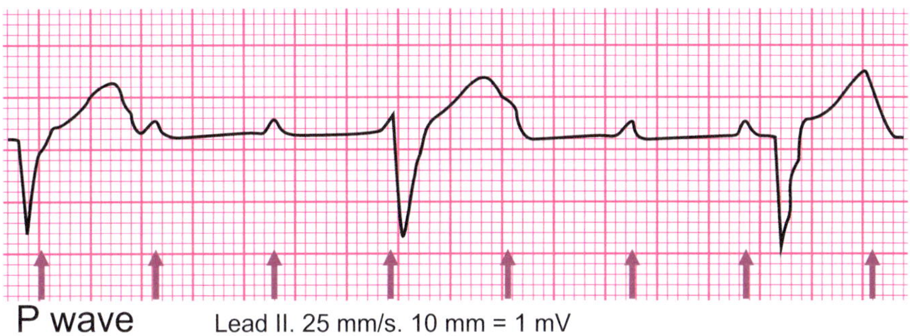


**Fig. 13.28** Complete AV block

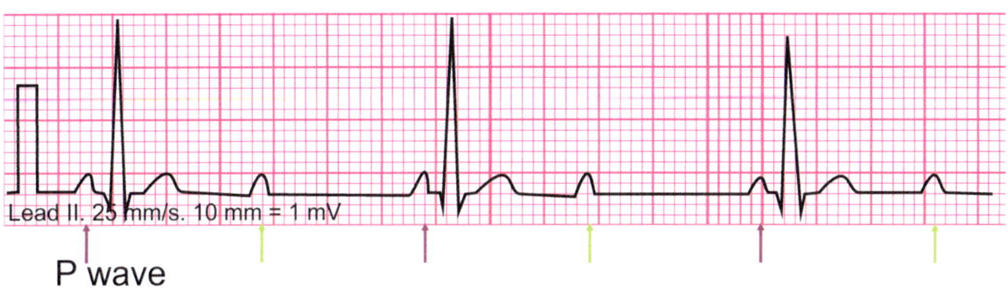


**Fig. 13.29** Mobitz type II second degree AV block. Note that alternate P waves are blocked (green arrow). This is 2:1 AV block. For every 2 P waves, there is 1 QRS complex

10. The patient has developed complete heart block. The P waves are marked in Fig. 13.30.

    The patient is symptomatic with complete heart block. Urgent temporary pacemaker should be inserted and after stabilization permanent pacemaker should be implanted if block is irreversible.

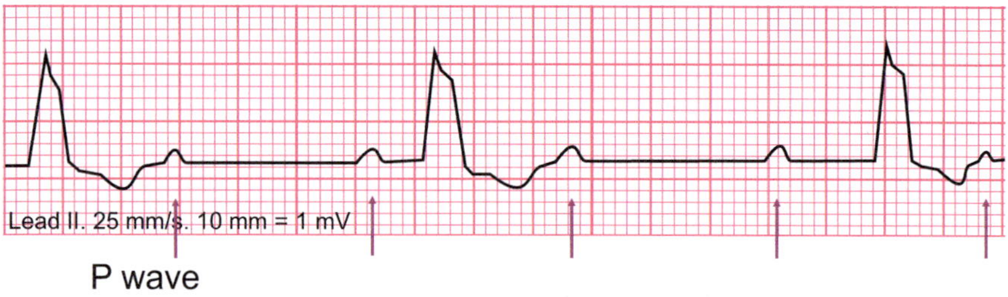


**Fig. 13.30** Complete heart block. Note that atrial rate is more than the ventricular rate and there is no fixed P-R interval. This indicates atrioventricular dissociation. Besides this also note the wide QRS complexes which indicate ventricular origin of these complexes

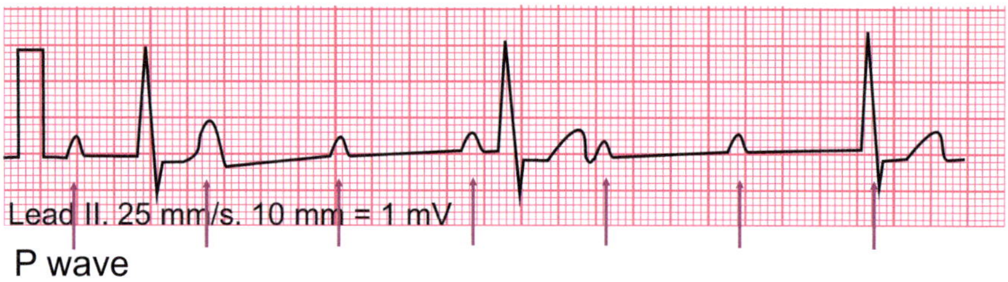


**Fig. 13.31** Complete AV block

11. The conduction abnormality is Mobitz type I second degree AV block (Wenckebach block). Note the progressive increase in the P-R interval of the first and second PQRS complexes. After this the third P wave is blocked. It is not followed by QRS complex.
12. The conduction disturbance is complete heart block. All the P waves are marked in Fig. 13.31. Note that there is no correlation between the P waves and QRS complexes (atrioventricular dissociation). Wide and bizarre QRS complexes with slow ventricular rate suggest that they are arising from a focus in ventricular myocardium. All the P waves are marked with arrows. There are seven P waves. The seventh P wave is hidden in the QRS complex.

    This patient will also need an urgent temporary pacemaker followed by a permanent pacemaker implantation if block is irreversible.

# Chapter 14
# Bundle Branch Block

**Learning Objectives**
After studying this chapter, the reader will learn about:

- Right bundle branch block
- Left bundle branch block

Bundle branch block is a type of intraventricular conduction defect. Intraventricular conduction defect means abnormality of conduction through the intraventricular conduction system distal to bundle of His. The block may be at the level of right bundle branch, left bundle branch, left anterior fascicle, left posterior fascicle or at the level of peripheral Purkinje fibres. In this chapter, bundle branch blocks will be discussed.

In bundle branch block, there is partial or complete failure of conduction of impulse through either the left or the right or both the bundle branches. Primarily, there are two types of bundle branch blocks: right and left bundle branch block (Fig. 14.1).



T. K. Koley, *Rapid Review of ECG*,
https://doi.org/10.1007/978-981-99-9116-7_14

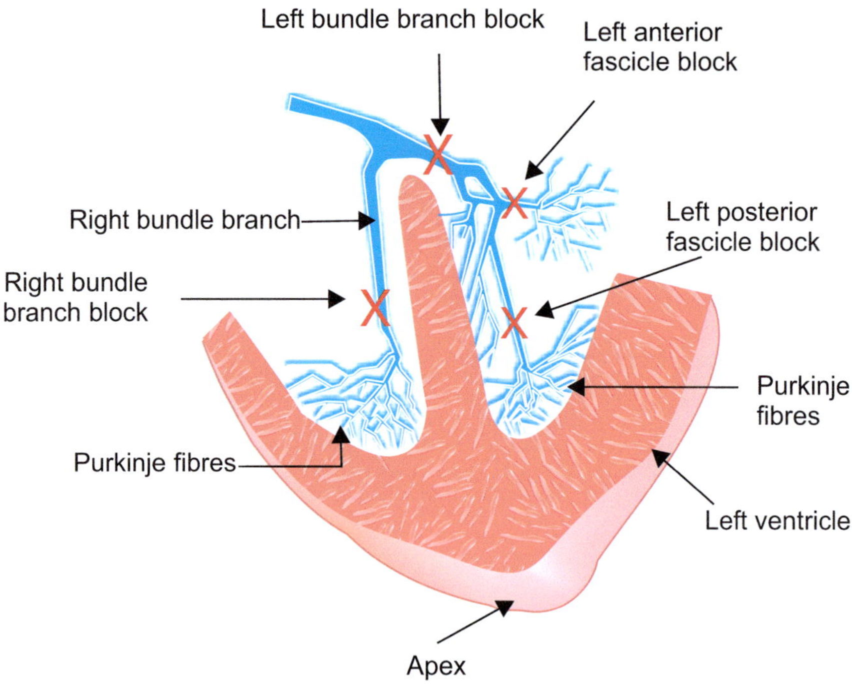


**Fig. 14.1** Diagram of bundle branch blocks

## 14.1 Right Bundle Branch Block

In right bundle branch block (RBBB), there is delay or interruption in conduction of impulse through the right bundle branch (Fig. 14.2). Due to block in conduction, there is delay in activation of the right ventricle, and it is represented in ECG by a wide QRS complex. The other important feature of RBBB is the presence of a second positive wave in lead V1, which is known as R' wave.

RBBB is a common ECG finding and alone it is not suggestive of any disease, because it is frequently present in normal persons also. It may be transient or permanent in the same or serial tracings of ECG depending upon the cause. Acute exacerbation of COPD or acute pulmonary embolism can lead to a transient RBBB. It may be a rate related phenomenon also. The various causes of RBBB are enumerated in Box 14.1.

The ECG manifestations of complete RBBB are the following:

- In lead V1 or V2, there is wide, slurred QRS complex with rsR' or rSR' pattern (Figs. 14.3 and 14.4). This is also called 'M' pattern (rabbit ear).

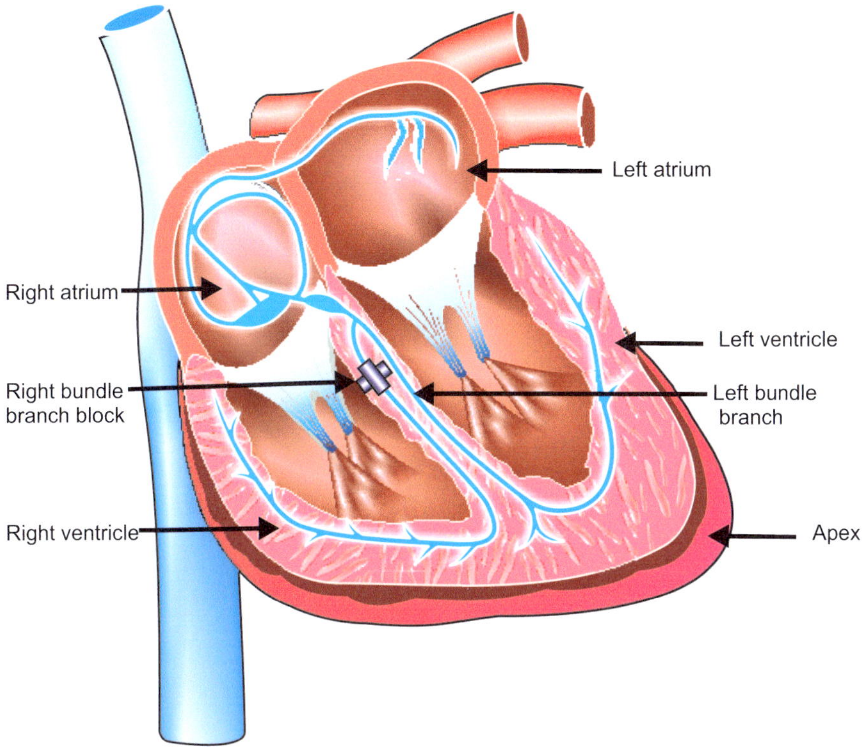


**Fig. 14.2** Right bundle branch block

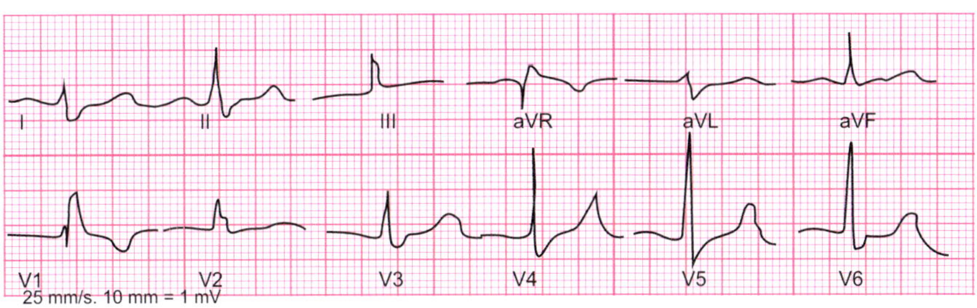


**Fig. 14.3** Right bundle branch block. Note the rsR' complex in lead V1

- QRS duration is more than 0.12 s.
- In lead V1 or V2, S-T segment depression and T wave inversion may be seen.
- VAT is more than 0.06 s in lead V1 or V2.

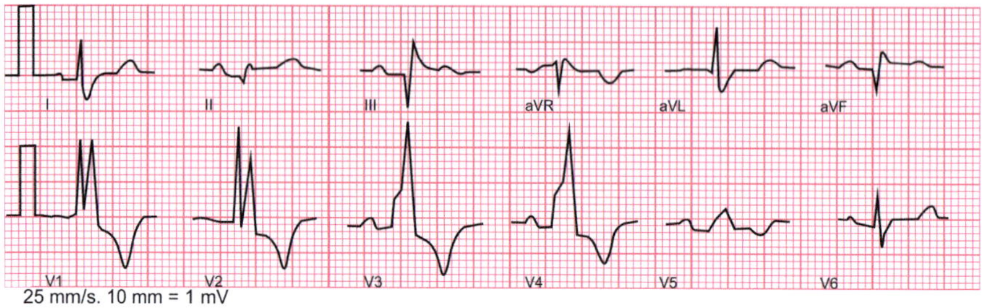


**Fig. 14.4** Right bundle branch block. Note the RSR' complex in lead V1 (M pattern)

- In leads I, aVL, V5 and V6, a wide slurred S wave may be present.
- There is a small r wave in lead V1 and a small q wave in lead V6.

**Box 14.1 Causes of RBBB**

Present in normal persons without heart disease
Coronary artery disease
Congenital
Cardiomyopathies
Acute massive pulmonary embolism
ASD (ostium primum type)
Ebstein's anomaly
Associated with right ventricular hypertrophy
Cardiac contusion
Idiopathic

**Tips and Tricks**

- Look for wide QRS complex with rSR' pattern in lead V1 to make a diagnosis of RBBB.
- There will be 'M' pattern in lead V1 and 'W' pattern in lead V6.
- The QRS becomes wide due to the extra time it takes for complete ventricular depolarization due to conduction block in right bundle branch.
- Do not jump into making a diagnosis of heart disease on diagnosing RBBB. It is commonly seen in normal healthy persons.
- No specific treatment is required.

### *14.1.1 Genesis of rsR' Complex in Lead V1*

The electrical impulse comes via bundle of His and at the beginning there is activation of the ventricular septum via the left to right septal vector. The vector is directed towards lead V1, resulting in a small r wave in lead V1 (Fig. 14.5).

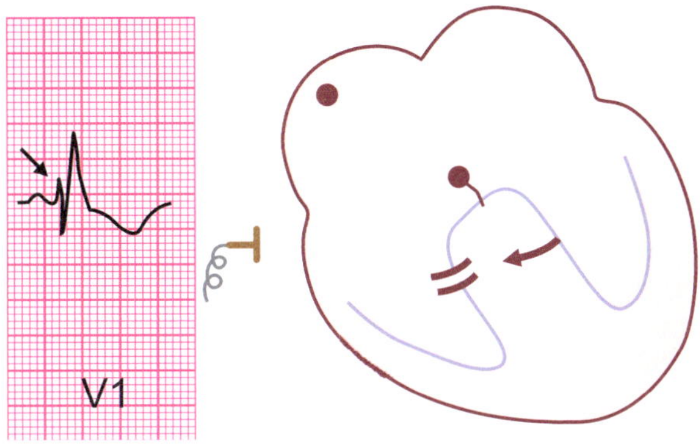


**Fig. 14.5** Genesis of r wave (arrow) of rsR' complex in lead V1

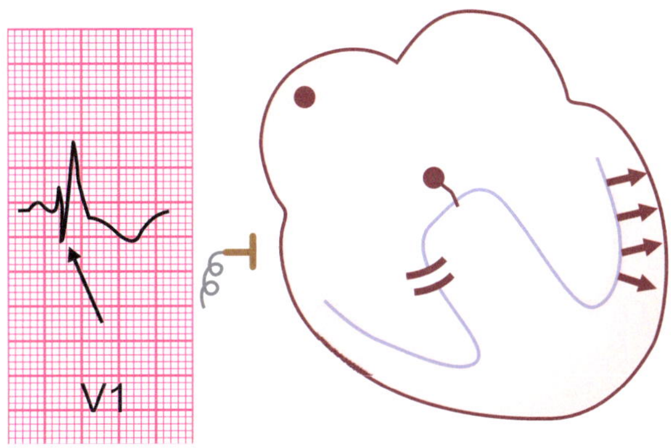


**Fig. 14.6** Genesis of s wave (arrow) of rsR' complex in lead V1

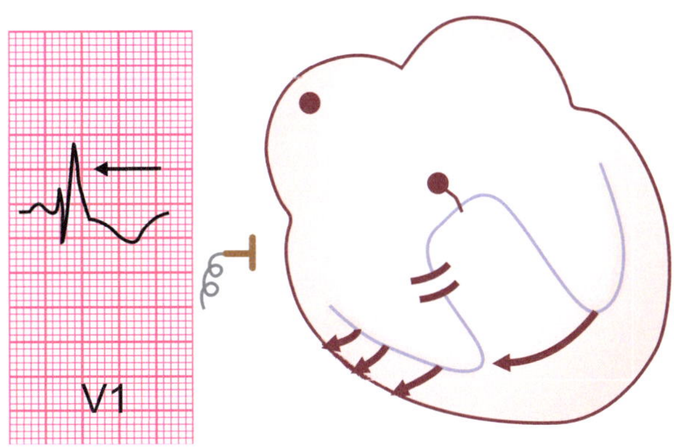


**Fig. 14.7** Genesis of R' wave (arrow) of rsR' complex in lead V1

Since the impulse cannot pass through the right bundle, it passes via the left bundle and depolarizes the left ventricle. The vector is directed away from lead V1 resulting in s wave (Fig. 14.6).

The impulse then passes round the blocked right bundle into the right ventricle. The impulse instead of passing through the Purkinje fibres passes through the ventricular myocardium. As a result, there is delay in right ventricular activation. This vector is directed towards lead V1 resulting in the R' wave (Fig. 14.7). Because of delay in ventricular depolarization (especially right ventricular delay), there is wide QRS complex.

### 14.1.2 Incomplete RBBB

In incomplete RBBB, the QRS duration is between 0.11 s and 0.12 s and the VAT in lead V1 is less than 0.06 s. There is diminution of S wave in lead V2 with slurring in the upstroke of S wave and it is the earliest feature of incomplete RBBB. Diminution of S wave may be the only feature of incomplete RBBB sometimes.

With further delay in conduction, there is development of a small r wave in lead V2 which results in a rsr' complex. With further increase in block, there may be development of rsR' complex in lead V2. Incomplete RBBB may be due to right ventricular hypertrophy or strain. Besides the delay in conduction, incomplete RBBB may be also due to increase in length of the right bundle in right ventricle dilatation due to volume overload, in conditions like cor pulmonale, atrial septal defect, etc.

Thus, it can be said that the development of incomplete RBBB can be studied by observing the following two changes in lead V2:

1. Progressive loss in amplitude of S wave.
2. Development and gradual increase in amplitude of r' or R' wave with final widening of this deflection.

### 14.1.3 Distinguishing Features of RBBB and RVH

Often it becomes difficult to differentiate between RBBB and RVH. Complete or incomplete RBBB may be a feature of RVH and it may be impossible to diagnose RVH in presence of RBBB. The following features help to distinguish between the two conditions:

- In RVH, the QRS duration is less than 0.12 s and in RBBB it is more than 0.12 s.
- In RVH, there is tall R wave in lead V1, whereas in RBBB there is rSR' complex in lead V1.
- In RVH, the VAT in lead V1 is usually between 0.03 and 0.05 s, while in RBBB, VAT is more than 0.06 s in lead V1.

### 14.1.4 RBBB in Presence of LVH

The ECG changes of LVH are present in leads V4–V6 and leads I and aVL. The features of RBBB are also present (rsR' complex in lead V1).

## 14.2 Left Bundle Branch Block

In left bundle branch block (LBBB), there is delay or complete block of transmission of impulse through the left bundle branch (Fig. 14.8). The conduction delay leads to incomplete LBBB and complete block produces complete LBBB. LBBB may be found in almost all types of cardiac disease and always it indicates some organic heart disease unlike RBBB. It may be transient or permanent. It may commonly be observed in conditions that cause LVH like hypertension or aortic stenosis. It is uncommon in congenital heart disease. LBBB may be transient or permanent in the same tracing or in serial tracings. Transient LBBB occurs after myocardial infarction or after consumption of drugs like digitalis, acute myocarditis, heart failure, etc. Permanent LBBB indicates organic heart disease. LBBB may be related to heart rate. The various causes of LBBB are enumerated in Box 14.2.

The ECG manifestations of complete LBBB are the following:

- In lead V5 or V6, there is wide, slurred, bizarre QRS complex. QRS duration is more than 0.12 s. There may be rsR' pattern (M pattern) in leads V5 or V6 (Figs. 14.9 and 14.10). In incomplete LBBB, the QRS duration is between 0.10 and 0.12 s.
- In leads V5 or V6, VAT is prolonged to more than 0.09 s.

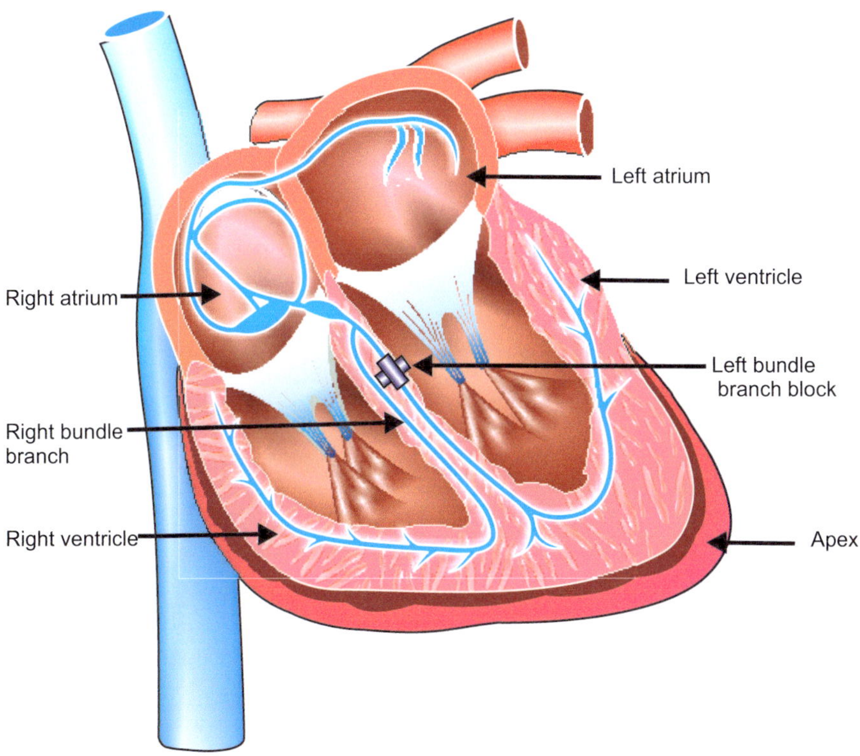


**Fig. 14.8** Left bundle branch block

**Box 14.2 Causes of LBBB**
Coronary artery disease
Myocarditis
Hypertensive heart disease
Acute myocarditis
Aortic valve disease
Cardiomyopathies
Degenerative disease of the conducting system

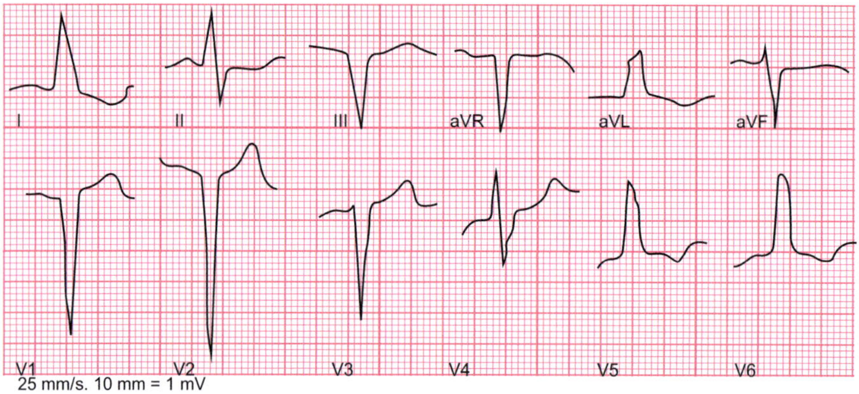


**Fig. 14.9** Left bundle branch block

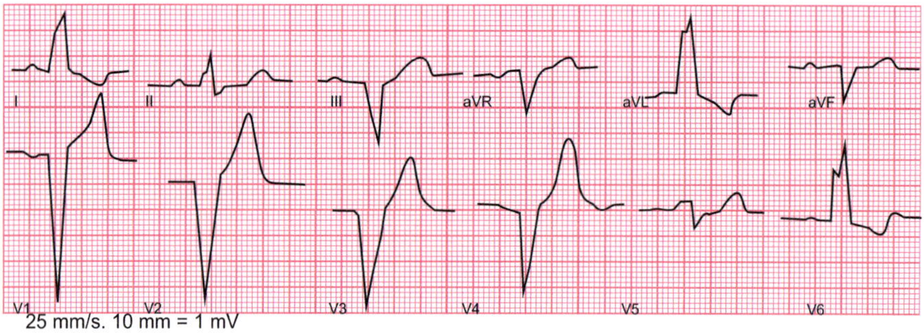


**Fig. 14.10** Left bundle branch block. This ECG is taken from a 62-year-old gentleman suffering from a long-standing hypertension with coronary artery disease. Note the widening of QRS complex and the notching of the R wave in leads aVL and lead V6

- Q or q wave is absent in leads V5 or V6. Presence of q wave signifies myocardial infarction.
- QS wave in lead V1 may show a small notch, giving the wave a characteristic 'W' pattern.
- The S-T segment and T wave are directed opposite to the QRS deflection. Hence, in lead V5 or lead V6, S-T segment is depressed and the T wave is inverted. Complete LBBB often mimics anterior wall myocardial infarction (pseudo-anterior wall infarction).

**Tips and Tricks**

- Look for wide QRS complex with rSR' pattern in lead V5 (M pattern) and 'W' pattern in lead V1 to make a diagnosis of LBBB.
- LBBB, unlike RBBB is always an indicator of heart disease, usually of the left ventricle.
- LBBB in presence of severe chest pain may be due to acute myocardial infarction.
- LBBB in asymptomatic patient does not require any treatment.

### *14.2.1 Genesis of rsR' Complex in Lead V6*

The electrical impulse reaches up to the bundle of His by the normal pathway of conduction. After this the impulse is not able to enter into the left bundle hence it enters into the right bundle first and activates the septum. This vector is oriented from right to left and hence produces a small r wave in lead V6. This is exactly the opposite of what happens in RBBB (Fig. 14.11).

The impulse then enters into the right ventricle and activates it. The net vector is moving away from the lead V6 resulting in s wave. Because of thin right ventricular wall, this s wave may not go below the base line and merely may produce a notch in the R wave (Fig. 14.12).

The impulse then bypasses the blocked left bundle and enters into the left ventricle and activates it. The net vector is directed towards the lead V6 resulting in R' wave (Figs. 14.13 and 14.14).

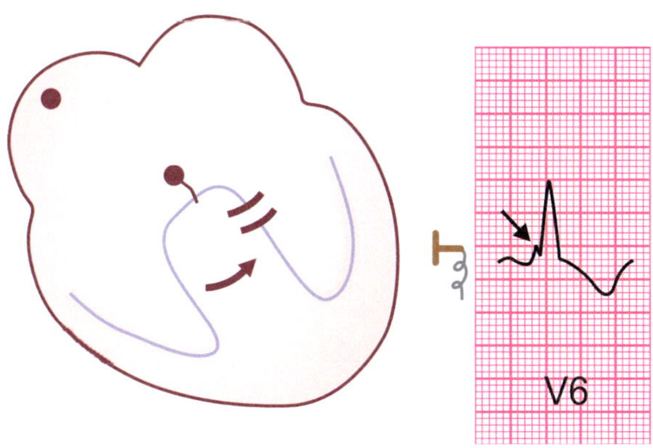


**Fig. 14.11** Genesis of r wave (arrow) of rsR' complex in lead V6

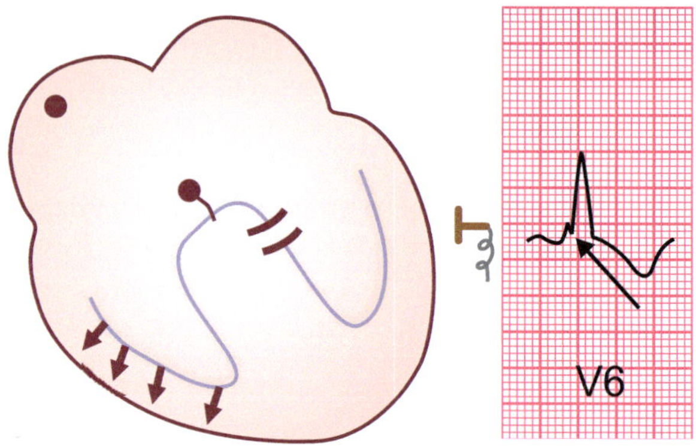


**Fig. 14.12** Genesis of s wave (arrow) of rsR' complex in lead V6

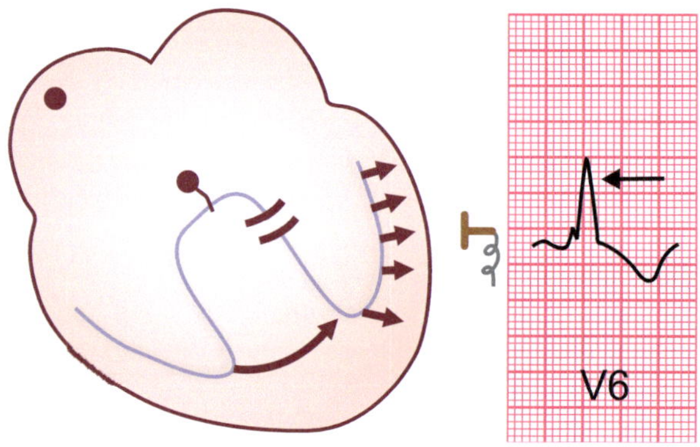


**Fig. 14.13** Genesis of R' wave (arrow) of rsR' complex in lead V6

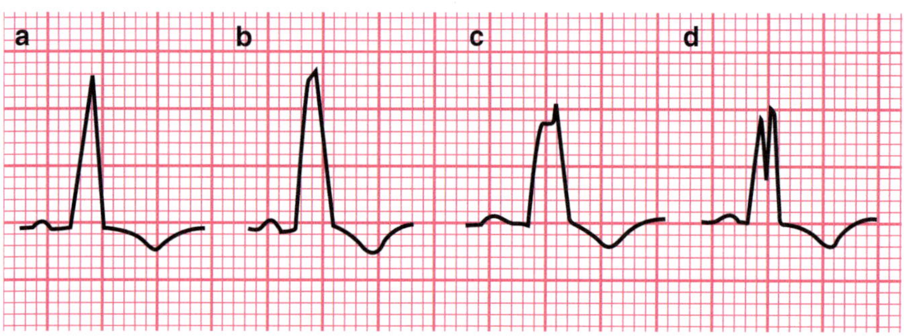


**Fig. 14.14** Types of rsr' complexes in lead V6. The rsR' complex in lead V6 may show only widening of QRS complex with T wave inversion (**a**) or it may show a notch in R wave with T wave inversion (**b**) and (**c**) or it may show a typical M pattern (**d**)

### 14.2.2 Distinguishing Features of LBBB and LVH

LBBB is often present in association with LVH. It is very important to distinguish between these two conditions. The main thing that one should look for is the initial q wave in leads V5, V6 and aVL. The presence of q wave rules out LBBB or indicates associated myocardial infarction. The other feature that one should look for is the feature of left atrial enlargement. If it is present, it indicates the presence of LVH. The voltage criteria for the diagnosis of LVH are not valid in presence of LBBB.

### 14.2.3 Incomplete Left Bundle Branch Block

In incomplete LBBB, there is delayed conduction through the left bundle. The features of incomplete LBBB are the following:

- Small q wave in lead V5 or V6 disappears and there is a tall R wave.
- Small r wave in lead V1 disappears and there is a big QS complex.
- Gradually, the other features of complete LBBB appear, but the width of QRS complex is less than 0.12 s and VAT is less than 0.09 s.

**Self-Assessment Questions**

1. RBBB may be rate dependent. True or false?
2. LBBB may occur transiently. True or false?
3. In RBBB, there is widening of QRS complex. True or false?
4. LBBB is characterized by a wide R wave in lead V6. True or false?
5. RVH and RBBB cannot be distinguished on the basis of QRS duration. True or false?
6. **In absence of structural heart diseases, which of the following is more common?**

   a. RBBB b. LBBB c. LAHB d. LPHB

7. **rSR' pattern is seen in lead V1 with S-T depression and T wave inversion. It suggests:**

   a. LBBB b. RBBB c. LAHB d. First degree AV block

8. **ECG shows rsR' pattern in lead V6 and there is T wave inversion. Which of the following type of block is suggested?**

   a. AV block b. SA block c. Bifascicular block d. LBBB

9. **The duration of QRS complex in complete LBBB is more than:**

   a. 0.08s b. 0.10 s c. 0.11 s d. 0.12 s

10. **LBBB is seen in which of the following condition:**

    a. Ebstein's anomaly b. Ostium primum ASD c. Acute massive pulmonary embolism d. Hypertensive heart disease

**Case Studies**

1. A 35-year-old gentleman was undergoing medical check-up for recruitment in army. His ECG (Fig. 14.15) is given below. Identify the conduction disturbance.
2. A 65-year-old gentleman came for medical check-up. He has history of hypertension. Examine the 12-lead ECG (Fig. 14.16) given below. Identify the abnormality. Give two important points in favour of your diagnosis.

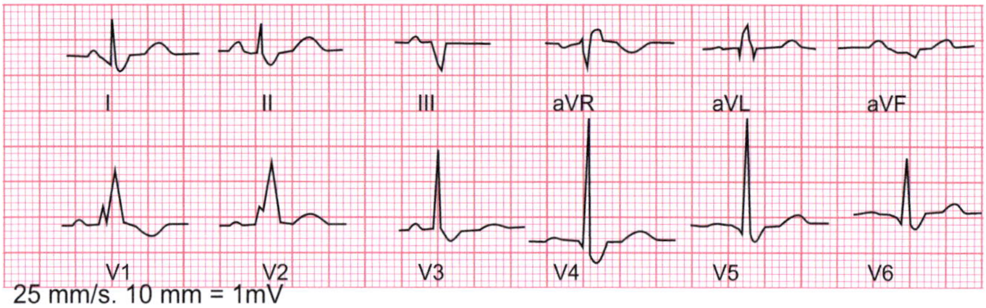


**Fig. 14.15** Identify the conduction disturbance

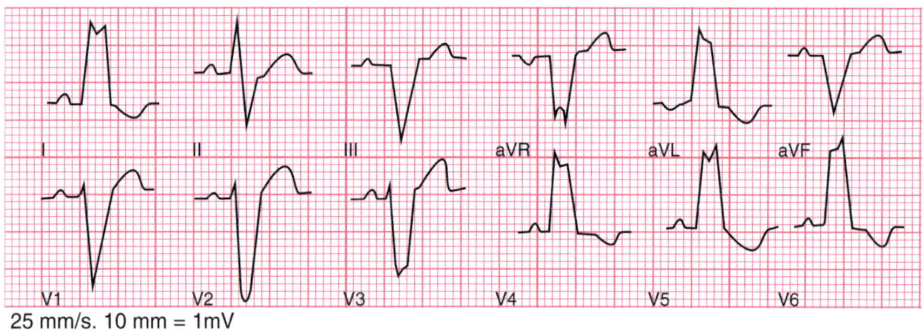


**Fig. 14.16** Identify the ECG abnormality

**Answers**

1. True  2. True  3. True  4. True  5. False  6. a  7. b  8. d  9. d  10. d

**Case Studies**

1. The conduction abnormality is RBBB.

   - There is rsR' complex in lead V1.
   - Duration of QRS complex in lead V1 is 0.14 s and there are S-T segment and T wave changes in lead V1.
   - Note the wide s wave in lead V6.

   RBBB is frequently seen in normal healthy persons and no active intervention is required.
2. The conduction abnormality is LBBB. The two most important points in favour of the diagnosis are wide QRS complex in lead V6 (more than 0.12 s) with S-T, T changes and presence of notch in QRS complexes of lead V5 and lead V6, which signify RsR' complexes. Also note the absence of q waves in these leads. QRS axis is deviated to left.

   LBBB in older age group may serve as an important marker for cardiovascular disease or death. This patient should be properly investigated and treated. If coexisting heart failure is detected, he may need cardiac resynchronization therapy. In asymptomatic individuals, no further therapy is needed but regular follow-up is essential.

# Chapter 15
# Fascicular Block

**Learning Objectives**
After studying this chapter, the reader will learn about:

- Left anterior fascicular block
- Left posterior fascicular block
- Bilateral bundle branch block
- Trifascicular block

## 15.1 Fascicular (Divisional) Blocks

The left bundle branch divides into two fascicles: anterior and posterior fascicles. When one of the fascicles is blocked, the impulse is conducted through the other fascicle. Since the conduction is very rapid through the fascicles, the fascicular block does not prolong the QRS duration.

### *15.1.1 Left Anterior Fascicular Block*

Left anterior fascicular block also called left anterior hemiblock (LAHB) is more common than the block of the posterior fascicle. The anterior fascicle is supplied by a single artery and it is long and thin, whereas the posterior fascicle has dual blood supply and it is short and thick. The impulse passes via the posterior fascicle of the left bundle and then anterior fascicle is activated by the Purkinje fibres distal to the site of the block. The various causes of LAHB are enumerated in Box 15.1. The ECG manifestations of LAHB are the following:


T. K. Koley, *Rapid Review of ECG*,
https://doi.org/10.1007/978-981-99-9116-7_15

**Box 15.1 Causes of LAHB**
Coronary artery disease
Left ventricular hypertrophy
Hypertension
Cardiomyopathy
Aortic stenosis

- Left axis deviation of QRS axis. The QRS axis lies between −30° and −90°.
- There are deep S waves in lead II and III and the depth of S wave in lead III is more than the depth of S wave in lead II (Fig. 15.1).
- The QRS duration is not prolonged (less than 0.12 s).
- In lead I, there is a tall R wave after the prominent q wave.
- The normal q wave in lead I and a VL becomes prominent.
- Prominent initial r waves in lead II, III and aVF.

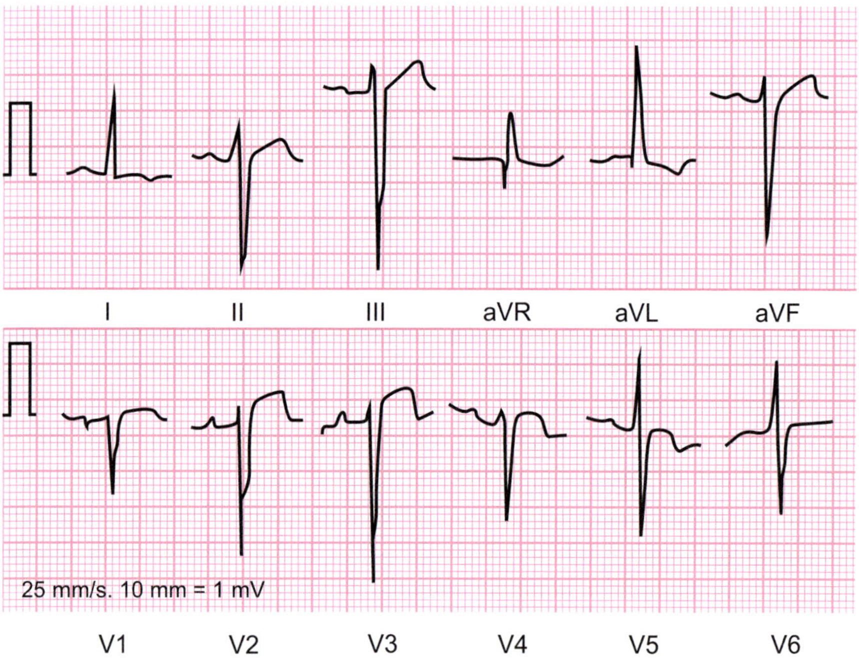


**Fig. 15.1** Anterior wall myocardial infarction with left anterior hemiblock

- The normally present small q waves tend to disappear in leads V5 and V6.
- In lead V5 and lead V6, the R wave height tends to diminish.
- In lead V5 and lead V6, the S wave becomes prominent and there may be terminal slurring.

**Tips and Tricks**
- If you come across an ECG showing left axis deviation, think of possibility of LAHB.
- Next check the depths of S waves in leads II and III to further confirm the diagnosis. The depth of S wave in lead III is more than the depth of S wave in lead II.

### *15.1.2 Left Posterior Fascicular Block*

Left posterior fascicular block also called left posterior hemiblock (LPHB) is due to the lesion in the posterior fascicle of the left bundle. Here the impulse is blocked at the left fascicle, and hence, the impulse travels via the anterior fascicle and then via the interconnected Purkinje fibres, the impulse travels via the posterior fascicle distal to the block. It is not very common. The ECG manifestations are the following:

- The QRS axis is deviated to right (beyond 120°).
- There are prominent R waves in leads II, III and aVF, and the R wave in lead III is the tallest among them (Fig. 15.2).
- In lead l and aVL, there are prominent S waves.
- There is a small but prominent q wave in lead II, III and aVF.
- In lead I, there is a small but prominent r wave.
- The T wave may be inverted in lead II, III and aVF.

**Tips and Tricks**
- It is important to rule out possibility of right ventricular hypertrophy and myocardial infarction before making a diagnosis of left posterior hemiblock.
- Look for right axis deviation and the height of R waves in leads II, III and aVF and the R wave in lead III is the tallest among them.

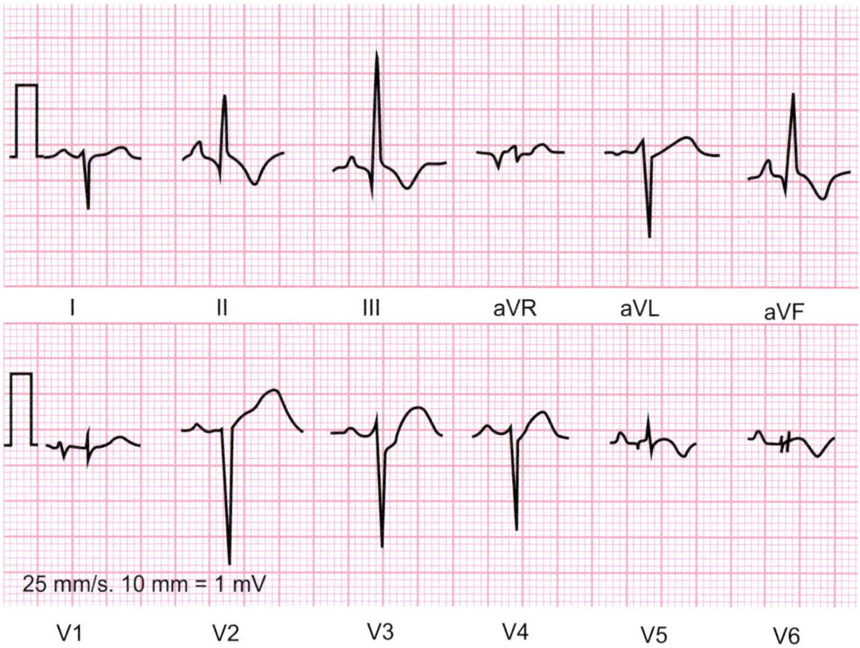


**Fig. 15.2** Left posterior fascicular block. It is always important to rule out right ventricular hypertrophy. This patient had come with chest pain and the chest leads show features of anterior wall myocardial infarction

### *15.1.3 Bilateral Bundle Branch Block*

Bilateral bundle branch block also called bifascicular block means block in conduction in both the right and the left bundle. The different types of bilateral bundle branch block are the following:

- RBBB with LAHB: Chest leads show RBBB pattern and left axis deviation in standard leads (Fig. 15.3). It is a common type of bifascicular block, often observed in myocardial infarction.
- RBBB with LPHB: There is RBBB with right axis deviation. It is a very rare combination, and the initial 0.08 s determines the axis and the divisional block.

Trifascicular block is a combination of RBBB with either LAHB or LPHB with first degree AV block (prolonged P-R interval).

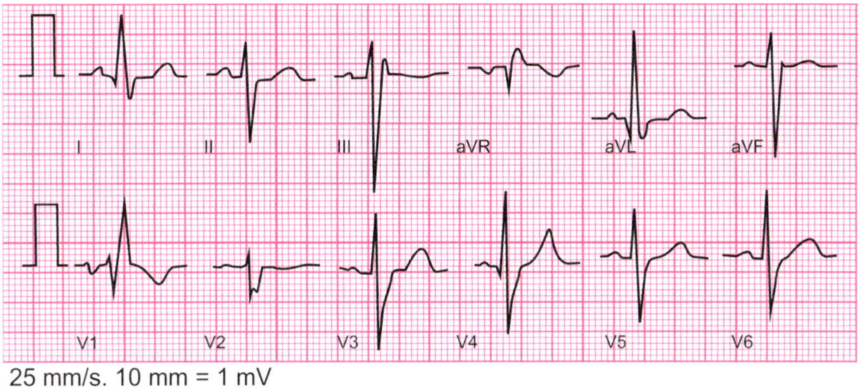


**Fig. 15.3** Right bundle branch block with left anterior hemiblock. Note the broad QRS complex in lead V1 with S-T segment, T wave change. There are also deep S waves in leads II and III and the depth of S wave in lead III is more than that of lead II. Hence, this is a bifascicular block

## Self-Assessment Questions

1. In LAHB, the QRS axis is normal. True or false?
2. In LPHB, R waves are recorded in lead II and lead III. True or false?
3. The presence of LAHB in an ECG can cause left axis deviation. True or false?
4. LPHB is characterized by a delay in the conduction of the left anterior fascicle of the bundle branches. True or false?
5. Bifascicular block is characterized by the presence of conduction block in both right and left bundle simultaneously. True or false?
6. **Which ECG finding is commonly associated with LAHB?**

   a. Right axis deviation b. Left axis deviation c. Prolonged P-R interval d. Shortened Q-T interval

7. **Which ECG finding is commonly associated with LPHB?**

   a. Right axis deviation b. Left axis deviation c. Prolonged P-R interval d. Tall R waves in leads V1 and V2

8. **The combination of LAHB and RBBB is known as:**

   a. LPHB b. Bifascicular block c. LBBB d. Anterior fascicular block

9. **Which ECG finding is characteristic of bifascicular block?**

   a. Prolonged Q-T interval b. CHB c. Wide QRS complex d. Delta wave

10. **Which ECG finding is commonly associated with bifascicular block and may indicate an increased risk of progression to complete heart block?**

    a. Q-T interval shortening b. S-T segment depression c. Prolonged P-R interval d. T wave inversion

**Case Studies**

1. A 60-year-old gentleman came for routine evaluation. He has past history of hypertension, diabetes and dyslipidaemia. He is asymptomatic. Examine the 12-lead ECG (Fig. 15.4) given below. Identify the abnormality. Give two important points in favour of your diagnosis.
2. A 50-year-old gentleman came for medical check-up. He has past history of hypertension for 25 years. He has taken irregular treatment for hypertension. He was asymptomatic. On examination, his blood pressure was 170/90 mmHg, pulse rate was 88/min, heart sounds were normal and chest was clear. His ECG is given in Fig. 15.5. What is your diagnosis?

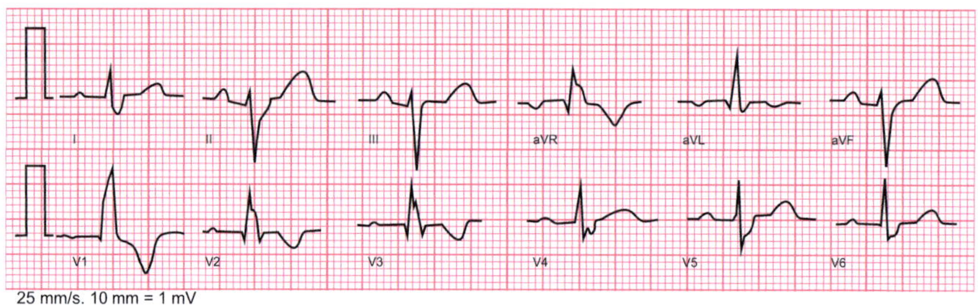


**Fig. 15.4** Identify the ECG abnormality

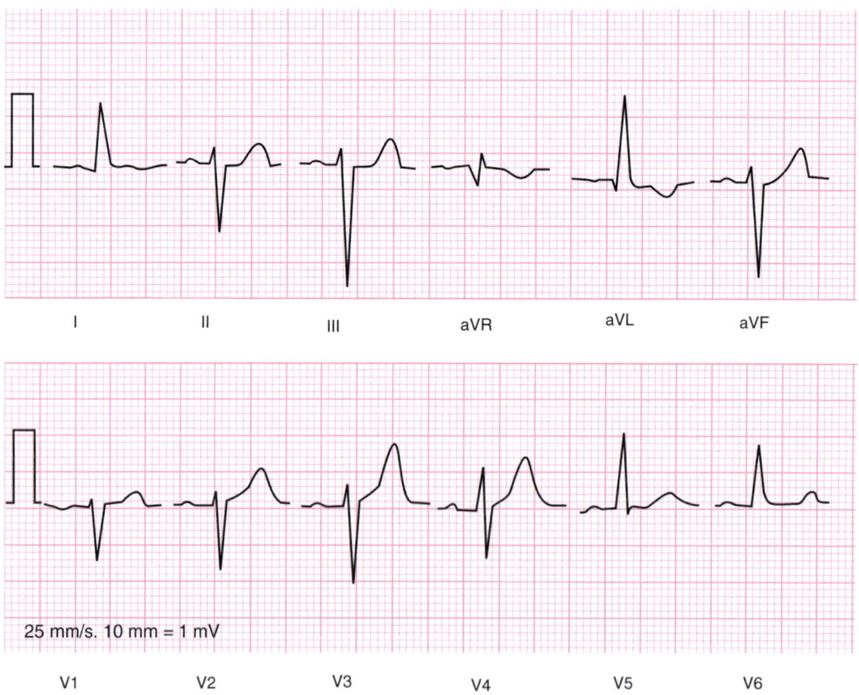


**Fig. 15.5** Identify the ECG abnormality

**Answers**

1. False 2. True 3. True 4. False 5. True 6. b. 7. a. 8. b. 9. c. 10. c.

**Case Studies**

1. The conduction abnormality is RBBB with LAHB. This is a bifascicular block. There is wide QRS complex in lead V1 with S-T, T changes with slurred s waves in leads V5 and V6. These are diagnostic of RBBB. LAHB is diagnosed by presence of S waves in lead II and lead III. The depth of S wave in lead III is more than the depth of S wave in lead II. Besides this if we consider lead I and lead aVF, there is left axis deviation.

   Asymptomatic bifascicular block usually does not require any treatment. There is modest evidence and weak consensus for cardiac pacemaker in this condition. Any provoking medication should be withdrawn. However, he should be advised regular cardiac check-up.
2. The ECG shows left axis deviation. There are prominent S waves in lead II and lead III. The depth of S wave in lead III is more than the depth of S wave in lead II. The QRS duration is normal. Hence, the diagnosis is LAHB.

   Patients of LAHB are at higher risk of cardiovascular morbidity and mortality. In this patient most likely it is due to long standing uncontrolled hypertension. Hypertension should be treated with appropriate antihypertensive. He should also be advised regular follow-up.

# Part IV
# Coronary Artery Disease

# Chapter 16
# Myocardial Ischaemia

**Learning Objectives**
After studying this chapter, the reader will learn about:

- Myocardial ischaemia
- S-T segment abnormalities
- T wave abnormalities
- U wave abnormalities

ECG is an inexpensive, most accessible and non-invasive diagnostic tool to evaluate patients presenting with clinical features suggestive of myocardial ischaemia or myocardial infarction. It provides us with reliable information regarding various important factors for the management of the patient like extent and location of the site of ischaemia/infarction, heart rate and disturbances of impulse formation and conduction.

## 16.1 Myocardial Ischaemia

Myocardial ischaemia occurs due to inadequate blood supply to the myocardium to meet its requirement. The commonest cause of myocardial ischemia is atherosclerosis induced blockage of coronary blood vessels. However, in other conditions like severe LVH (aortic stenosis) where the coronary artery is normal, there may be relative ischaemia and angina pectoris. The various causes of myocardial ischaemia are enumerated in Box 16.1.


T. K. Koley, *Rapid Review of ECG*,
https://doi.org/10.1007/978-981-99-9116-7_16

**Box 16.1 Causes of Myocardial Ischaemia**
Atherosclerosis
Severe aortic stenosis
Polycythaemia
Anaemia
Thyroid disorders
Syphilitic aortitis

The electrocardiographic manifestations of myocardial ischaemia are mainly observed in S-T segment and T waves. The changes are however not specific of myocardial ischaemia because they can be seen in other conditions including LVH, pericarditis and myocarditis. Hence, the ECG changes need to be correlated with clinical findings to make the right diagnosis. The main ECG features are:

- S-T segment changes
- T wave changes
- U wave changes

### *16.1.1 S-T Segment Changes*

Analysis of S-T segment change is the most important aspect in diagnosis of myocardial ischaemia. S-T segment change is the commonest electrocardiographic change seen in this condition. The characteristic ECG features of myocardial ischaemia are the various types of changes observed in S-T segment. This is an abnormality of ventricular repolarization. S-T segment abnormality may be of two types:

(a) Depression of S-T segment
(b) Elevation of S-T segment

#### 16.1.1.1 Depression of S-T Segment

Due to myocardial ischaemia, there is injury of subendocardial area of ventricle. S-T segment depression is the ECG manifestation of this injury. Due to injury, the S-T segment vector is directed opposite to the surface of the ventricle, i.e. towards the cavity. Hence, the leads overlying the area will record S-T segment depression. S-T segment depression is seen prominently during a period of ongoing angina.

It may be transient but sometimes it may be a permanent feature also. It is often considered that more the depression, more severe is the disease and worse is the prognosis. S-T segment depression may be of three types:

1. Downsloping S-T segment depression
2. Horizontal S-T segment depression
3. Upsloping S-T segment depression

### Downsloping S-T Segment Depression

Downsloping S-T segment depression reflects severe coronary insufficiency. Both the proximal and distal part of S-T segment are depressed and depression in distal part is more than that of proximal part (Figs. 16.1 and 16.2).

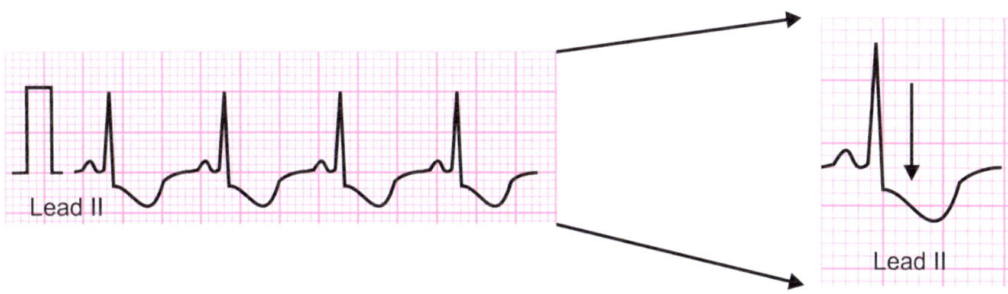


**Fig. 16.1** Downsloping S-T segment depression. Note that both the proximal and distal part of the S-T segment are depressed and the distal part is more depressed than the proximal part

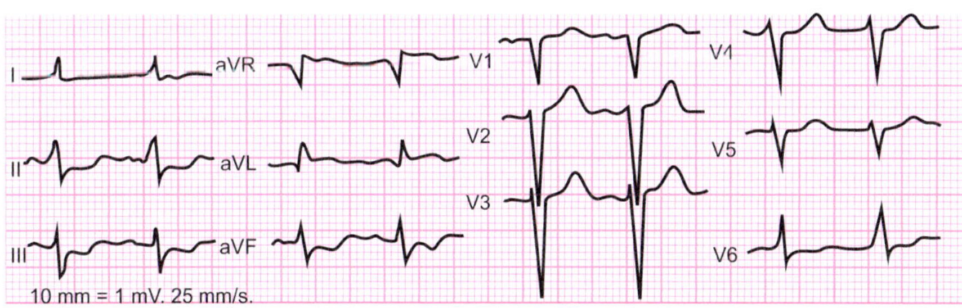


**Fig. 16.2** Inferior wall myocardial ischaemia. This ECG is recorded from a 55-year-old gentleman suffering from severe chest pain. He had history of diabetes mellitus for last 10 years. ECG revealed downsloping S-T segment depression in leads II, III and aVF

### Horizontal S-T Segment Depression

Horizontal S-T segment depression means the depression of both the proximal and distal part of S-T segment (Fig. 16.3). Almost the entire S-T segment does not touch the isoelectric line. The J point is depressed more than 1 mm below the isoelectric line. Hence, the S-T segment is depressed at the very beginning and merges with the proximal limb of T wave. The S-T segment remains depressed 1 mm or more below the baseline 80 ms after the J point.

### Upsloping S-T Segment Depression

In upsloping S-T segment depression, only the proximal part of S-T segment (near its junction with QRS complex) is depressed (Fig. 16.4). It does not always reflect myocardial ischaemia. However, it needs to be interpreted carefully in the presence of ongoing chest pain. It may be observed in sinus tachycardia.

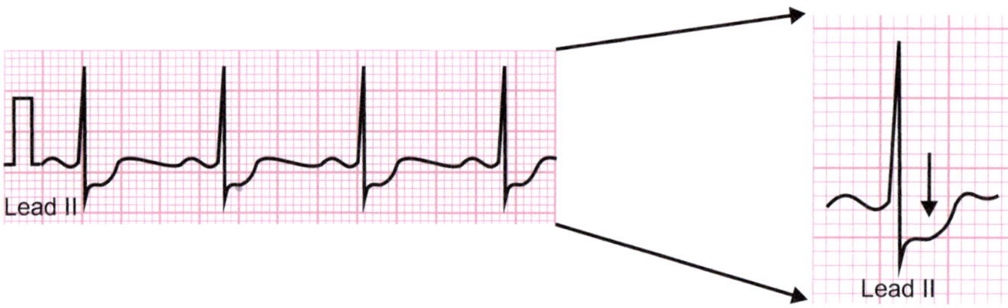


**Fig. 16.3** Horizontal S-T segment depression. Note that both the proximal and distal part of the S-T segment are depressed below the baseline

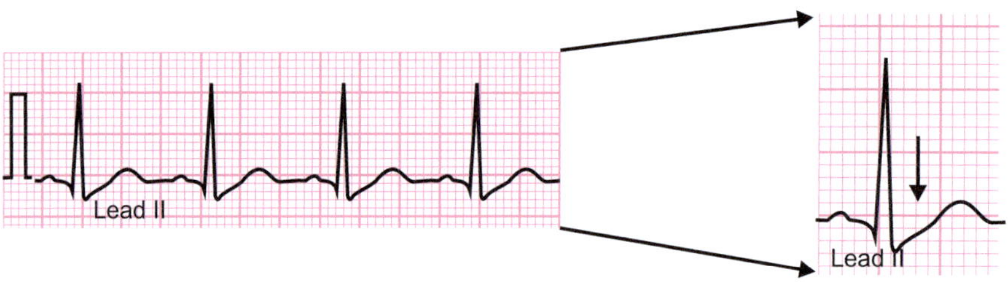


**Fig. 16.4** Upsloping S-T segment depression. Note that the proximal part of the S-T segment is depressed but the distal part is not depressed and it is approaching the baseline

**Tips and Tricks**

- Minor degrees of S-T segment depression, in the absence of any symptoms is often normal.
- ECG changes of unstable angina often become normal after relief of chest pain.

#### 16.1.1.2 Elevation of S-T segment

The most dangerous but least common S-T segment change of myocardial ischaemia is S-T segment elevation which points more towards myocardial infarction. It represents transmural ischaemia. S-T segment elevation is observed in Prinzmetal's angina (coronary vasospasm). J point is elevated. The S-T segment elevation is accompanied by a tall and widened T wave. The elevated S-T segment tends to be concave upward (Fig. 16.5). The S-T segment usually becomes isoelectric when chest pain subsides. It is a feature of transmural epicardial injury. Various ECG features of Prinzmetal's angina are enumerated in Box 16.2.

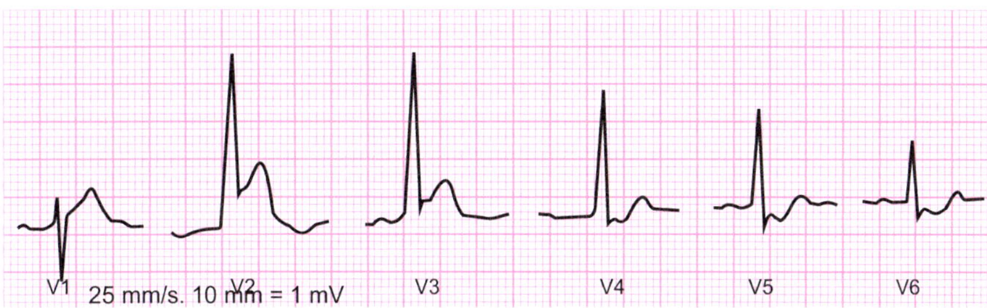


**Fig. 16.5** Prinzmetal's angina. This ECG is recorded from a 45-year-old gentleman suffering from severe chest pain. ECG shows increased amplitude of R waves and S-T segment elevation in leads V2 and V3 with tall and widened T waves. There is S-T segment depression in leads V4–V6. It was due to coronary artery spasm

**Box 16.2 ECG Features of Prinzmetal's Angina**

S-T segment elevation
Increase in amplitude of R wave
Decrease in depth of S wave
Inversion of U wave
Ventricular premature beats
AV block

The important causes of S-T segment depression are enumerated in Box 16.3.

**Box 16.3 Depression of S-T Segment**
Myocardial ischaemia
Subendocardial infarction
Digitalis effect
Digitalis toxicity
Myocarditis
Cardiomyopathy
Cerebrovascular accident

### *16.1.2 T Wave Abnormalities*

T wave inversion is the characteristic ECG finding of myocardial ischaemia. The inverted T wave has symmetrical limbs with a narrow, pointed nadir (arrowhead appearance). T wave inversion of ischaemia needs to be differentiated from other causes of T wave inversion. In strain pattern (LVH), the T wave is inverted but it is asymmetric. In digitalis effect, the T wave is inverted but it is asymmetrical and the nadir is blunted (Fig. 16.6).

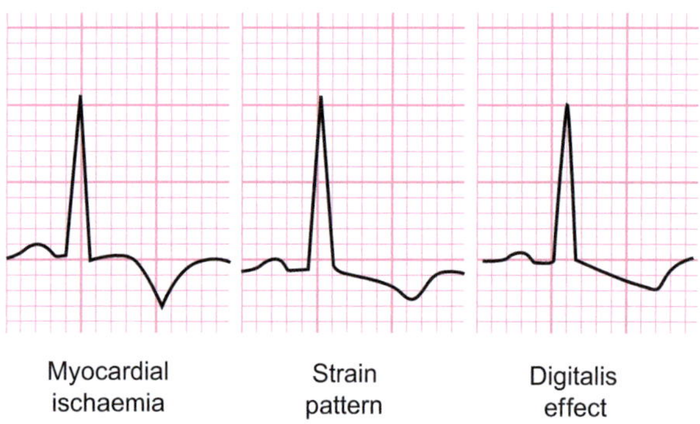


**Fig. 16.6** Three types of T wave inversion. Note the arrowhead appearance in myocardial ischaemia, the asymmetry of T wave in strain pattern and the reverse check sign in digitalis effect

### 16.1.3 U Wave Abnormalities

Inverted U waves are observed in myocardial ischaemia. Inversion of U wave is also seen in hypertensive heart disease. The various ECG criteria for diagnosis of myocardial ischaemia are enumerated in Box 16.4.

**Box 16.4 ECG Criteria of Myocardial Ischaemia**

Downsloping or horizontal S-T segment depression equal to or greater than 1 mm at 80 ms after J point
S-T segment and J point elevation (Prinzmetal's angina)
Symmetric T wave inversion
Inversion of U wave

**Self-Assessment Questions**

1. Myocardial ischaemia is represented by pathological q waves. True or false?
2. Downsloping S-T segment depression is one of the most important diagnostic ECG features of myocardial ischaemia. True or false?
3. Symmetric T wave inversion is a feature of myocardial ischaemia. True or false?
4. **For diagnosis of myocardial ischaemia, S-T segment should be depressed for at least:**

   a. 1 mm or more below the baseline 80 ms after the J point
   b. 0.1 mm or more below the baseline 80 ms after the J point
   c. 10 mm or more below the baseline 80 ms after the J point
   d. 100 mm or more below the baseline 80 ms after the J point

5. **Which of the following ECG changes are normally associated with Prinzmetal's angina:**

   a. Arrhythmia b. S-T segment elevation c. S-T segment depression d. Shortened P-R interval

6. **Which one of the following is typical feature of myocardial ischaemia?**

   a. Horizontal S-T segment depression b. Upsloping S-T segment depression c. Prolonged Q-T interval d. Prolonged P-R interval

7. **Which one of the following is not an ECG feature of myocardial ischaemia?**

   a. T wave inversion b. Upsloping S-T segment depression c. Downsloping S-T segment depression d. Horizontal S-T segment depression

### Case Studies

1. A 65-year-old gentleman presented with chest pain and sweating in the emergency department. Examine the 12-lead ECG (Fig. 16.7) done in the emergency department and answer the following questions:

   a. Can you identify the abnormality?
   b. Is the R wave progression normal in chest leads?
   c. What is your diagnosis?

2. Examine the ECG (Fig. 16.8) and point out the abnormalities. What is you diagnosis?
3. A 75-year-old lady presented with dyspnoea and sweating. She denied any history of chest pain. She had been suffering from diabetes and dyslipidaemia for last 15 years. Examine her ECG (Fig. 16.9) and make your diagnosis. What is the main point in favour of your diagnosis?
4. A 55-year-old gentleman came to the emergency department with history of chest discomfort for last two hours. He has history of hypertension, diabetes and dyslipidaemia for past 10 years. On examination he was found to be in moderate discomfort. His pulse was 110/min, blood pressure was 150/94 mmHg, chest was clear and heart sounds were normal. His ECG is given in Fig. 16.10. What is your diagnosis? How will you treat this patient?

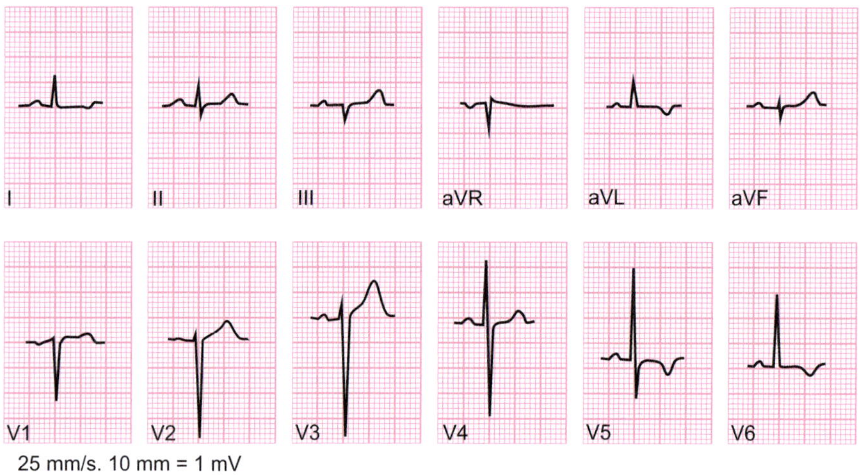


**Fig. 16.7** Identify the ECG abnormality

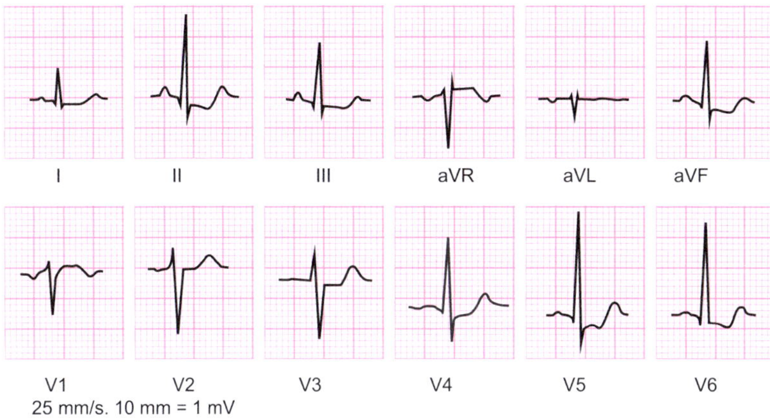


**Fig. 16.8** Identify the ECG abnormality

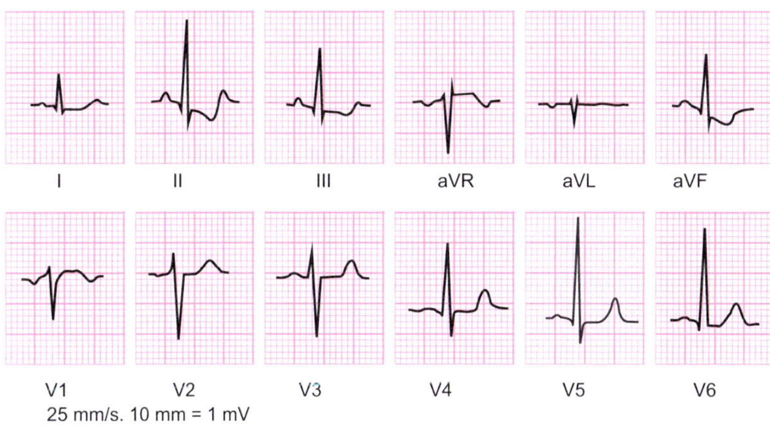


**Fig. 16.9** Identify the ECG abnormality

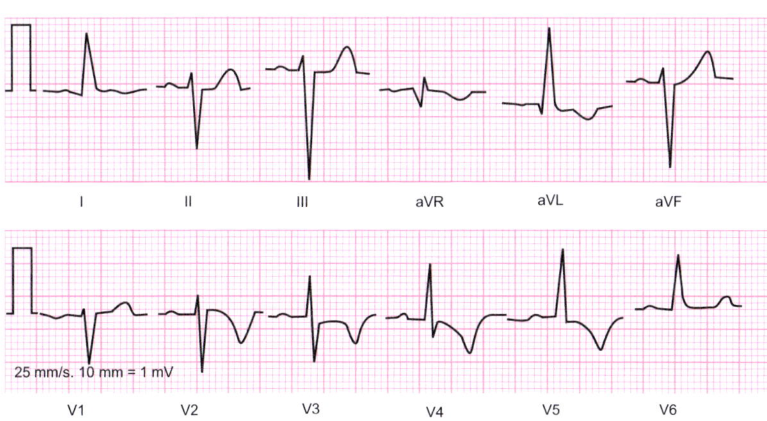


**Fig. 16.10** Identify the ECG abnormality

**Answers**

1. False 2. True 3. True 4. a 5. b 6. a 7. b

**Case Studies**

1. a. There are T wave inversions in leads I, aVL, V5 and V6.
   b. R wave progression is normal in chest leads.
   c. Diagnosis is lateral wall ischaemia.
2. The abnormalities are S-T segment depression in leads II, III, aVF, V4, V5 and V6. Diagnosis is inferior and lateral wall myocardial ischaemia.
3. The diagnosis is inferior wall ischaemia.

   The main point in favour of diagnosis is downsloping S-T segment depression in leads II, III and aVF.
4. The patient has history suggestive of acute coronary syndrome. The ECG shows left axis deviation with deep S waves in lead II and lead III and the depth of S wave in lead III is more than that in lead II. This makes it a case of LAHB. In anterior wall there is S-T segment depression with T wave inversion in leads V2–V5. There is T wave inversion in lead I and lead aVL also. Hence, the final diagnosis is anterior wall myocardial ischaemia with LAHB.

   The patient should be immediately treated with oxygen, nitrates, heparin, antiplatelet therapy and statin. Cardiac monitoring should be started. If chest pain persists and cardiac biomarkers are elevated, he may need coronary angiography.

# Chapter 17
# Myocardial Infarction

**Learning Objectives**
After studying this chapter, the reader will learn about:

- Myocardial infarction
- Zone of necrosis, injury and ischaemia
- Evolution of myocardial infarction
- Localization of myocardial infarction

Myocardial infarction occurs due to disruption of the blood supply to a part of myocardium, resulting in myocardial necrosis. The most common cause is total occlusion of a coronary artery due to rupture of an atherosclerotic plaque (Fig. 17.1). Myocardium may be spared if there is good collateral circulation. Most often the left ventricle is infarcted; however, the right ventricular infarction is not uncommon.

The ECG is the most valuable and initial investigation in patients presenting with chest pain to rule out myocardial infarction. Similar ECG changes may be observed in other diseases such as pericarditis, ventricular aneurysms and so in all cases, a medical history should be taken properly before interpreting the ECG. A single ECG recording might not show the infarct related changes, but multiple ECG tracings are frequently needed to make the right diagnosis.

ECG is the main diagnostic tool of the decision-making pathway that divides patients with acute coronary syndrome who show S-T segment elevation (S-T segment elevated myocardial infarction, STEMI) and those without S-T segment elevation (non S-T segment elevation myocardial infarction, NSTEMI). This



T. K. Koley, *Rapid Review of ECG*,
https://doi.org/10.1007/978-981-99-9116-7_17

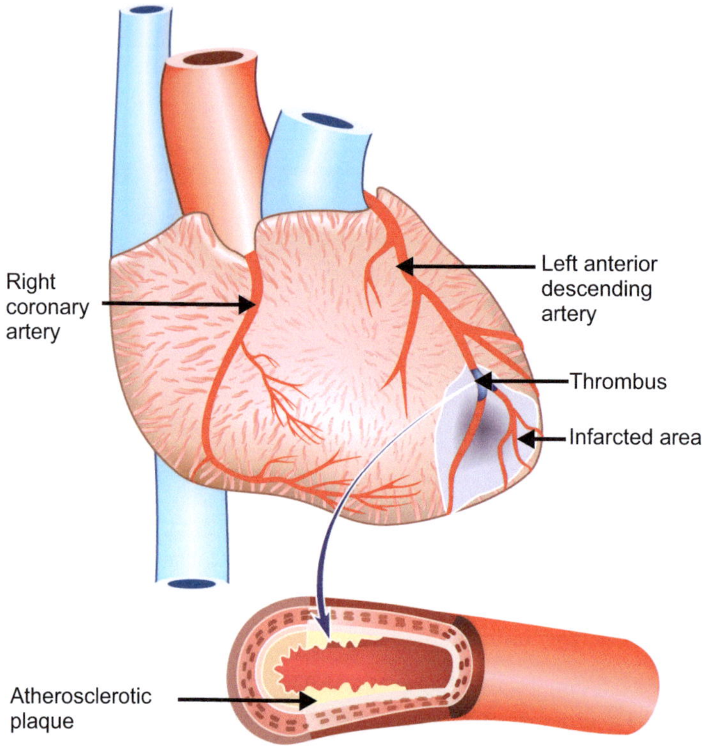


**Fig. 17.1** Myocardial infarction

distinction is extremely important because of the time urgency of reperfusion in patients with STEMI. The terminologies like Q wave MI, non Q wave MI, subendocardial infarction, transmural infarction are less widely used, as the latest diagnostic classification of acute coronary syndrome based on S-T segment elevation correlates more accurately with the pathophysiology of infarction and determines early management.

## 17.1 Zones of Necrosis Injury and Ischaemia

A fully evolved case of myocardial infarction has three pathological zones. There is a central zone of necrosis (Figs. 17.2 and 17.3) which is surrounded by a zone of injury; this in turn is surrounded by a zone of ischaemia.

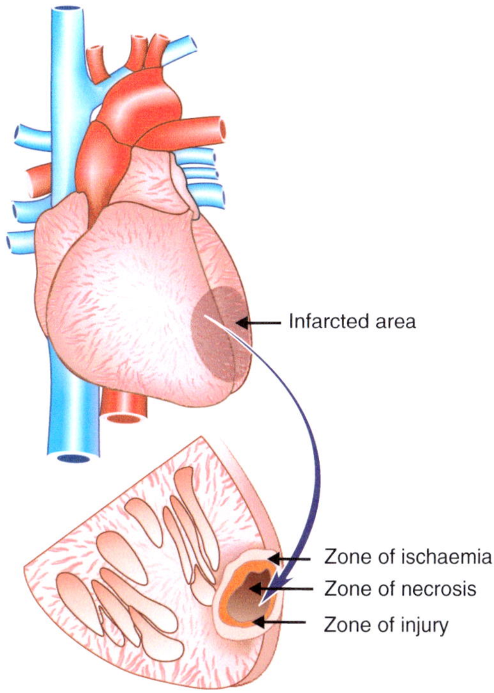


**Fig. 17.2** Three zones of myocardial infarction

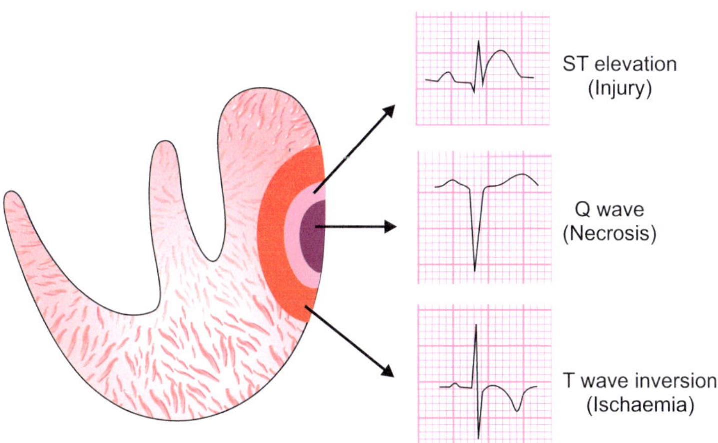


**Fig. 17.3** ECG manifestation of three zones of myocardial infarction

### 17.1.1 Myocardial Necrosis

The necrosed myocardium is dead tissue, which cannot be depolarized. Hence it is electrically inert and produces an electrical window. The lead over the window records the electrical activity of the healthy myocardium through the window. At first, the wavefront generated by depolarisation of interventricular septum will be directed away from the electrode. Next there will be depolarization of the distant free wall. This will again generate a wavefront moving away from the electrode. The QRS vector is thus directed completely away from the necrosed myocardium. Hence, the cardinal features of myocardial necrosis in ECG are Q waves (Fig. 17.4) and loss of amplitude of R waves. It is represented by QS complex. It is a totally negative complex.

The pathological Q wave needs to be differentiated from physiological q wave. The pathological Q wave is more than 0.04 s in duration and more than 4 mm in depth or more than 25% deep than the height of R wave (Fig. 17.5). Q waves of 0.04 s duration are often detected in lead III and occasionally in lead aVL, and the Q:R ratio is more than 25%. As a result, infarction should not be diagnosed solely on the basis of lead III. An abnormal Q wave can appear as soon as two hours after the onset of chest discomfort and is usually completely developed within twelve hours after the onset of myocardial infarction.

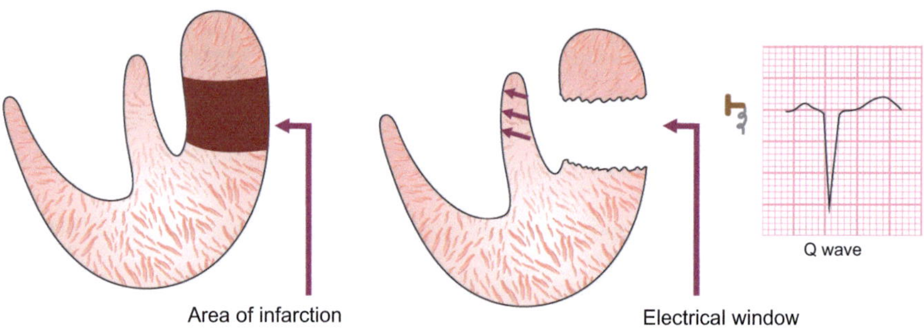


**Fig. 17.4** Genesis of Q wave

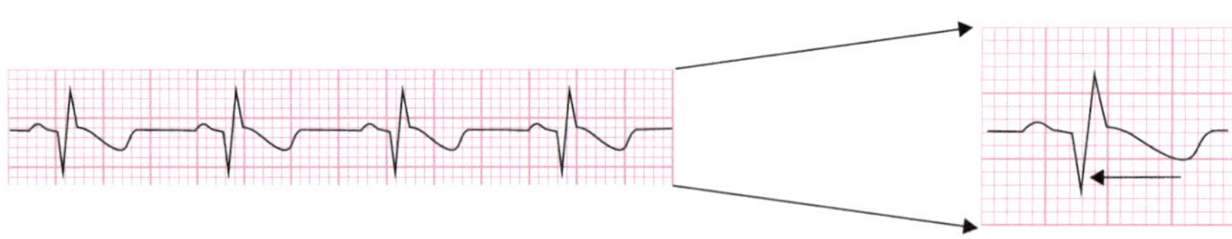

**Fig. 17.5** Pathological Q wave. Note the depth and width of the Q wave (arrow)

**Tips and Tricks**

- Narrow and even deep Q waves in the inferior and lateral leads are often seen in normal persons.
- Q wave in lead III but not in lead aVF is often normal.
- Q waves often do not develop if patient is treated promptly by thrombolysis or PCI (percutaneous coronary intervention).

### *17.1.2 Myocardial Injury*

Myocardial injury involves a wedge shaped section of myocardium, which does not repolarize completely. It is manifested in ECG by S-T segment elevation. This is often the first ECG change of myocardial infarction. The S-T segment is elevated and is convex or curved upward. The lead oriented to the injured epicardial surface records S-T segment elevation and the lead oriented to the uninjured surface records S-T segment depression (cavity lead aVR). S-T segment elevation is commonly recorded since most of the infarctions are transmural infarctions. According to the Minnesota Code, the S-T segment elevation must be of new onset, ≥1 mm in one or more of the following leads: I, II, III, aVL, aVF or leads V5 and V6, or ≥2 mm in one or more of the following leads: leads V1–V4 to be considered for making a diagnosis of myocardial infarction. However, an S-T segment elevation of ≥1 mm or more in two or more adjacent leads is usually sufficient to make a diagnosis of acute coronary syndrome. To make a correct diagnosis of STEMI, along with the ECG criteria one must always look for the clinical features of myocardial infarction or else it will lead to an overdiagnosis of STEMI.

### *17.1.3 Myocardial Ischaemia*

Symmetrical, deep and pointed T wave inversion is the typical ECG feature of myocardial ischaemia. The term 'coronary T' or 'Pardee T' means inverted T wave with isoelectric S-T segment, which has upward convexity. The term 'cove plane T' means T wave inversion in a lead with S-T segment elevation with convexity upwards.

An electrode oriented towards the infarcted myocardium will record all the three changes of myocardial infarction.

## 17.2 Evolution of Myocardial Infarction

There are three phases during the evolution of myocardial infarction, which can be recorded by ECG. They are:

1. The hyperacute phase
2. Fully evolved phase
3. Chronic stable phase

### *17.2.1 Hyperacute Phase*

Hyperacute phase develops within the first few hours after onset of myocardial infarction. It is an important stage in the development of infarction that takes place before the fully evolved phase. The patient is at risk for developing potentially fatal ventricular fibrillation during this stage. This period is crucial since the patient will benefit greatly from thrombolytic therapy at this time. The ECG manifestations are the following:

1. Tall and wide T waves
2. Tall R waves
3. Increased VAT
4. Slope elevation of S-T segment

Hyperacute phase is characterized by an increase in the magnitude of the T wave (Figs. 17.6 and 17.7). The T wave becomes symmetrical and pointed. Besides this, the T wave is also influenced by the abnormality of the preceding S-T segment. The transition of the S-T segment to T wave becomes straightened. It results in a wide T wave. The S-T segment is elevated with a slope which is either straight upwards towards the apex of the tall T wave or concave upwards. In this phase, Q wave and T wave inversion are absent. In leads opposite the infarct site, there is reciprocal S-T segment depression.

**Tips and Tricks**

- Sometimes tall and peaked T waves are normal as well.

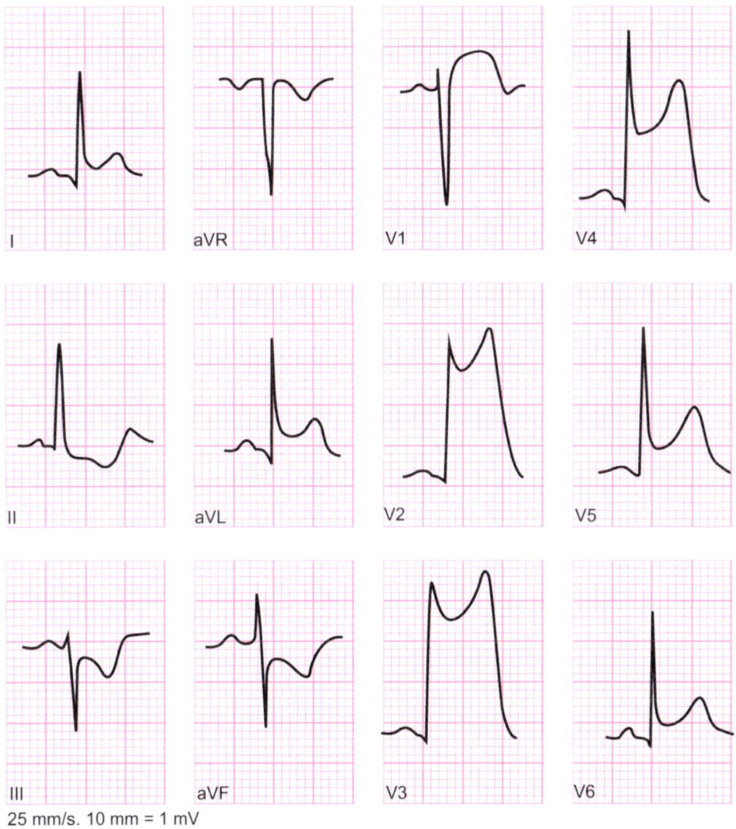


**Fig. 17.6** Hyperacute anterior wall myocardial infarction. Hyperacute infarction is indicated by tall R waves with slope elevation of T waves in leads V2–V4. There is reciprocal depression of S-T segment in leads II, III and aVF. The S-T segment in lead V1 is also elevated with convexity upwards

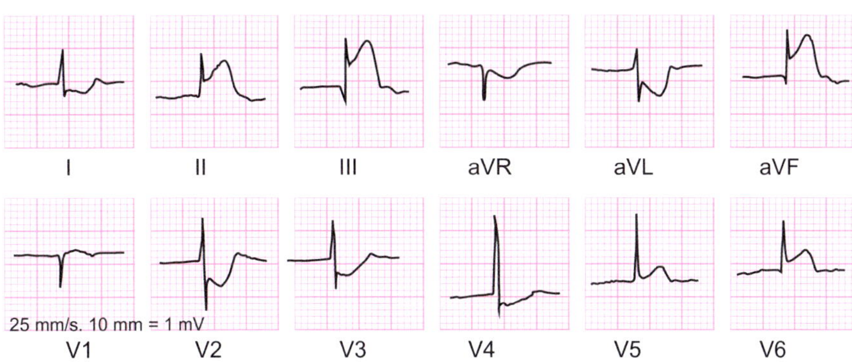


**Fig. 17.7** Hyperacute inferior wall myocardial infarction. Hyperacute infarction is indicated by tall R waves with slope elevation of T waves in leads II, III and aVF. There is reciprocal depression of S-T segment in leads I, aVL and V2–V4. The S-T segment in leads V5 and V6 is also elevated. This patient is developing lateral wall infarction also

### *17.2.2 Fully Evolved Phase*

The fully evolved phase of myocardial infarction has three main features: pathological Q waves, S-T segment elevation with convexity upwards and deep and symmetrical T wave inversion. Often the patient arrives late at the hospital after chest pain and the ECG taken at that time reflects the fully evolved phase of myocardial infarction; the hyperacute phase is frequently missed due to late presentation.

### *17.2.3 Chronic Stable Phase*

After the fully evolved phase, ECG changes gradually resolve. First, the S-T segment becomes isoelectric, but the T wave remains inverted. After a several hours, the T wave becomes upright. Q waves usually persist and remain markers of old myocardial infarction. The terms old myocardial infarction and chronic myocardial infarction are often used interchangeably. After 1 year, about 30% of ECGs are no longer diagnostic of myocardial infarction. Various phases of evolution are shown in Fig. 17.8.

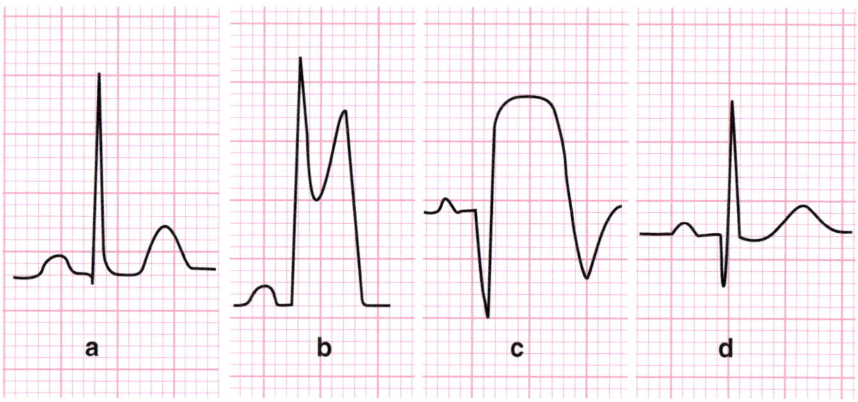


**Fig. 17.8** Various phases of evolution of myocardial infarction. (**a**) Normal PQRST complex. (**b**) Hyperacute phase. (**c**) Fully evolved phase. (**d**) Chronic stable phase

## 17.3 Localization of Myocardial Infarction

Myocardial infarction mainly involves the left ventricle. Sometimes the right ventricle and atrium are also involved. Coronary arteries that develop occlusion due to atherosclerosis or undergo coronary spasm can be predicted by leads showing S-T, T changes as shown in Box 17.1.

**Box 17.1 Prediction of Blockage of Coronary Artery**

| Leads showing S-T, T change | Coronary artery blocked |
|---|---|
| Leads V1–V4 | Left anterior descending coronary artery |
| Leads I, aVL, V5 and V6 | Left circumflex coronary artery |
| Leads II, III and aVF | Right coronary artery |

### *17.3.1 Left Ventricular Infarction*

Myocardial infarction mainly affects the left ventricle. Right ventricle infarction is not very common. For localization of infarction of left ventricle (Fig. 17.9), the following regions are taken into consideration:

1. Anterior wall
2. Inferior wall
3. Posterior wall

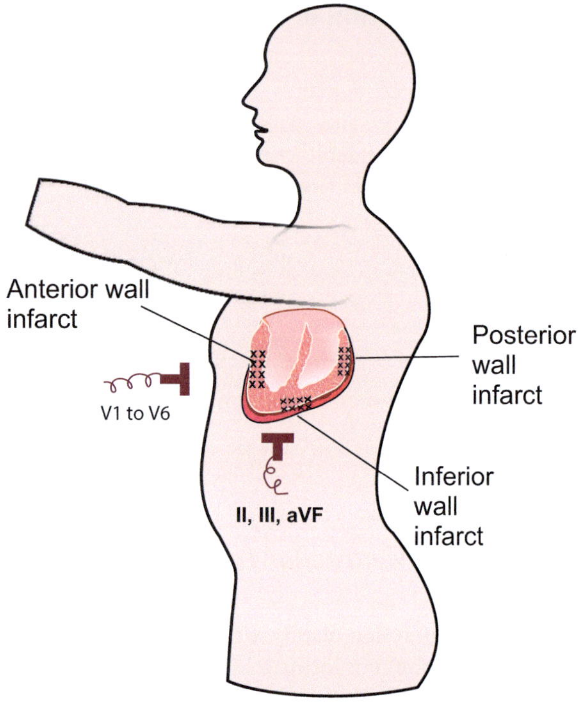


**Fig. 17.9** Illustration of anterior, inferior and posterior wall myocardial infarction

#### 17.3.1.1 Anterior Wall Myocardial Infarction

Anterior wall myocardial infarction is due to occlusion of left anterior descending artery. The proximal occlusion leads to infarction of a large area of left ventricle. The conducting system is also often affected. The anterior wall infarction (Figs. 17.10, 17.11 and 17.12) may be arbitrarily subdivided into the following types:

1. Extensive anterior wall infarction: The ECG changes are located in leads I, aVL and V1–V6.
2. Anteroseptal infarction: The ECG changes are located in leads V1–V4.
3. Anterolateral infarction: The ECG changes are located in leads I, aVL, V5 and V6.
4. Apical infarction: The ECG changes are located in leads V5 and V6.

In anterior wall infarction, reciprocal changes (S-T segment depression) are seen in leads II, III and aVF.

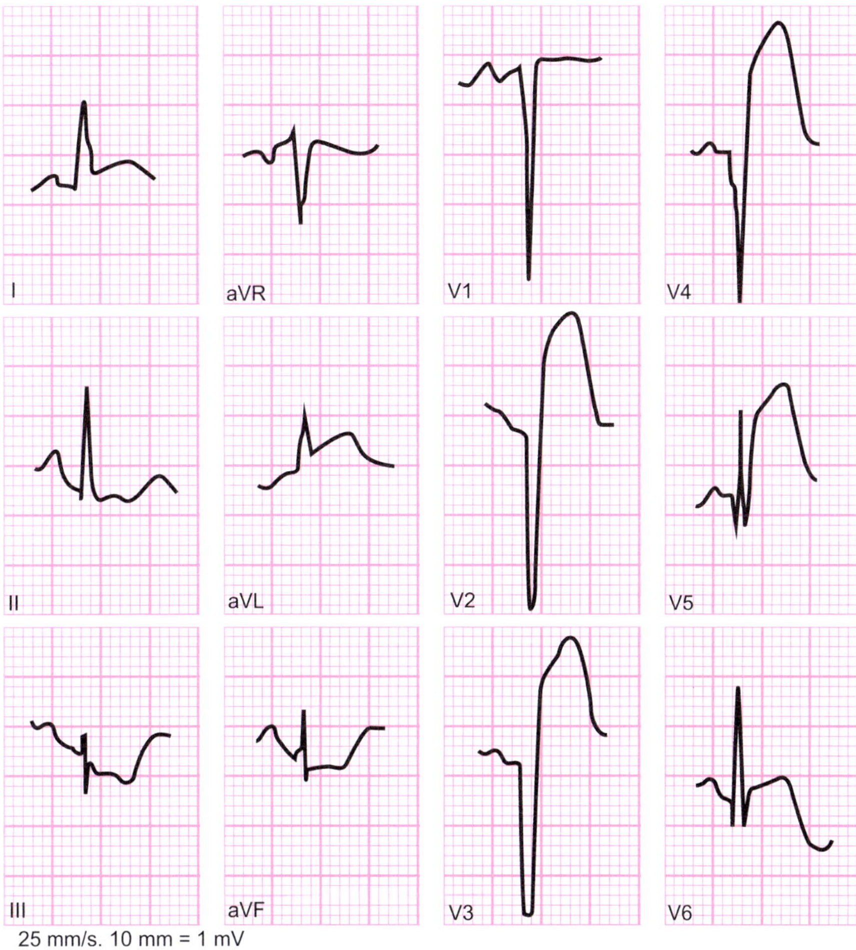


**Fig. 17.10** Extensive anterior wall myocardial infarction. This ECG is recorded from a 55-year-old lady suffering from severe chest pain with left ventricular failure. She was also suffering from uncontrolled diabetes mellitus. Note the S-T segment elevation with convexity upwards in leads V2–V6. Note that there is a rising trend of S-T segment in leads I and aVL

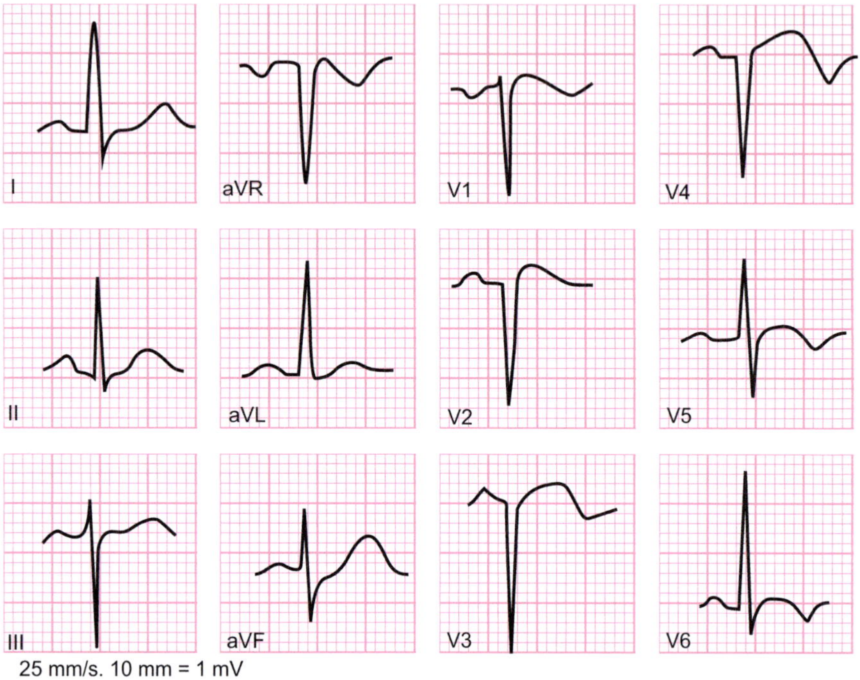


**Fig. 17.11** Anterior wall myocardial infarction. This ECG is recorded from a 67-year-old gentleman suffering from severe chest pain with vomiting, sweating and left ventricular failure. He was suffering from diabetes mellitus and hypercholesterolaemia. Note the S-T segment elevation with convexity upwards in leads V2–V6. Note that there is a rising trend of S-T segment in lead V1 also

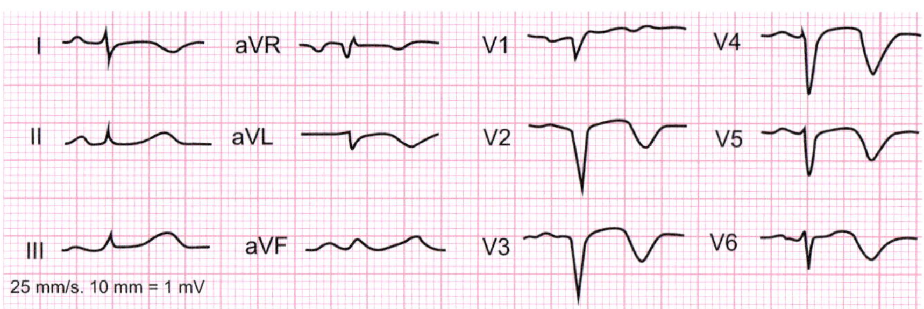


**Fig. 17.12** Recent anterior wall myocardial infarction. This ECG is recorded from a 56-year-old gentleman suffering from severe chest pain with vomiting and sweating. Note the slightly upward curving S-T segment with deep T wave inversion in leads V2–V6

#### 17.3.1.2 Inferior Wall Myocardial Infarction

An inferior wall myocardial infarction is usually caused by occlusion of right coronary artery. The characteristic ECG changes are located in leads II, III and aVF (Figs. 17.13 and 17.14). S-T segment elevation and T wave inversion in leads II, III and aVF may produce reciprocal changes in the form of S-T segment depression and tall T waves in leads I, aVL and V1 to V6.

Patients with inferior wall infarction often develop sinus bradycardia, sinus arrest and heart block. Inferior wall infarction is often associated with a right ventricular, lateral wall or posterior wall infarction. Hence, in patients suffering from inferior wall infarction, thoroughly one must try to look for infarctions at these sites as well.

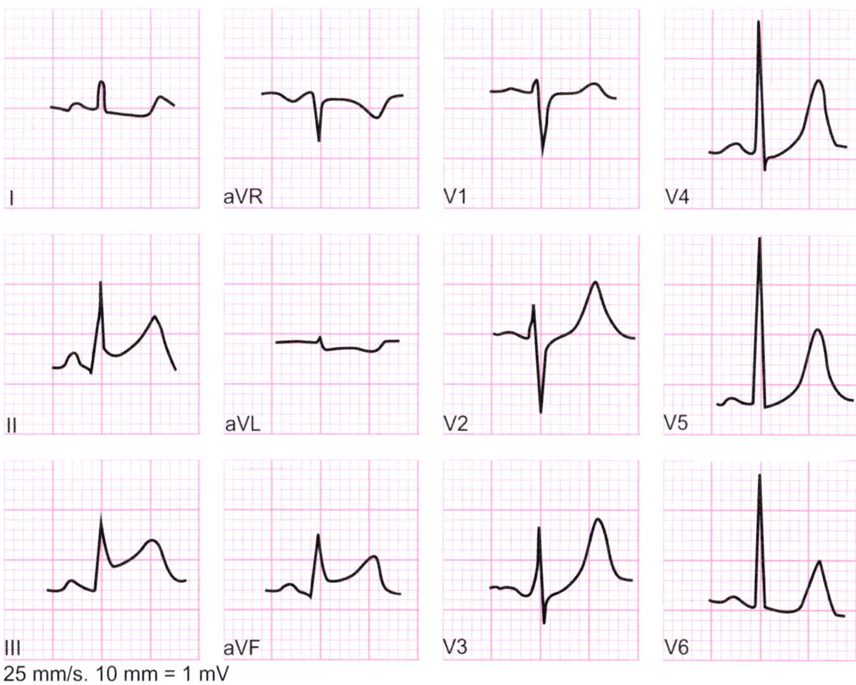


**Fig. 17.13** Hyperacute inferior wall myocardial infarction. This ECG is recorded from a 73-year-old gentleman suffering from severe chest pain with vomiting and sweating. He was also suffering from diabetes mellitus. Note the slope elevation of S-T segment in leads II, III and aVF. This is a very early stage of infarction

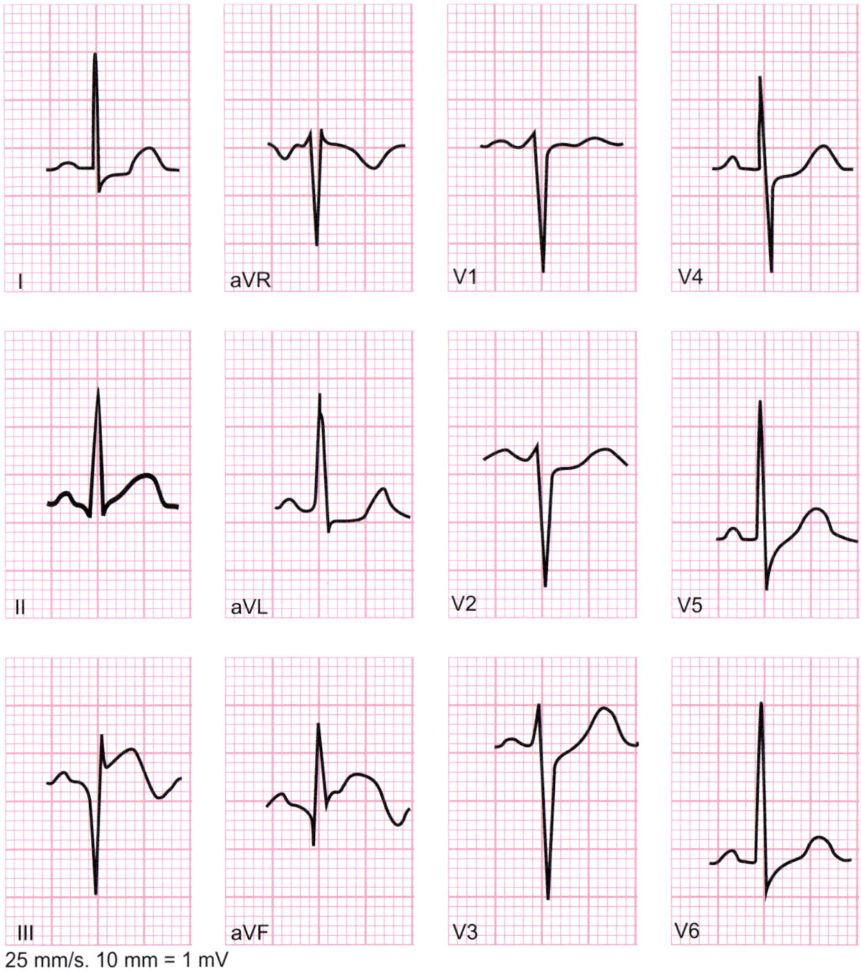


**Fig. 17.14** Acute inferior wall myocardial infarction. This ECG is recorded from a 74-year-old gentleman suffering from severe chest pain with vomiting, sweating and palpitation. He was also suffering from diabetes mellitus and hypertriglyceridaemia. Note the S-T segment elevation with convexity upwards in leads II, III and aVF

### 17.3.1.3 Posterior Wall Myocardial Infarction

Posterior wall myocardial infarction is usually associated with inferior wall infarction. It rarely occurs alone. Occlusion of right coronary artery or left circumflex artery leads to posterior wall myocardial infarction. None of the leads of the conventional 12 lead ECG is directly oriented towards the posterior wall of the heart. Hence, the leads opposite to the posterior wall, i.e. anterior wall will record the inverse or the mirror image changes. Thus the changes are recorded in leads V1–V3, especially lead V2 (Fig. 17.15). The changes in lead V2 are:

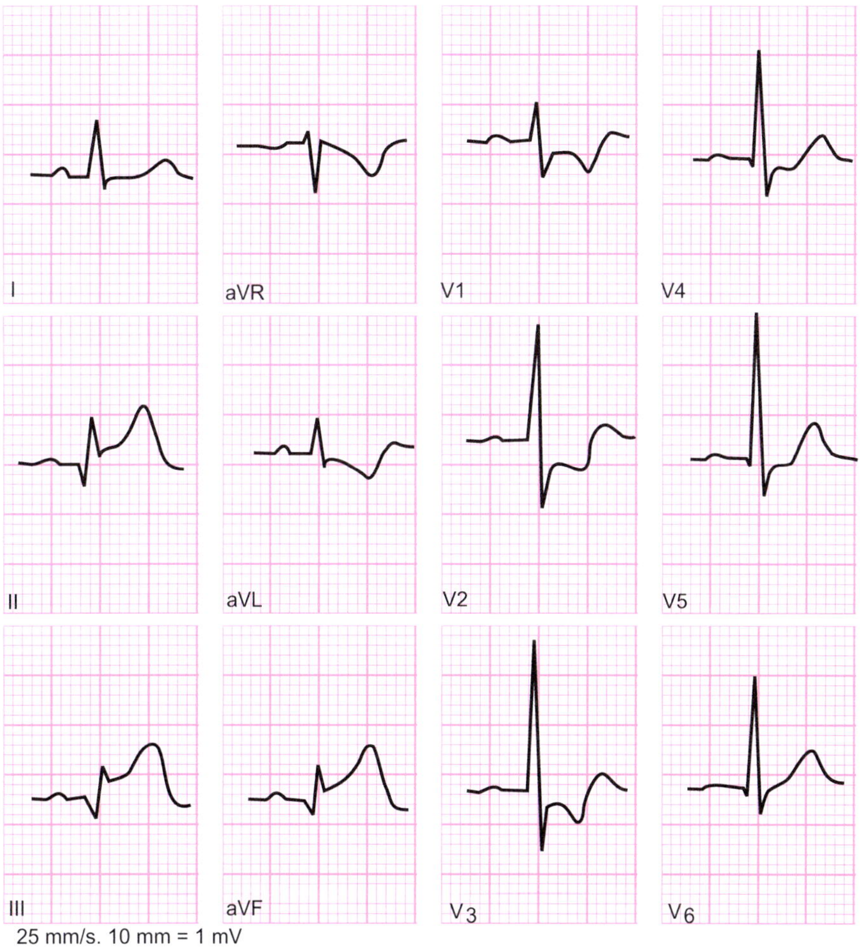


**Fig. 17.15** Posterior and inferior wall infarction. This ECG is recorded from a 72-year-old gentleman suffering from chest pain with vomiting and sweating. Note the tall R and T waves in leads V1 and V2 indicative of posterior wall infarction. There are Q waves with T wave inversion in leads II, III and aVF indicative of inferior wall infarction

1. Tall and slightly wide R wave, which is mirror image of QS complex.
2. Depressed and concave upward S-T segment (mirror image of convex upwards S-T segment elevation).
3. Upright, tall and wide T wave (mirror image of inverted T wave).

The height of the R wave in lead V1 and/or V2 more than the depth of the S wave in these leads is a strong indicator of posterior wall myocardial infarction. While there are S-T segment depression in the leads V1 and V2, a true posterior lead will record S-T segment elevation. Posterior wall infarctions are often associated with AV conduction defects and changes in sinus rate and rhythm.

### 17.3.2 Right Ventricular Infarction

Right ventricular myocardial infarction is caused by proximal occlusion of right coronary artery. Isolated right ventricular infarction is very rare. It is usually associated with inferior wall infarction. Right ventricular infarction should be suspected in presence of inferior wall infarction, if the following changes are recorded:

1. S-T segment elevation in lead V1 and lead V4R (Fig. 17.16).
2. S-T segment depression in lead V2 is 50% or less than the magnitude of S-T segment elevation in lead aVF.
3. S-T segment elevation in leads V1–V4 but the maximum elevation will be in lead V1 and the elevation decreases from lead V1 to lead V4. Q waves will be absent in these leads.
4. S-T segment elevation in lead V1 and S-T segment depression in lead V2.

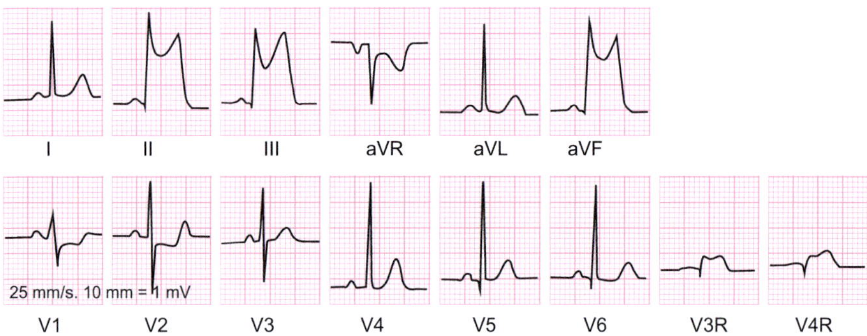


**Fig. 17.16** Inferior and right ventricular infarction. Note the tall R waves in leads II, III and aVF with slope elevation of S-T segment indicative of hyperacute inferior wall infarction. There is S-T segment elevation in leads V3R and V4R, which indicates right ventricular infarction

**Tips and Tricks**

- Sometimes patient presents with severe chest pain and sweating, but ECG turns out to be normal. In such patients, start preliminary treatment for ACS but repeat ECG after a few minutes.
- Serial ECG is often required to make a diagnosis of myocardial infarction if the initial ECG is normal.
- One can do an ECG with chest electrodes placed a bit up or down if the initial ECG is normal in presence of chest pain.
- In young patients, do not ignore chest pain. ACS is not uncommon in young people.
- In young patients, always look for chest wall tenderness. It is often simple costochondritis instead of ACS.

**Self-Assessment Questions**

1. Pathological Q wave is less than 25% of the height of the R wave. True or false?
2. Zone of myocardial injury is surrounded by the zone of myocardial necrosis in acute myocardial infarction. True or false?
3. Tall and wide T waves are seen in hyperacute phase of myocardial infarction. True or false?
4. Myocardial necrosis is represented in ECG by prolonged P-R interval. True or false?
5. Poor progression of R wave amplitude in anterior wall is a feature of anterior wall myocardial infarction. True or false?
6. **Convex S-T segment elevation is seen in all of the following condition EXCEPT:**

   a. Constrictive pericarditis b. Ventricular aneurysm c. Myocardial infarction d. Coronary artery spasm

7. **ACS includes all EXCEPT:**

   a. Unstable angina b. Non-S-T segment elevation myocardial infarction (NSTEMI) c. S-T segment elevation myocardial infarction (STEMI) d. Ventricular aneurysm.

8. **In inferior wall STEMI, all of the following are seen in inferior leads, EXCEPT:**

   a. S-T segment elevation b. Q waves c. Prominent U waves d. Inversion of T waves.

9. **A 60-year-old gentleman presented with history of chest pain with radiation to left arm, sweating and vomiting for last one hour. ECG revealed S-T segment elevation in leads V3–V6. There was deep symmetric inversion of T waves and 5 mm deep q waves in these leads. The patient has developed:**

   a. Inferior wall myocardial infarction b. Anterior wall myocardial infarction c. Posterior wall myocardial infarction d. Right ventricular myocardial infarction

10. **A 73-year-old patient is having an ECG to evaluate myocardial infarction. Which part of the ECG complex would you focus on to identify myocardial infarction?**

    a. P-R interval b. P wave c. QRS complex and S-T segment d. T wave

11. **The ECG changes of myocardial infarction due to complete occlusion of left anterior descending artery are seen in leads:**

    a. Leads II, III and aVF b. Leads aVL and lead I c. Leads V1–V4 d. Leads V1 and lead V4R

12. **S-T segment elevation with concavity upwards is seen in:**

    a. Ventricular aneurysm b. Pericarditis c. Inferior wall MI d. Anterior wall MI.

**Case Studies**

1. Examine the 12-lead ECG given in Fig. 17.17 and answer the following questions:

    a. Is there any S-T segment elevation in leads II, III and aVF?
    b. Is there any abnormal Q wave in leads II, III and aVF?
    c. Is there any reciprocal S-T segment change in any of the 12 leads?
    d. What is your diagnosis?
    e. Name two conditions in which S-T segment is elevated.

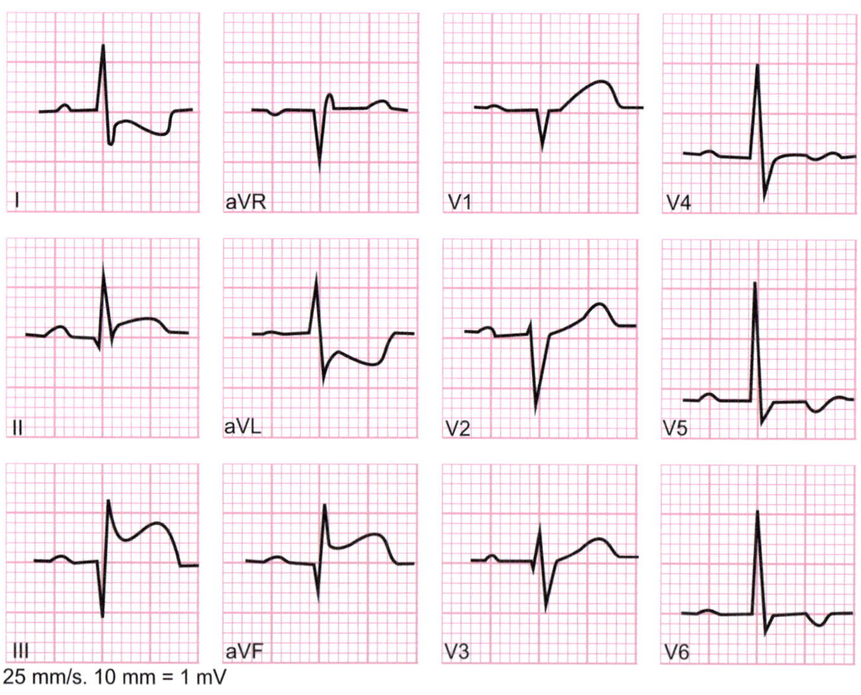


**Fig. 17.17** Identify the ECG abnormality and interpret it

2. Examine the 12-lead ECG given in Fig. 17.18 and answer the following questions:

    a. Name the leads showing S-T segment elevation.
    b. Is the R wave progression normal in chest leads?
    c. What is your diagnosis?

3. A 72-year-old gentleman, chronic smoker, suffering from diabetes for 23 years presented with severe chest pain, sweating and vomiting. He has past history of hypertension and dyslipidaemia. He was in severe chest pain. The pain was radiating to left shoulder. Patient was sweating and had two episodes of vomiting. Blood pressure was 110/76 mmHg and pulse rate was 126/min. Cardiac examination revealed elevated JVP and an S4 gallop. Lungs are clear. The ECG (Fig. 17.19) was done one hour after onset of chest pain. Examine the ECG and answer the following questions.

    a. What is your diagnosis?
    b. What is the main point in favour of your diagnosis?

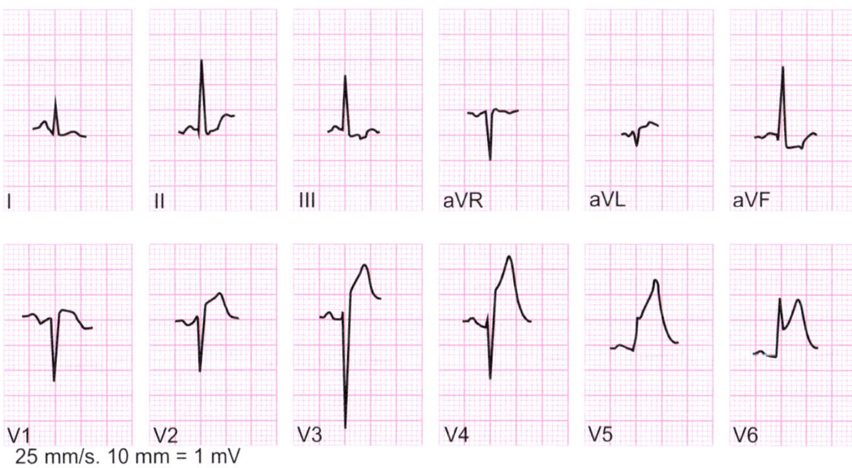


**Fig. 17.18** Identify the ECG abnormality and interpret it

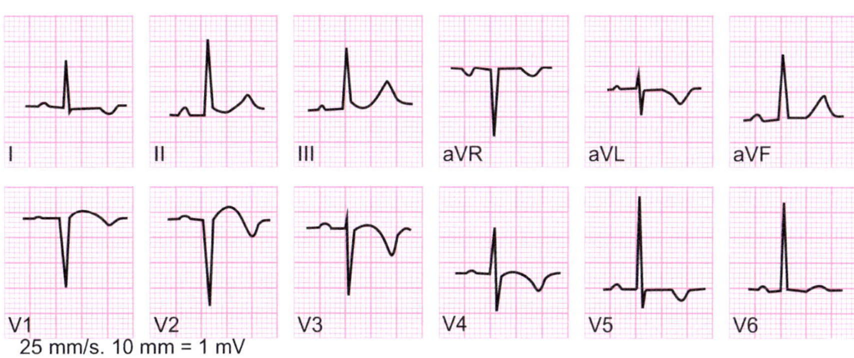


**Fig. 17.19** Identify the ECG abnormality and interpret it

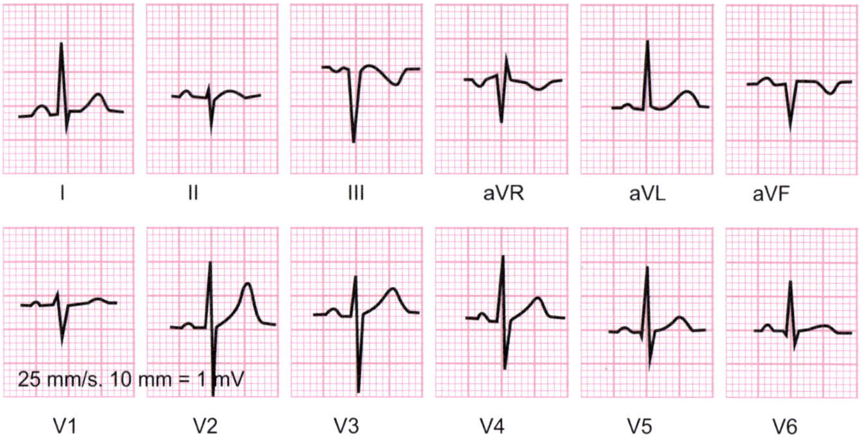


**Fig. 17.20** Identify the ECG abnormality and interpret it

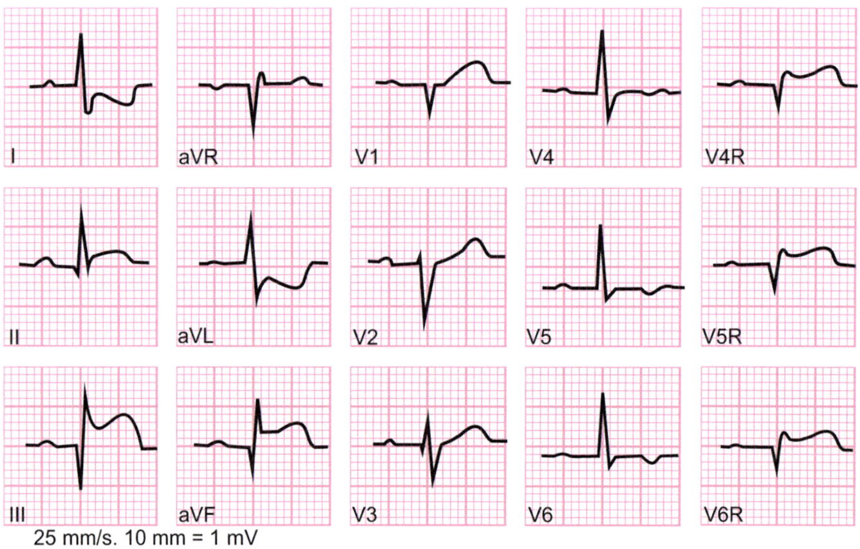


**Fig. 17.21** Identify the ECG abnormality and interpret it

c. Which important investigation will help you to confirm your diagnosis?
d. How will you differentiate this S-T segment elevation from that of acute pericarditis?

4. Examine the 12-lead ECG (Fig. 17.20) and make your diagnosis. What is the main point in favour of your diagnosis?
5. A 68-year-old gentleman came with history of retrosternal chest pain for last one hour radiating to lower jaw. He had two episodes of vomiting. On examination, his pulse rate was 106/min and blood pressure was 84/60 mmHg. Heart sounds were normal and chest was clear. Examine the ECG (Fig. 17.21) and make your

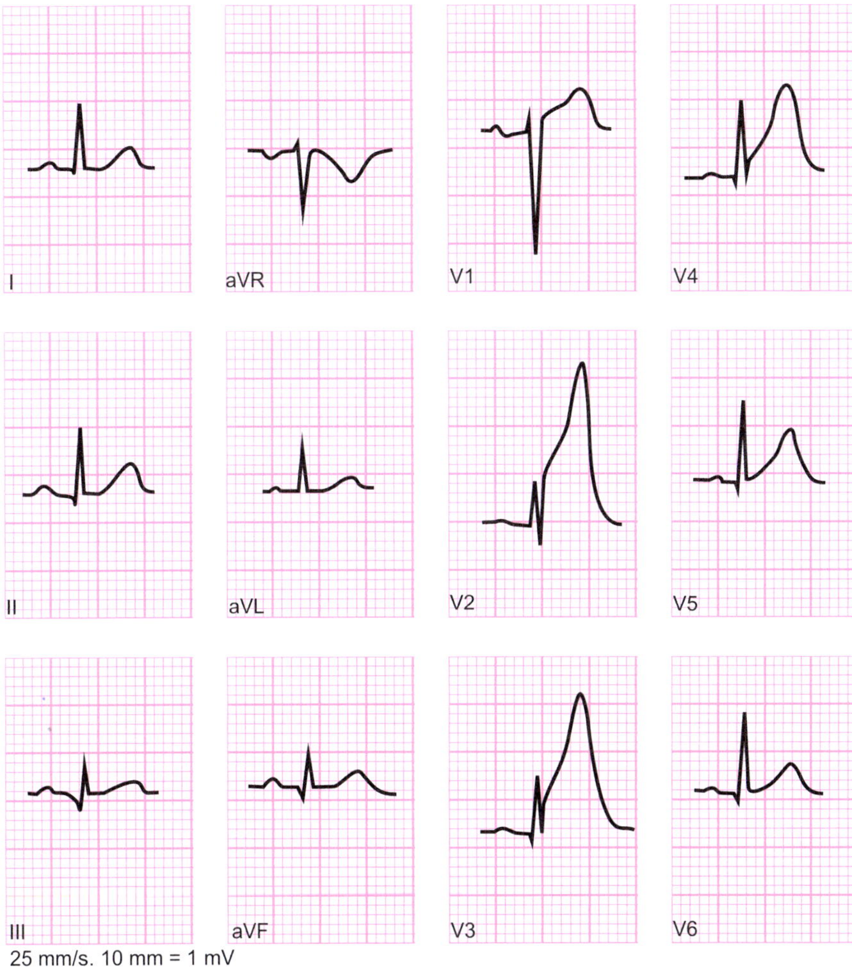


**Fig. 17.22** Identify the ECG abnormality and interpret it

diagnosis. What are the points in favour of your diagnosis? What are the abnormalities in lead I and lead aVL?

6. A 50-year-old patient came to the casualty with history of retrosternal chest pain for one and half hours with radiation of pain to left arm. He also had two episodes of vomiting. Describe the abnormalities seen in his ECG (Fig. 17.22).

**Answers**

1. False 2. False 3. True 4. False 5.True 6. a 7. d 8. c 9. b 10. c 11. c 12. b

**Case Studies**

1. a. S-T segments are elevated in leads II, III and aVF with maximum elevation in lead III.
   b. Pathological Q waves are present in leads III and aVF.

c. Reciprocal changes in the form of S-T segment depression are present in leads I and aVL. Besides this T wave inversion is also present in leads V5 and V6.
d. S-T segment elevation in inferior leads indicates inferior wall STEMI.
e. In acute pericarditis and ventricular aneurysm, S-T segment is elevated.

2. a. S-T segments are elevated in leads V1–V6.
   b. There is poor progression of R wave in chest leads.
   c. Diagnosis is anterior wall STEMI, hyperacute phase.
3. a. Diagnosis is anterior wall STEMI.
   b. The main point in favour of diagnosis is convex upwards S-T segment elevations in leads V1 and V2. Besides this, there are T wave inversions in leads I, aVL, V3, V4 and V5.
   c. Cardiac enzymes like Troponin I, Troponin T and CK MB will help to confirm the diagnosis.

   The history and clinical examination suggest acute coronary syndrome. ECG has revealed STEMI. This patient should ideally be sent to cardiac catheterization laboratory without even waiting for cardiac biomarkers test so that primary angioplasty can be done at the earliest.

   If facility for primary angioplasty is not available, he should be administered fibrinolytics. Additionally, he should receive nitrates, antiplatelets, heparin and statins. The prognosis is best if primary angioplasty can be performed in this condition.

   d. In acute pericarditis, S-T segment is elevated with concavity upwards, whereas in STEMI, S-T segment is elevated with convexity upwards.
4. The diagnosis is old inferior wall myocardial infarction. The main point in favour of diagnosis is presence of pathological Q waves in leads III and aVF.
5. The diagnosis is inferior wall and right ventricular STEMI. The main points in favour of diagnosis are S-T segment elevations in leads II, III, aVF, V4R, V5R and V6R. There are S-T segment depression in leads I and aVL. These are reciprocal changes.

   Management of this patient is different from other cases of myocardial infarction. In RVMI, there is decreased right heart function leading to decreased left ventricular preload, decreased cardiac output leading to systemic hypotension. Ideally, he should be given a fluid challenge of 500 mL of crystalloid fluid. Treatment with nitrates may be harmful as drop in preload will further worsen right ventricular dysfunction. Primary percutaneous coronary intervention (PCI) is the best option, but thrombolytic therapy is an option where facility for PCI is absent.

   It is important to remember that arrhythmias ranging from bradycardia to complete heart block may arise in patients with RVMI.
6. There are S-T segment elevations in leads V1 to V4. Besides this, there are tall and wide T waves in leads V2–V4. There is also a rising tendency of S-T segment in leads V5 and V6. The patient is suffering from anteroseptal STEMI (hyperacute phase). Most likely, if ECG is recorded half an hour later, it will reveal S-T segment elevations in leads V5 and V6 as well and the true extent of anterior wall damage will be seen.

   Urgent PCI is needed in this patient. Statin, nitrates, antiplatelet therapy and heparin should be stared as early as possible.

# Part V
# Cardiac Arrhythmias

# Chapter 18
# Sinus Rhythm

**Learning Objectives**
After studying this chapter, the reader will learn about:

- Normal sinus rhythm
- Sinus tachycardia
- Sinus bradycardia
- Sinus arrhythmia

The normal cardiac rhythm depends on the spontaneous generation of the impulse by the SA node and its proper conduction through the conducting system of the heart. Disturbance in any of the two (generation or conduction of impulse) will lead to the rhythm disturbances. The SA node acts as the pacemaker of the heart as it has the fastest inherent rate of impulse generation (on average 70–80 bpm). There are several other potential pacemakers of the heart also. These are present in atria, AV junctional area, bundle branches, Purkinje fibres, etc. If SA node fails to generate the impulse, the other structures will take up the pacemaker function. The rates of inherent discharge of these other pacemakers are slow. Thus, the usual rate of discharge of AV node is 60 bpm, of Bundle of His is 50 bpm and of ventricular myocardium is 30–45 bpm.

The pacemaker activity depends on various factors like autonomic nervous system, potassium concentration, calcium concentration, etc. Besides these physiologic factors there are several other factors like temperature, hypoxia, cardiac dilatation, local injury, hypercapnia, etc. which influence the pacemaker activity. The effect of all these factors on the automaticity of the heart is beyond the scope of this book and the readers are advised to read books on cardiac physiology to understand them.

The rate of conduction is influenced by the rate of depolarization (phase 0 of action potential) of the cardiac cells. A decrease in rate may decrease the rate of conduction and lead to a block. This is usually a unidirectional block that stops conduction in one direction while permits conduction in the opposite direction. It may thus favour reentry and lead to coupling of beats or reentry tachyarrhythmias.



T. K. Koley, *Rapid Review of ECG*,
https://doi.org/10.1007/978-981-99-9116-7_18

Concealed conduction means an impulse partly penetrates a part of the conduction system (usually AV node) but is not conducted and this effect is not seen at that time, but is seen in the disturbance produced in the next conducted beat. The effect is best seen in ventricular premature complex. The ectopic beat via retrograde penetration resets the SA node, resets its timing and leads to compensatory pause.

## 18.1 AV Node Electrophysiology

AV junction area is made up of the following parts:

(a) Area of junction of atria and AV node
(b) AV node proper
(c) Area of junction of AV node and His bundle

The cells of the AV node proper do not have automaticity and hence never act as the pacemaker of the heart, but this area has the property of slowing down the conduction that contributes a large part of P-R interval. The other two areas have the property of automaticity and may act as the pacemaker in pathologic conditions.

## 18.2 Normal Sinus Rhythm

Normal sinus rhythm reflects the normal electrical activity of the heart. The SA node is the pacemaker of the heart and the rate of discharge is governed by the sympathetic and parasympathetic system. The normal sinus rate of discharge is between 60 and 100 bpm. This is the normal heart rate. Whenever the impulse originates at a normal rate and rhythm from the SA node, it is called sinus rhythm. This is seen in ECG by the normal P wave followed by the normal QRST complexes. The P-R interval and QRS complex are normal (Figs. 18.1 and 18.2).

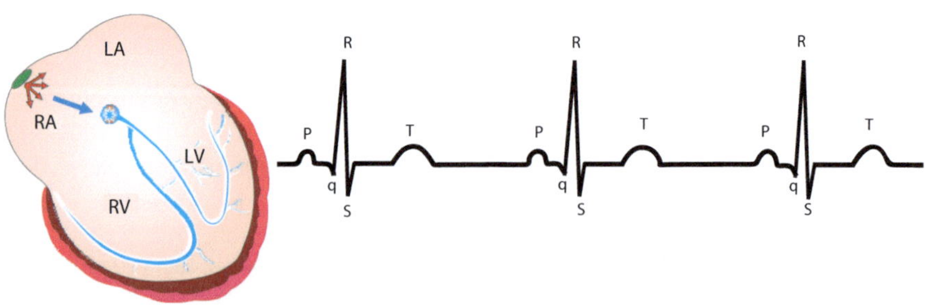


**Fig. 18.1** Illustration of genesis of normal sinus rhythm. The impulse originates at SA node at a rate between 60 and 100 bpm and travels via the normal conducting system to the ventricles

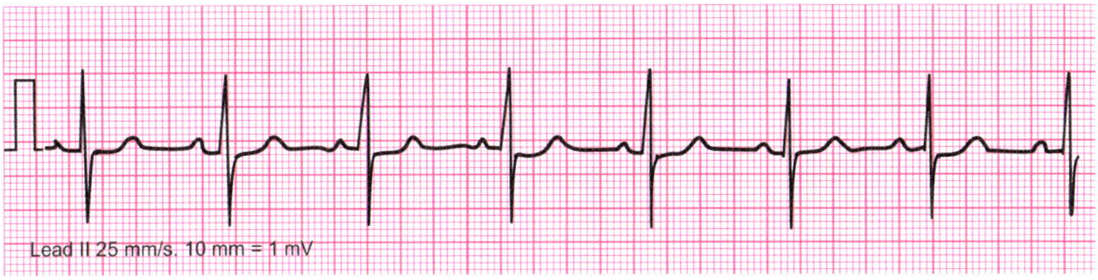


**Fig. 18.2** Normal sinus rhythm. The rhythm is regular and the heart rate is 72 bpm. The P-R interval and QRS duration are normal

**Tips and Tricks**

- Look for a smooth, rounded and upright P wave preceding every QRS complex in lead II to diagnose SA nodal origin of the impulse. If the rhythm is regular and occurs at a rate of 60–100 bpm, it is sinus rhythm.

## 18.3 Sinus Tachycardia

Sinus tachycardia is a normal response of the heart to the demand for excess blood flow (e.g. exercise, exertion, etc.). When the SA node generates impulse at a rate greater than 100 bpm, it is called sinus tachycardia. P, QRS and T waves are normal but are in rapid succession. In adults, usually, sinus tachycardia does not exceed 160 bpm. The P-R interval and QRS duration are normal (Fig. 18.3). It is a physiological response to exercise, anxiety, etc. It can occur due to fever, thyrotoxicosis, cardiac failure, myocarditis, shock, drugs (adrenaline, atropine), etc. If sinus tachycardia does not occur in conditions like fever, exercise, thyrotoxicosis, it may be due to underlying SA nodal disease like sick sinus syndrome. The various causes of sinus tachycardia are enumerated in Box 18.1.

**Box 18.1 Causes of Sinus Tachycardia**
Exercise, emotion, pain
Anxiety
Thyrotoxicosis
Fever
Excessive tea and coffee consumption
Atropine and adrenaline administration
Heart failure
Shock
Hypoxia
Pulmonary embolism
Myocardial infarction

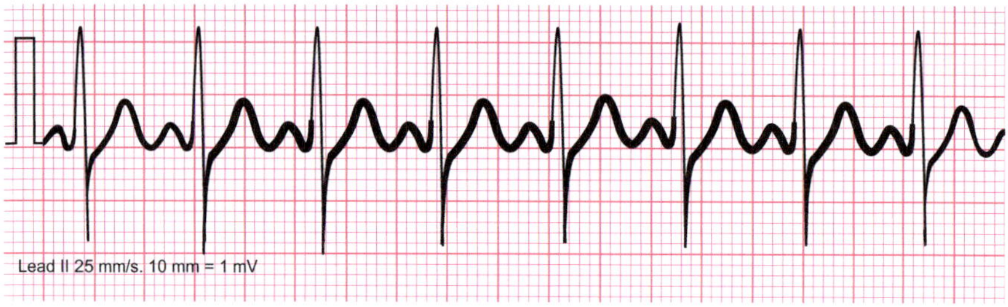


**Fig. 18.3** Sinus tachycardia. The heart rate is 125 bpm

## 18.4 Sinus Bradycardia

Sinus bradycardia is a normal body response to relaxation, sleep, etc. When the SA node generates impulse at a rate less than 60 bpm, it is called sinus bradycardia. P, QRS and T waves are normal but are in slow succession. The various causes of sinus bradycardia are summarized in Box 18.2. Sinus bradycardia is a manifestation of SA nodal dysfunction but the common causes like hypothyroidism, beta-blocker therapy, etc. should be ruled out in the beginning (Figs. 18.4 and 18.5).

**Box 18.2 Causes of Sinus Bradycardia**

Athletes
Deep sleep
Beta-blockers
Raised intracranial tension
Hypothermia
Obstructive jaundice
Diseases of SA node
Digitalis effect
Inferior wall myocardial infarction
Sick sinus syndrome

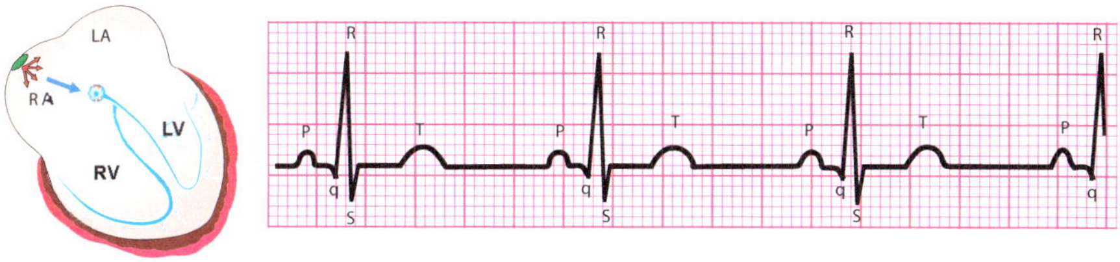


**Fig. 18.4** Illustration of genesis of sinus bradycardia. The impulse arises at the SA node and travels via the normal conducting system at a rate less than 60 bpm

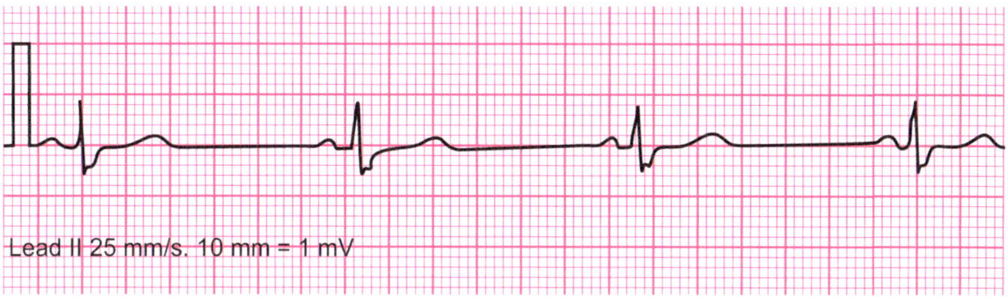


**Fig. 18.5** Sinus bradycardia

## 18.5 Sinus Arrhythmia

In sinus arrhythmia the impulse originates at the SA node but in an irregular manner. It is characterized by alternating periods of fast and slow discharge of SA node. This is usually associated with the phases of respiration and hence called respiratory sinus arrhythmia. The slow rate occurs at the end of expiration and the faster rate occurs at the end of inspiration (Fig. 18.6). The heart rate may be normal (60–100 bpm). It is a normal physiological phenomenon and is prominent in young children. During inspiration there is increased venous return to heart, vagal tone decreases and heart rate increases. During expiration venous return decreases, vagal tone increases and heart rate decreases.

The P waves and QRS complexes are normal. The P-R interval and QRS duration are also normal. The difference between the longest and the shortest R-R interval is greater than 0.12 s. It is commonly associated with sinus bradycardia. Sinus arrhythmia is seen during carotid sinus compression and digitalis therapy. There is also a condition called non-respiratory sinus arrhythmia where the arrhythmia is not associated with phases of respiration.

**Tips and Tricks**

- To diagnose sinus arrhythmia, look for grouping of complexes in an irregular rhythm, where the rest of the features are similar to that of sinus rhythm

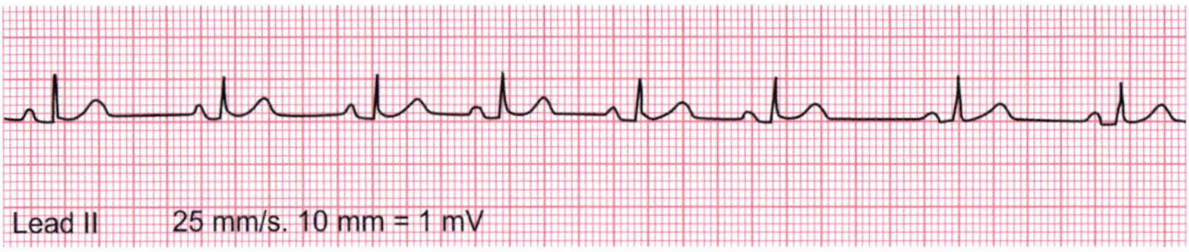


**Fig. 18.6** Sinus arrhythmia. There is grouping of complexes at the middle of the strip. The R-R intervals are smaller at the middle of the strip as compared to the R-R intervals of the complexes at the beginning and end of the strip. The difference between the longest and the shortest R-R interval is more than 0.12 s

## Self-Assessment Questions

1. Sinus tachycardia is characterized by a heart rate greater than 100 bpm. True or false?
2. In sinus bradycardia, the pacemaker lies in AV node. True or false?
3. Sinus tachycardia can occur as a physiological response to stress fever or exercise. True or false?
4. Sinus arrhythmia is characterized by an irregular heart rhythm that changes with respiration. True or false?
5. Sinus arrhythmia requires urgent treatment as it is considered an abnormal rhythm. True or false?
6. **Which of the following ECG findings is consistent with sinus rhythm?**

   a. Absence of P waves b. Irregular R-R intervals c. Wide QRS complex d. Consistent smooth and rounded P wave before each QRS complex

7. **Sinus bradycardia refers to:**

   a. Heart rate below 60 bpm b. Heart rate above 100 bpm c. Irregular heart rhythm d. Absence of P waves

8. **Characteristic ECG feature of sinus arrhythmia is:**

   a. Absence of P waves b. Irregular R-R intervals c. Long Q-T interval d. Inverted T waves

9. **In sinus tachycardia, the P wave morphology:**

   a. Remains unchanged b. Becomes inverted c. Widens d. Disappears

10. **Sinus bradycardia can be a normal ECG finding in**:

    a. Athletes b. Elderly individuals c. Individuals with hypertension d. Individuals with hyperthyroidism

## Case Studies

1. Analyze the rhythm strip given in Fig. 18.7.
2. Analyze the rhythm strip given in Fig. 18.8.
3. Analyze the rhythm strip given in Fig. 18.9
4. Analyze the rhythm strip given in Fig. 18.10.

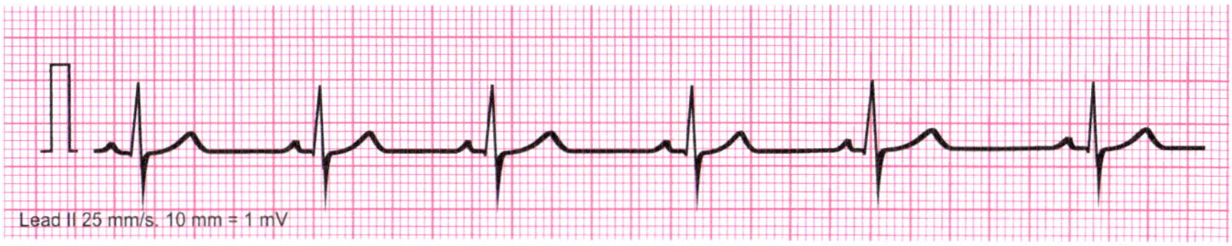


**Fig. 18.7** Analyze the rhythm strip

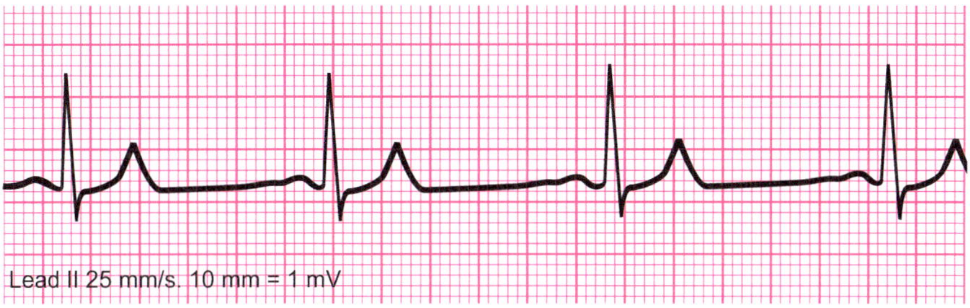


**Fig. 18.8** Analyze the rhythm strip

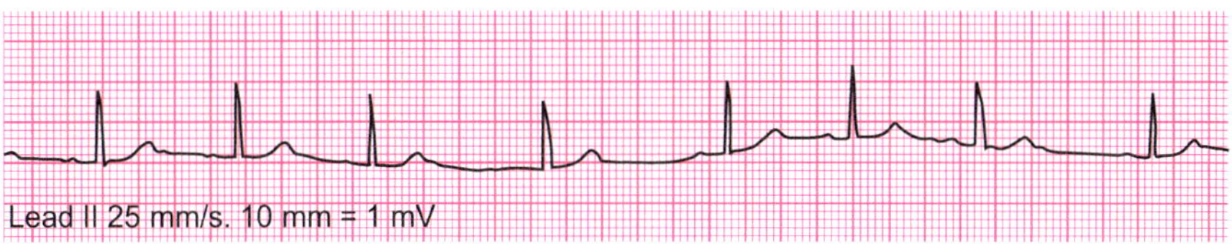


**Fig. 18.9** Analyze the rhythm strip

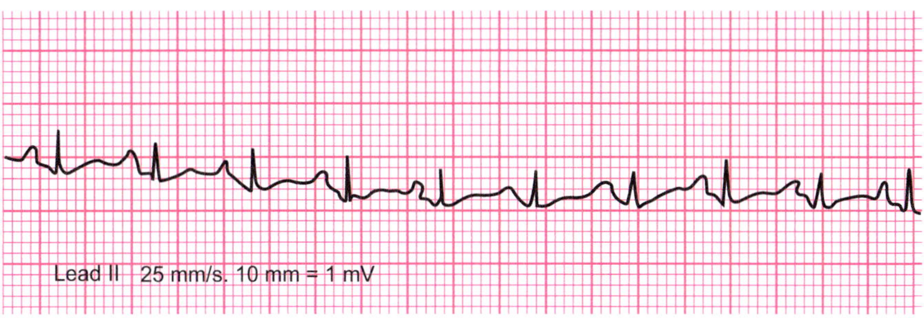


**Fig. 18.10** Analyze the rhythm strip

**Answers**

1. True 2. False 3. True 4. True 5. False 6. d 7. a 8. b 9. a 10. a

**Case Studies**

1. Complete analysis of ECG (Fig. 18.7):

   - Rhythm: Sinus rhythm, irregular.
   - P wave: Smooth, round, upright and every P wave is followed by QRS complex.
   - P-R interval: 0.16 s.
   - QRS duration: 0.08 s.
   - S-T segment: Isoelectric.
   - T wave: Normal.
   - Q-T interval: 9 × 0.04 s = 0.36 s.
   - Special feature: The difference between the shortest R-R interval and longest R-R interval is more than 0.12 s.

   Diagnosis: Sinus arrhythmia
2. Complete analysis of ECG (Fig. 18.8):

   - Rate: Heart rate is less than 60 bpm (53 bpm).
   - Rhythm: Sinus rhythm, regular.
   - P wave: Smooth, round, upright and every P wave is followed by QRS complex.
   - P-R interval: 0.16 s.
   - QRS duration: 0.08 s.
   - S-T segment: Isoelectric.
   - T wave: Normal.
   - Q-T interval: 10 × 0.04 s = 0.40 s.
   - Special feature: Nil.

   Diagnosis: Sinus bradycardia.
3. Complete analysis of ECG (Fig. 18.9):

   - Rhythm: Sinus rhythm, irregular.
   - P wave: Smooth, round, upright and every P wave is followed by QRS complex.
   - P-R interval: 0.16 s.
   - QRS duration: 0.08 s.
   - S-T segment: Isoelectric.
   - T wave: Normal.
   - Q-T interval: 8 × 0.04 s = 0.32 s.
   - Special feature: The difference between the shortest R-R interval and longest R-R interval is more than 0.12 s. There is increased heart rate during inspiration and slowing of heart rate during expiration. The heart rate is 70 bpm by six second method.

   Diagnosis: Sinus arrhythmia.

4. Complete analysis of ECG (Fig. 18.10):

   - Rate: Heart rate is 150 bpm.
   - Rhythm: Sinus rhythm, regular.
   - P wave: Smooth, round, upright and every P wave is followed by QRS complex.
   - P-R interval: 0.12 s.
   - QRS duration: 0.06 s.
   - S-T segment: Isoelectric.
   - T wave: Upright.
   - Q-T interval: 0.24 s.
   - Special feature: Nil.

   Diagnosis: Sinus tachycardia.

# Chapter 19
# Atrial Arrhythmias

**Learning Objectives**
After studying this chapter, the reader will learn about:

- Atrial extrasystoles
- Wandering atrial pacemaker
- Paroxysmal atrial tachycardia
- Atrial flutter
- Atrial fibrillation

Arrhythmias originate from either atria, atrioventricular (AV) junction or in ventricles. Any part of atria or ventricles can be activated and act as pacemaker. Rhythm originating from AV node is often called nodal rhythm or junctional rhythm.

Sinus rhythm, atrial rhythm and junctional rhythm are called supraventricular rhythm. In these three conditions, the electrical impulse follows the His bundle and normal pathway of conduction in the ventricles. Hence the QRS complex is normal in all these three types of rhythms. However, in ventricular rhythms the pacemaker is situated in the ventricles and the impulse does not follow the normal pathway of conduction resulting in broad QRS complex. Depolarization and repolarization are affected resulting in T wave abnormalities also. In this chapter, the atrial rhythm disturbances will be covered.

**Tips and Tricks**
- Supreventricular rhythms have narrow QRS complex (QRS interval < 0.12 s).
- In supraventricular rhythm, QRS complex can be broad if there is coexisting WPW syndrome, RBBB or LBBB.
- Ventricular rhythms have broad QRS complex (QRS interval > 0.12 s and often more than 0.14 s).



T. K. Koley, *Rapid Review of ECG*,
https://doi.org/10.1007/978-981-99-9116-7_19

## 19.1 Atrial Arrhythmias

Atrial arrhythmias originate from an ectopic focus in the atria. The main feature is the different morphology of the P wave from the sinus P wave as it originates from a different focus. The P wave may be pointed, notched or inverted. If the atrial rate is very fast, P wave may not be visible or it may be superimposed on preceding T wave or there may be saw tooth appearance or a wavy baseline.

There are mainly five types of atrial rhythm disturbances. They arise from ectopic focus either in atrium or in AV node.

- Atrial extrasystoles
- Wandering atrial pacemaker
- Paroxysmal atrial tachycardia
- Atrial flutter
- Atrial fibrillation

### *19.1.1 Atrial Extrasystoles*

Atrial extrasystoles, also called atrial premature complexes (PAC) are atrial premature beats. The premature atrial contraction is an early (premature in timing) beat that originates from an ectopic atrial focus that discharges before the next sinus beat and thus interrupts the rhythm. They arise from atrial muscle (not from SA node) and the wave front passes in the atria through abnormal pathway resulting in abnormal, bizarre P′ wave. The P′ wave may be hidden in the preceding T wave resulting in alteration of contour of the T wave. The QRS complex will be normal. The impulse may originate from anywhere in either atrium (Figs. 19.1 and 19.2).

Atrial premature beats are commonly observed in normal persons. They may occur due to emotional disturbance, excess tea, coffee or tobacco consumption, etc. Almost any type of heart disease can lead to ectopic atrial beats. Digitalis is a known cause of atrial extrasystoles. The various causes of atrial extrasystoles are enumerated in Box 19.1. Three or more than three consecutive atrial extrasystoles at

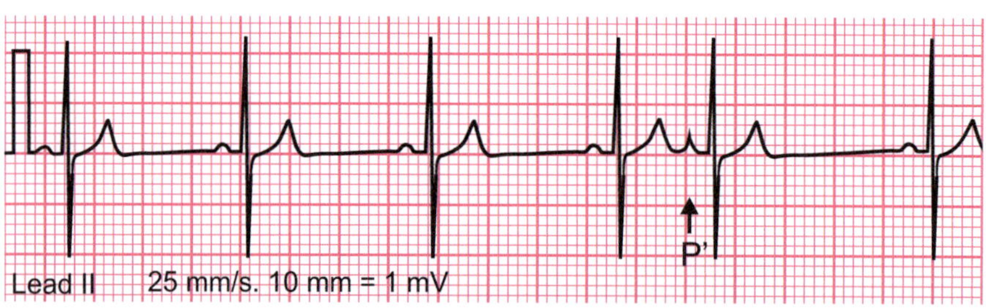


**Fig. 19.1** Atrial extrasystoles. The P′ wave is shown with arrow which has a different configuration from the sinus P waves. Also note the incomplete pause after the atrial extrasystoles. The QRS complex following the P′ wave is similar to rest of the QRS complexes

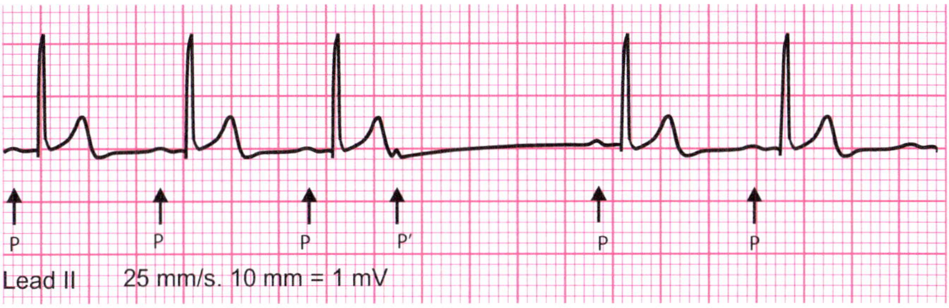


**Fig. 19.2** Nonconducted atrial extrasystole. Note the premature P′ wave and absent QRS complex after it

a rate of more than 100–250 bpm constitute atrial tachycardia. Frequent multifocal atrial extrasystoles may precipitate atrial fibrillation.

The characteristics of atrial extrasystoles are the following:

The P′ wave occurs earlier than the anticipated P wave. It may be upright, biphasic, inverted, flattened, notched, pointed or may be lost in preceding T wave.

The QRS complex following the P′ wave is usually normal and similar to the QRS complex of the sinus beat.

The compensatory pause following the atrial extrasystole is incomplete. This means that the total duration of the pre- and post-extrasystolic R-R interval is less than twice the normal R-R interval.

The P′-R interval may be normal, short or prolonged.

The fate of the ectopic atrial impulse may be of several types. These are:

The ectopic impulse may be normally conducted to the ventricles resulting in a normal QRS complex.

The impulse may arrive when one of the bundles has not recovered. Then the impulse will travel through only one of the bundles resulting in bundle branch block pattern. There may be left anterior of left posterior hemiblock pattern also.

Some of the ectopic impulse may be so premature that they arrive when the AV node or the ventricles are in their refractory phase. In this condition, the impulse will be blocked and QRS complex will be absent (Fig. 19.2). This is nonconducted premature atrial extrasystole.

There may be abnormal intraventricular conduction resulting in bizarre QRS complex. This is aberrant intraventricular conduction. If successive beats are conducted in aberrant manner rapidly, it may resemble ventricular tachycardia.

**Box 19.1 Causes of Atrial Extrasystoles**

Normal phenomenon
Excessive tea, coffee and tobacco consumption
Coronary, thyrotoxic, rheumatic, hypertensive heart disease
Drugs: Digitalis, adrenaline, thyroxin
Pulmonary embolism
Hypokalaemia
Hypomagnesaemia

**Tips and Tricks**

- To diagnose atrial extrasystole, just check the P wave regularity.
- If you find a P wave premature in timing with an abnormal morphology followed by a normal morphology QRS complex, think of atrial extrasystole.
- It does not require any specific treatment. Alcohol, tea, coffee, adrenergic stimulants should be avoided.

### *19.1.2 Wandering Atrial Pacemaker*

Wandering pacemaker, as the name suggests is characterized by origin of impulses from SA node as well as from various other foci located in various parts of atria and AV junction. This leads to various types of P′ waves with variation in rhythm and changing P′-R intervals. At least three different types of P wave morphologies must be identified before making a diagnosis (Figs. 19.3 and 19.4). This arrhythmia can occur in normal persons and in various types of heart diseases like acute rheumatic fever, myocarditis, digitalis toxicity, sick sinus syndrome, etc. The main ECG features are:

- P waves are of different morphologies.
- P-P and R-R intervals may vary.
- QRS duration is normal.
- Heart rate is normal or there may be bradycardia.
- P-R interval is usually normal but may vary.

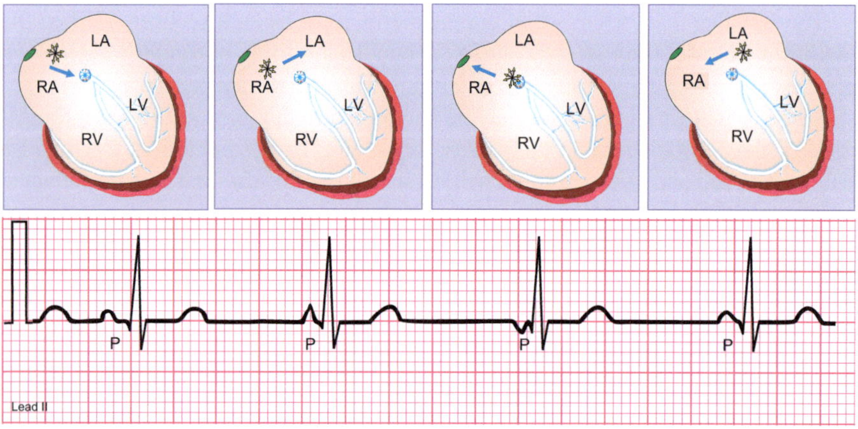


**Fig. 19.3** Illustration of genesis of wandering atrial pacemaker. Note the different foci of origin of the P waves in upper panel that results in different morphologies of P waves, as shown in lower panel

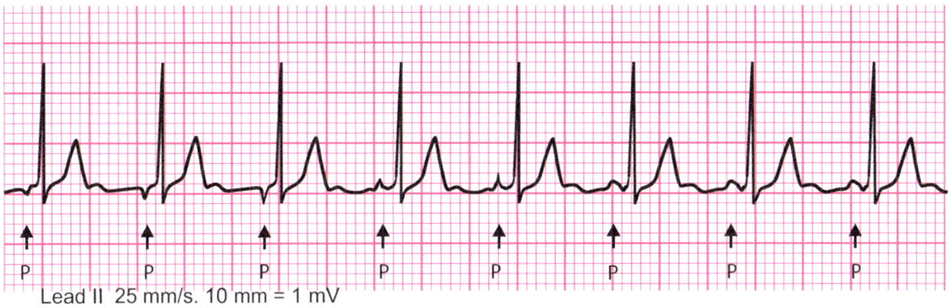


**Fig. 19.4** Wandering atrial pacemaker. Note the different morphologies of P waves

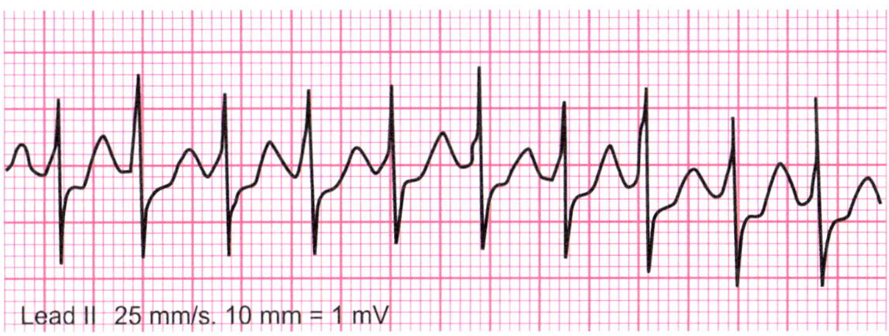


**Fig. 19.5** Paroxysmal atrial tachycardia

### *19.1.3 Paroxysmal Atrial Tachycardia*

Paroxysmal atrial tachycardia (PAT) is manifested electrocardiographically by three or more than three atrial extrasystoles at a regular rate of 160–230 bpm. It is also known as paroxysmal supraventricular tachycardia (PSVT). The tachycardia occurs in bursts, i.e. it starts abruptly and ends abruptly. Since it occurs intermittently, it is called paroxysmal. It is associated with a normal or nearly normal QRS complex. The QRS complex may be widened if there is intraventricular conduction defect. The P′ wave is difficult to identify as it is merged with the T wave of the preceding complex. If P′ waves are seen, they may be flattened, notched, pointed or biphasic. P-R interval is usually not measurable (Fig. 19.5).

PAT is often seen in persons in whom there is no evidence of heart disease. It is commonly associated with WPW syndrome. It occurs more commonly in patients with an accessory conduction pathway, coronary artery disease, mitral valve prolapse, digitalis toxicity, etc. PAT may last for a few seconds or may last for a few days. Patients usually complain of palpitation and they must be first reassured that they are not suffering from a catastrophic heart disease.

#### 19.1.3.1 Mechanism of PAT

There are two mechanisms to explain PAT:

- Ectopic: Impulse originates at a very rapid rate from an ectopic focus in the atria and each impulse is transmitted to the ventricle resulting in narrow QRS complex tachycardia.
- Re-entry: Re-entry means that an impulse after originating in atria travels into the ventricles and then re-enters the atria. The re-entry is facilitated by a closed circuit, which is formed by the AV nodal pathway and an accessory atrioventricular bypass tract or by two tracts that lie inside the AV node. The two pathways are interconnected and form a closed loop (Fig. 19.6). An ectopic atrial impulse first passes via one pathway during which the other pathway is in refractory state and then re-enters via the other pathway that has by then recovered

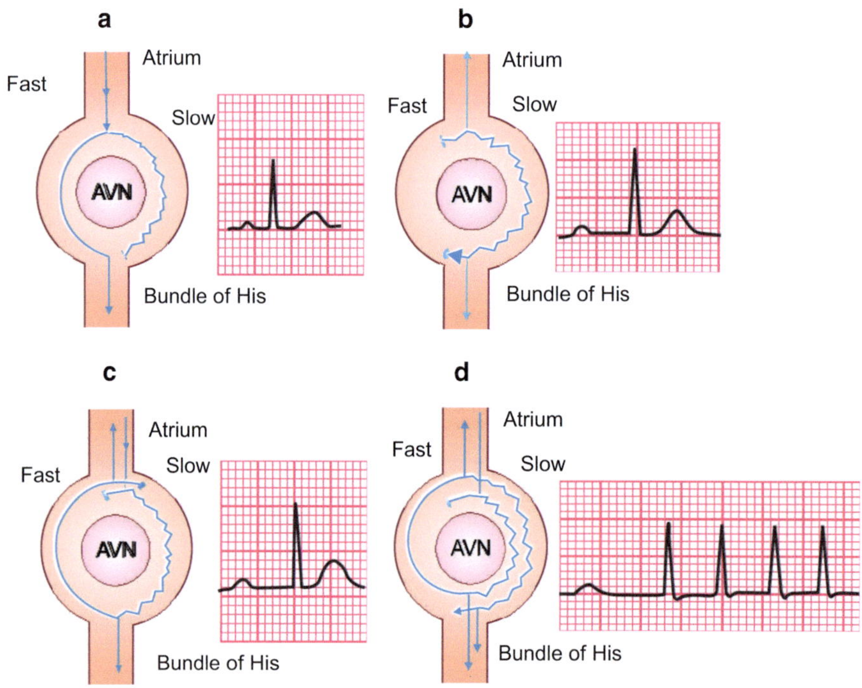


**Fig. 19.6** Mechanism of AV nodal re-entry and generation of PAT. (**a**) During sinus rhythm, the impulse is conducted over both the pathways but ECG reveals conduction over the fast pathway only and there is a normal P-R interval of 0.16 s. (**b**) A premature beat is blocked in the fast pathway and is slowly conducted over the slow pathway resulting in slightly longer P-R interval of 0.28 s. (**c**) A more premature impulse is blocked in the fast pathway and is conducted with increasing delay resulting in a P-R interval of 0.32 s. The re-entry is prevented by block in the slow pathway. (**d**) A still premature impulse initially conducts over the slow pathway and produces a P-R interval of 0.44 s and retrograde conduction occurs over the fast pathway and re-entry occurs resulting in sustained PAT

from refractory state. Thus, the cycle goes on and the ventricles are repetitively stimulated resulting in the narrow QRS tachycardia.

The heart rate is usually in the range of 120–160 bpm, if ectopic focus is the cause of PAT. If re-entry mechanism is involved, the heart rate may be around 160–220 bpm.

**Tips and Tricks**

- Narrow complex regular tachycardia and absent P waves indicate PAT.
- Vagal manoeuvres like carotid sinus massage, eye ball pressure or valsalva manoeuvre often terminate the arrhythmia.
- IV adenosine is the drug of choice for treatment. 6–12 mg IV is given to terminate the arrhythmia.

### *19.1.4 Atrial Flutter*

Atrial flutter originates from an ectopic atrial focus that discharges in a regular and rapid rate of 230–350 bpm. The P′ waves of atrial flutter produce a 'saw tooth' appearance of the base line (Figs. 19.7 and 19.8). The flutter wave (F wave) is best seen in leads II and V1. The flutter wave affects the baseline in such a way that there is no isoelectric line and T wave is partially or completely obscured by flutter waves. AV block of varying degrees (2:1, 3:1 or 4:1 block) exist and the ventricular rate is slower than the atrial rate. The QRS complexes are normal unless there is bundle branch block or aberrant ventricular conduction. If conduction ratio remains constant (e.g. 4:1), then ventricular rhythm will be regular, and if the conduction ratio varies (e.g. from 2:1 to 3:1 or 4:1), then ventricular rhythm will be irregular. When ventricular rate is less than 100 bpm, then atrial flutter is termed 'controlled', and when the ventricular rate is more than 100 bpm, then it is called 'uncontrolled'.

Atrial flutter may be seen in normal individuals, but usually, it is seen in patients suffering from coronary artery disease, rheumatic heart disease, thyrotoxicosis, pulmonary embolism, etc. Often flutter coexists with atrial fibrillation, which is called flutter-fibrillation.

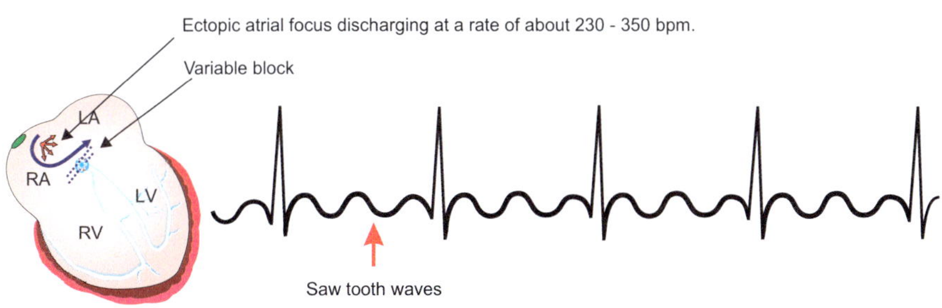


**Fig. 19.7** Illustration of genesis of atrial flutter. Note the saw tooth waves

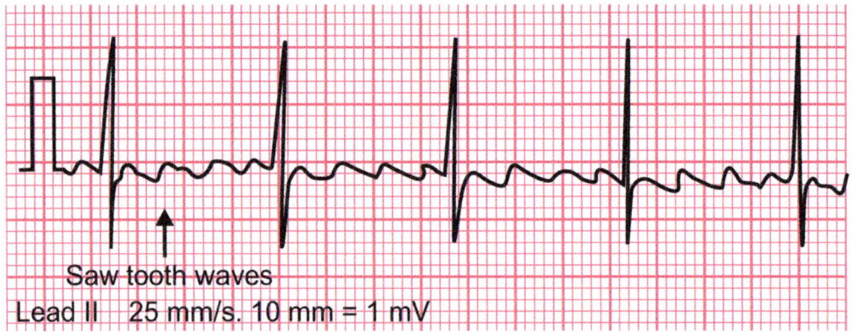


**Fig. 19.8** Atrial flutter with 4:1 conduction. Note the saw tooth waves (arrow)

There are two mechanisms responsible for atrial flutter. First there is a circus movement in a closed loop around the orifices of superior and inferior vena cava. This is the most likely mechanism. The second possible mechanism is the generation of very frequent impulses from an ectopic focus in the atria.

### *19.1.5 Atrial Fibrillation*

Atrial fibrillation (AF) occurs when multiple ectopic foci in atria (or via re-entry mechanism) discharges at a rate between 400 and 600 bpm. Atrial fibrillation is an absolutely irregular atrial rhythm. It is commonly observed in coronary artery disease, rheumatic heart disease, thyrotoxicosis, etc. It may also be seen in normal persons. Paroxysm of atrial fibrillation is seen in thyrotoxicosis and WPW syndrome. Sometimes it is not associated with any disease, which is called lone atrial fibrillation. The various causes of atrial fibrillation are enumerated in Box 19.2.

Patients usually suffer from palpitation and sometimes they may be asymptomatic also. However, continuous atrial fibrillation may lead to thrombus formation in the atrium, which may further lead to embolism. Besides this, long-standing atrial fibrillation may lead to hypertrophy of heart. So, always an attempt should be made to convert them into sinus rhythm. The prognosis lies in the underlying cardiac disease.

In atrial fibrillation, the depolarization and repolarization of the atria are disorganized and chaotic and hence at a given time part of atria is in excited state and part of it is in recovery state. These numerous impulses reach the AV node at irregular intervals at a very high frequency which overwhelms the AV node. AV node conducts some of these impulses and block most of them during its refractory state. These in turn excite the ventricles irregularly at a fairly rapid rate. This leads to irregular atrial and ventricular rhythm.

Atrial fibrillation is diagnosed by the following ECG features:

Irregularly irregular ventricular rhythm with normal QRS complexes. The ventricular rate is usually 120–160 bpm. This leads to varying R-R interval. Ventricular rate may be regular because of digitalis toxicity.

The P waves are replaced by fibrillatory waves (f waves) resulting in a wavy baseline. Atrial rate is 350–400 bpm. There is no identifiable P wave (Figs. 19.9 and 19.10).

**Box 19.2 Causes of Atrial Fibrillation**

Rheumatic fever
Mitral stenosis
Thyrotoxicosis
Drugs: Adrenaline, digitalis
Cor pulmonale
Excessive consumption of tea, coffee, alcohol
Constrictive pericarditis
Lone atrial fibrillation
Acute myocardial infarction
Sick sinus syndrome
Cardiac surgery
Pulmonary embolism
Paroxysmal atrial fibrillation in young people after consumption of alcohol—"Holiday Heart Syndrome"
Cardiomyopathy
Hypertensive heart disease

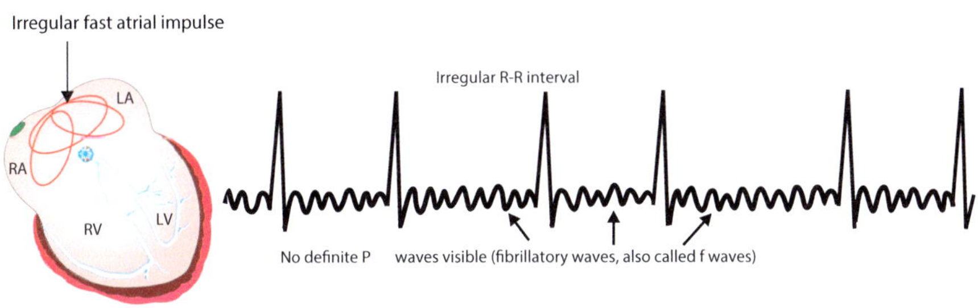


**Fig. 19.9** Illustration of genesis of atrial fibrillation

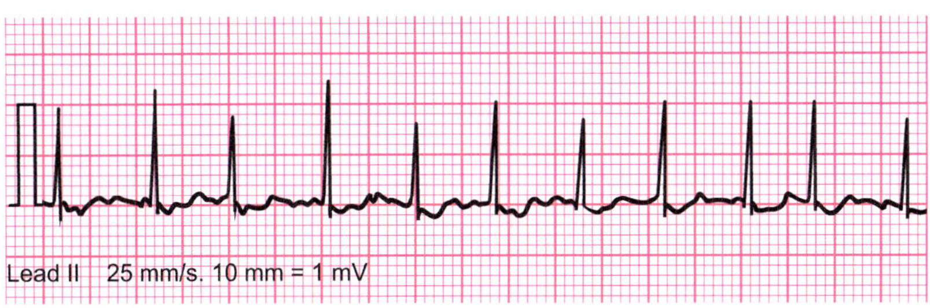


**Fig. 19.10** Atrial fibrillation. Note the irregularly irregular R-R interval. The P waves are replaced by fibrillatory waves (wavy baseline)

**Tips and Tricks**

- Narrow complex tachycardia, irregularly irregular rhythm and absent P wave indicate atrial fibrillation.
- In such a case if rhythm is regular, think of PAT.
- Vagal manoeuvres do not have any effect.
- In presence of severe cardiovascular compromise, electrical cardioversion (100Ws) is the main treatment.
- Treatment of underlying causes like thyrotoxicosis, pericarditis and CHF is equally important.

**Self-Assessment Questions**

1. Atrial extrasystoles, also known as premature atrial contractions (PACs), appear as abnormal P′ waves on the ECG. True or false?
2. Atrial fibrillation is characterized by the absence of P waves on the ECG. True or false?
3. Atrial extrasystoles are usually not followed by a compensatory pause on the ECG. True or false?
4. Atrial flutter is characterized by 'sawtooth' patterns on the ECG. True or false?
5. Mitral stenosis is an important cause of atrial fibrillation. True or false?
6. **Characteristic ECG feature of PAT is:**

   a. Presence of fibrillatory waves b. Prolonged Q-T interval c. Absence of QRS complexes d. Sudden onset and termination of tachycardia

7. **In atrial extrasystole, the abnormal P wave on the ECG appears:**

   a. Before the QRS complex b. Between the QRS complex and T wave c. After the QRS complex d. None of the above

8. **In AF, the ventricular rhythm on the ECG is typically:**

   a. Regular b. Irregularly irregular c. Both of the above d. None of the above

9. **ECG of wandering atrial pacemaker shows:**

   a. Wide QRS complex b. Irregularly irregular rhythm c. Presence of P waves with different morphologies d. Absence of P waves

10. **The treatment approach for PAT is:**

    a. Electrical cardioversion b. Medications to slow the heart rate c. Vagal manoeuvres d. All of the above

**Case Studies**

1. A 45-year-old gentleman came for medical check-up. He had no history of CAD, DM, HT. He was asymptomatic. His rhythm strip is given in Fig. 19.11. Analyse his rhythm strip. What is the treatment?

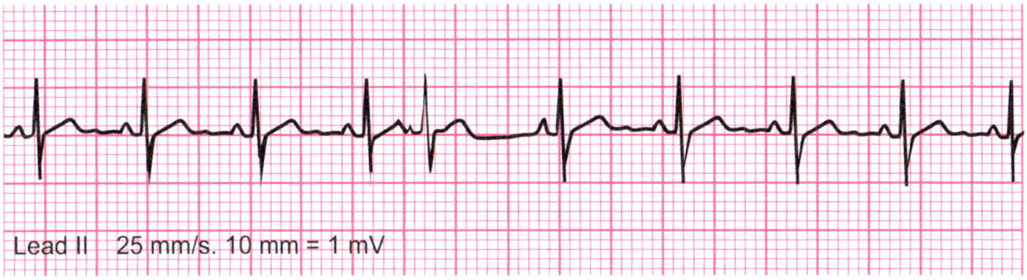


**Fig. 19.11** Analyse the rhythm strip

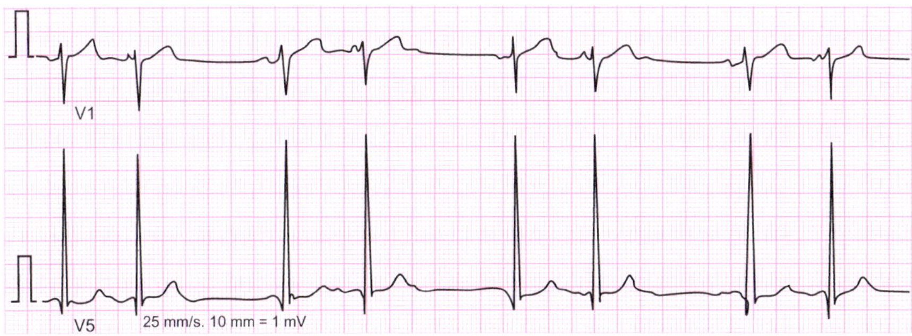


**Fig. 19.12** Analyse the rhythm strip

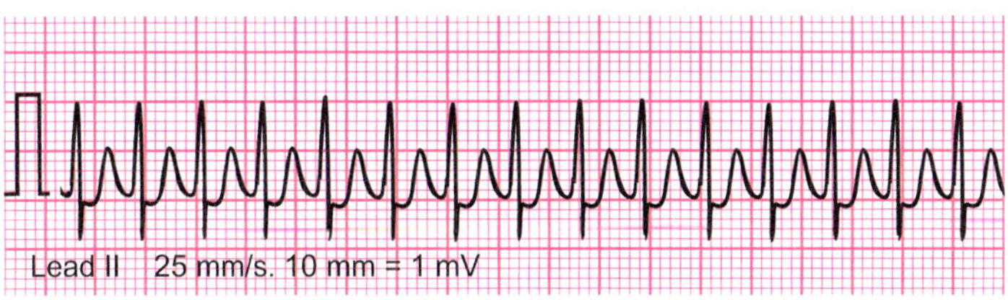


**Fig. 19.13** Analyse the rhythm strip

2. A 40-year-old lady suffering from hypothyroidism was taking 100 mcg of thyroxine daily. She had not checked her thyroid status for last one year. She complained of palpitation off and on for last 15 days. On examination she had fine tremor. Analyse her rhythm strip given in Fig. 19.12. What is your diagnosis? Which blood test will you advise?
3. A 35-year-old gentleman arrived in the casualty with history of sudden onset palpitation for last 10 min. Similar episode of palpitation occurred 3 months back which lasted for about 2 min. He ignored it and did not consult any physician. His blood pressure was 110/70 mmHg, pulse rate was approximately 170 bpm, regular with no special character. Analyse his rhythm strip given in Fig. 19.13. What is your diagnosis? How will you treat him?

4. A 50-year-old gentleman arrived in the casualty with history of severe palpitation. He did not suffer from palpitation in the past. He was mildly breathless. There was no chest pain. He has no history of CAD, DM and HT. His BP was 90/60 mmHg. Analyse his rhythm strip given in Fig. 19.14. What is the diagnosis? What is the best treatment?
5. This ECG was given for spot diagnosis in examination for final year medical students. Analyse the rhythm strip given in Fig. 19.15 and make your diagnosis. Name five conditions which can cause this.

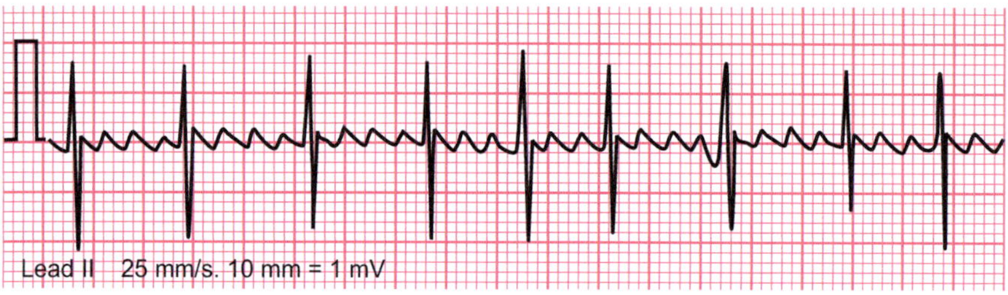


**Fig. 19.14** Analyse the rhythm strip

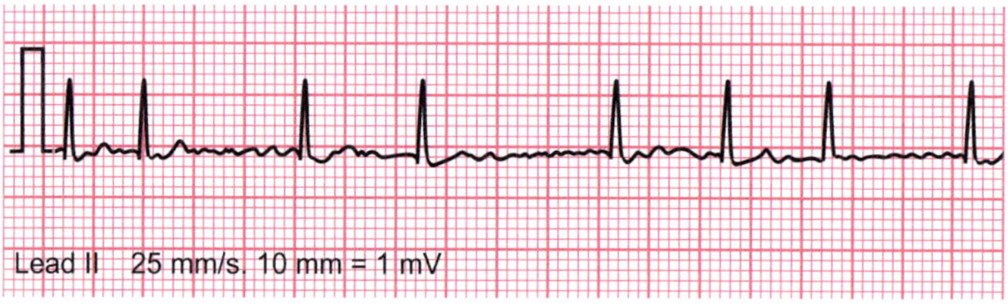


**Fig. 19.15** Analyse the rhythm strip

**Answers**

1. True 2. True 3. False 4. True 5. True 6. d 7. a 8. b 9. c 10. d

**Case Studies**

1. The rhythm strip in Fig. 19.11 shows an atrial extrasystole. The fifth P wave is different from other P waves. It is a P′ wave. It is followed by a narrow QRS complex which is premature in timing and it is followed by a pause. The pause is incomplete. Rest of the rhythm strip does not show any gross abnormality.

   He should be advised to reduce intake of tea and coffee. He should be further advised to avoid stress and anxiety. A mild sedative may be prescribed for about a week.
2. The rhythm strip in Fig. 19.12 shows atrial bigeminy. Every normal PQRST complex is followed by a premature PQRST complex. The P waves of these complexes are different from the normal P waves. The second, fourth, sixth and eighth complexes are premature atrial complexes or atrial extrasystoles. Also note the incomplete pause after the atrial extrasystoles. This alternating sinus beat and atrial extrasystole is known as atrial bigeminy.

   The patient should be advised to get a free T3, free T4 and TSH tests done at the earliest. Atrial bigeminy is most likely to be a side effect of thyroxine. Most likely she will respond to reduction in the dose of thyroxine.
3. The rhythm strip in Fig. 19.13 shows paroxysmal atrial tachycardia. Note the regular and rapid ventricular rate with absence of P wave and S-T segment depression. The ventricular rate is 250 bpm. This is a narrow complex tachycardia as the QRS duration is about 0.06 s. The rhythm is regular. Hence, a regular narrow complex tachycardia with absent P waves is diagnostic of paroxysmal atrial tachycardia.

   The patient is haemodynamically stable. He should be advised to perform vagal manoeuvre like valsalva manoeuvre. If it does not revert back to sinus rhythm, you can use IV adenosine which is the drug of choice for treatment. 6–12 mg IV is given to terminate the arrhythmia.

   Synchronized cardioversion with 50–100 joules is the main treatment for haemodynamically unstable patients of PAT.
4. The ECG in Fig. 19.14 shows atrial flutter with variable conduction. Carefully note the saw tooth waves which have replaced the baseline. There is no isoelectric line. The QRS complexes are narrow and irregular.

   The patient is not stable. He is suffering from hypotension. 25–50 joules DC cardioversion should be carried out under mild sedation. 100 joules may also be used as the initial shock strength as it is always successful and virtually never harmful.
5. The ECG in Fig. 19.15 shows atrial fibrillation. The P waves are not visible. The rhythm is irregularly irregular. The QRS complexes are narrow. The baseline is replaced by fibrillatory waves.

   Five conditions that can cause atrial fibrillation are: rheumatic fever, thyrotoxicosis, mitral stenosis, COPD and pulmonary embolism.

   Antiarrhythmic drugs, anticoagulants and catheter ablation are the main treatment options in atrial fibrillation. Rate control, rhythm control and prevention of stroke due to embolism are the main treatment goals.

# Chapter 20
# Junctional and Ventricular Arrhythmias

**Learning Objectives**
After studying this chapter, the reader will learn about:

- AV junctional rhythm
- Premature junctional complex
- Junctional rhythm
- Ventricular extrasystoles
- Ventricular tachycardia
- Ventricular flutter
- Ventricular fibrillation
- Idioventricular rhythm
- Accelerated idioventricular rhythm
- Ventricular asystole

## 20.1 AV Junctional/Nodal Rhythm

An impulse may originate from the AV junction instead of the SA node. It is called AV junctional/nodal rhythm. It must be kept in mind that the rhythm does not originate from the AV node proper because it has no property of generation of impulse. The impulse may be conducted to the atria and the ventricles or the impulse may be conducted to the ventricles only and the retrograde conduction to the atria may be blocked.

When the impulse is conducted to both the atria and the ventricles, the ventricular activation proceeds along the normal pathway resulting in normal QRS complex. The conduction to the atria occurs in a retrograde manner, i.e. the direction of depolarization is reversed resulting in inverted P waves in leads II, III and aVF and


T. K. Koley, *Rapid Review of ECG*,
https://doi.org/10.1007/978-981-99-9116-7_20

upright in lead aVR. This P wave may precede or follow or may be hidden in the QRS complex. This depends upon the relative velocity of the anterograde and retrograde conduction. This nodal rhythm may be in the form of AV nodal extrasystole, AV nodal escape beat, paroxysmal AV nodal tachycardia or idionodal tachycardia. In all these arrhythmias, the features are similar to that described in atrial arrhythmias except that the P waves will be inverted and may appear before, after or hidden in QRS complex.

### 20.1.1 Premature Junctional Complex

The ECG features of premature junctional complex (PJC) are similar to that of premature atrial complex except that the P′ wave will be inverted. It may appear before, after or hidden in the QRS complex (Fig. 20.1).

### 20.1.2 Junctional Rhythm

Junctional rhythm arises from AV junction at a rate between 40 and 60 bpm. This rhythm occurs when the discharge rate of SA node falls and the AV junction takes over as the dominant pacemaker (Figs. 20.2 and 20.3). The ECG features are:

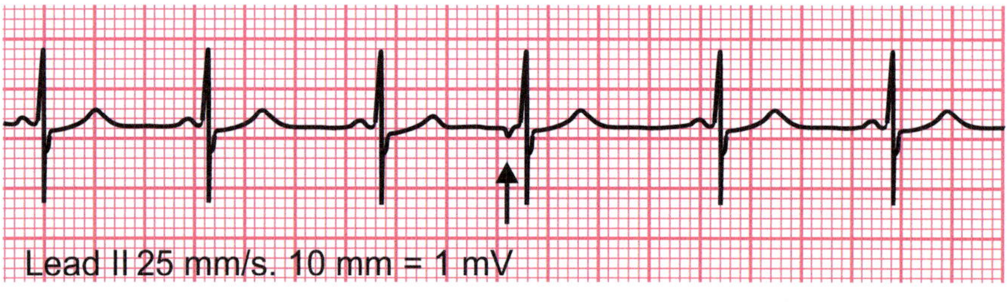


**Fig. 20.1** Premature junctional complex. Note the inverted P′ wave of fourth complex which is followed by a pause

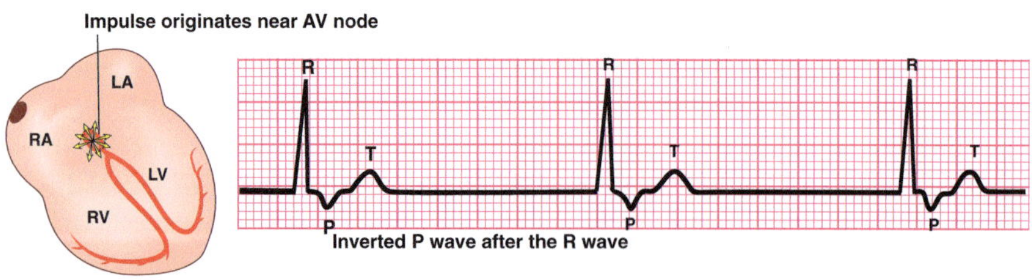


**Fig. 20.2** Illustration of genesis of junctional rhythm. The impulse originates near AV node and results in inverted P wave that appears after the R wave. The rate is between 40 and 60 bpm

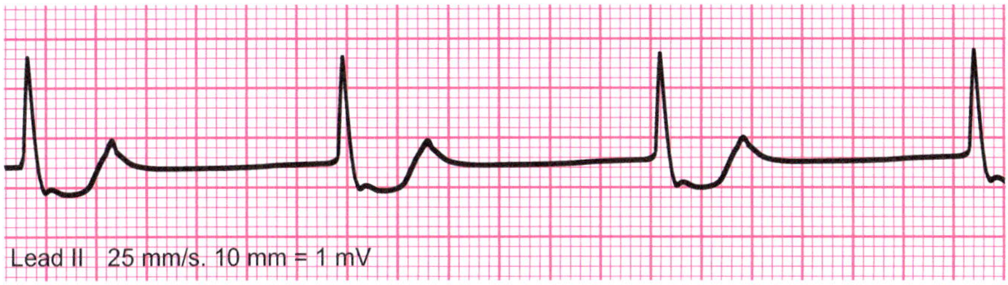


**Fig. 20.3** Junctional rhythm. Note that the P′ waves are not seen as they are hidden in the QRS complexes. The QRS complexes are of normal duration. The rate is 48 bpm

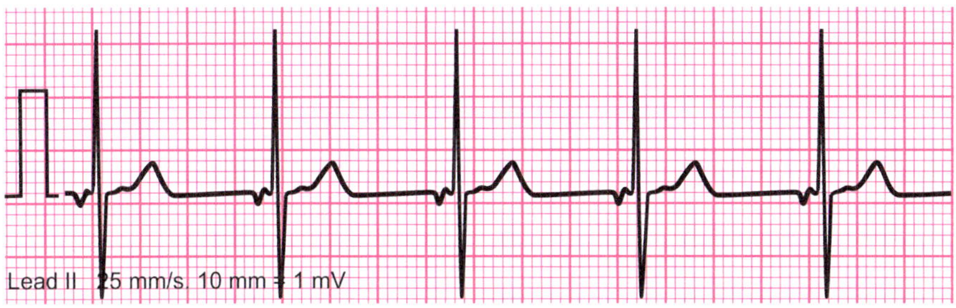


**Fig. 20.4** Accelerated junctional rhythm. Note the inverted P′ waves before QRS complexes and the heart rate is 79 bpm

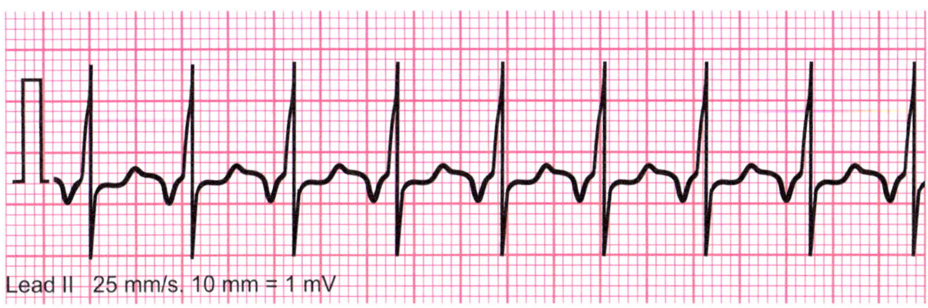


**Fig. 20.5** Junctional tachycardia. The heart rate is 136 bpm

- The P′ waves are inverted and either appear before, after or are hidden in QRS complexes.
- The QRS duration is normal.
- The P′-R interval will be less when P′ waves appear before the QRS complex.

A junctional rhythm is called accelerated junctional rhythm when the rate is between 60 and 100 bpm (Fig. 20.4). Rest of the ECG features are same. In junctional tachycardia, the rate is more than 100 bpm and rest of the ECG features are like junctional rhythm (Fig. 20.5).

**Tips and Tricks**

- You should suspect junctional origin of the rhythm if P wave is inverted or absent and the QRS complexes are of normal duration.

## 20.2 Ventricular Arrhythmia

Ventricular arrhythmias originate from the ventricles. The electrical impulse does not follow normal pathway and depolarizes one ventricle before the other. The ventricular arrhythmias are thought to be due to altered automaticity, triggered activity or re-entry. The common types of ventricular rhythm disturbances are the following:

- Ventricular extrasystoles
- Ventricular tachycardia
- Ventricular flutter
- Ventricular fibrillation
- Idioventricular rhythm
- Accelerated idioventricular rhythm
- Ventricular asystole

**Tips and Tricks**

- Ventricular origin of the rhythm should be suspected whenever there is broad QRS complex with T wave abnormality.

### *20.2.1 Ventricular Extrasystoles*

Ventricular extrasystoles also called ventricular premature complex (VPC) originate from the premature discharge of an ectopic focus either in right or left ventricle. It is the commonest ventricular arrhythmia. It is usually seen in almost all types of heart disease. Sometimes it may be seen in normal persons but in them one should carefully search for an underlying cardiac disease. The ventricular extrasystole may be unifocal (arising from single focus) or multifocal (arising from multiple foci). Ventricular extrasystoles occurring in pairs or at a frequent rate may lead to ventricular tachycardia or more serious ventricular fibrillation. If it occurs after myocardial infarction, it carries poor prognosis. Digitalis is a frequent cause of ventricular extrasystoles. The causes of ventricular extrasystoles are summarized in Box 20.1.

**Box 20.1 Causes of Ventricular Extrasystoles**
Coronary artery disease
Digitalis toxicity
Electrolyte imbalance
Acid base disturbance
Congestive heart failure
Hypoxia
Acute myocardial infarction
During or after reperfusion therapy or angioplasty
Cardiac surgery
Cardiomyopathy

The extrasystole arises from an irritable focus in the myocardium of the ventricle (Fig. 20.6). This impulse then activates the ventricles and this impulse does not depolarize the SA node and hence, the sinus rhythm is maintained. However, the next sinus beat after the extrasystole will not be able to activate the ventricles because they are in a refractory state. The ventricle will respond to the next sinus impulse. This will lead to a pause, which is known as compensatory pause. However, if the sinus rate is slow, then a ventricular extrasystole can occur between two normal sinus beats without any change in the R-R interval. This is known as 'interpolated beat'. Sometimes the ventricular extrasystole may be so premature that it coincides with the apex or distal limb of T wave of the preceding QRST complex. This is called 'R on T phenomenon' and indicates the highly excitable state of the ventricles and may lead to ventricular tachycardia or fibrillation.

Ventricular extrasystole is diagnosed by the following features:

The beat arises prematurely, i.e. it occurs earlier than the anticipated QRS complex.

The P wave is absent in the extrasystoles.

The QRS complex is wide, bizarre with the S-T segment and T wave in opposite direction to the dominant QRS deflection. The duration of QRS complex is more than 0.12 s.

The compensatory pause is complete, i.e. the R-R interval between the two sinus beats preceding and following the ventricular extrasystoles is double the R-R interval between two normal sinus beats (Figs. 20.7 and 20.8).

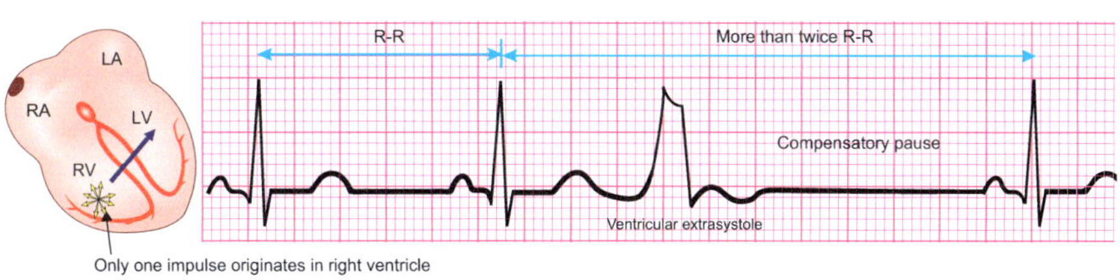


**Fig. 20.6** Illustration of genesis of ventricular extrasystole. Note that the impulse originates in the right ventricle and does not travel via the normal conducting system, thus producing the broad and bizarre QRS complex followed by compensatory pause

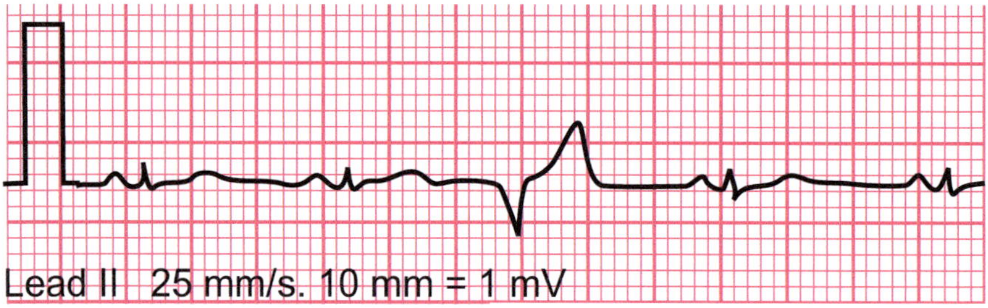


**Fig. 20.7** Ventricular extrasystole. Note the wide and bizarre QRS complex

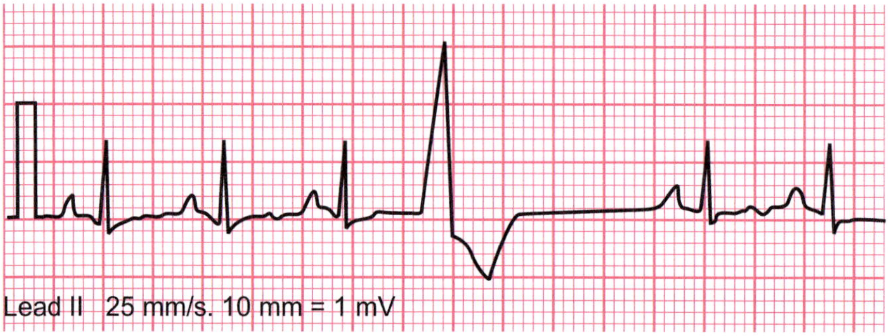


**Fig. 20.8** Ventricular extrasystole. Note the wide and bizarre QRS complex. Note also the complete compensatory pause

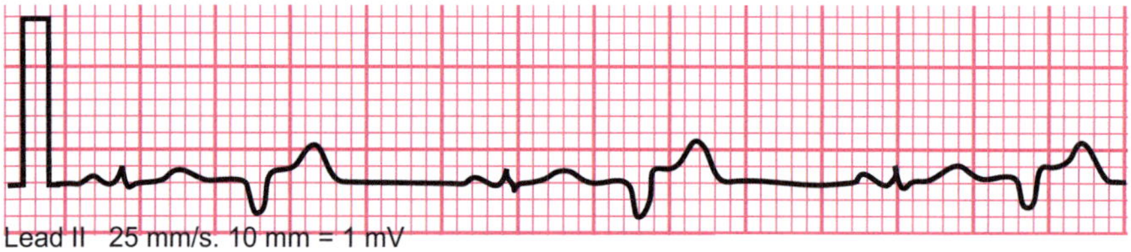


**Fig. 20.9** Ventricular bigeminy

When one ventricular extrasystole is present after every sinus beat, that is alternation of sinus beat and ventricular extrasystole, it is called ventricular bigeminy (Figs. 20.9 and 20.10). The classification used to assess the severity of ventricular extrasystoles is given in Box 20.2.

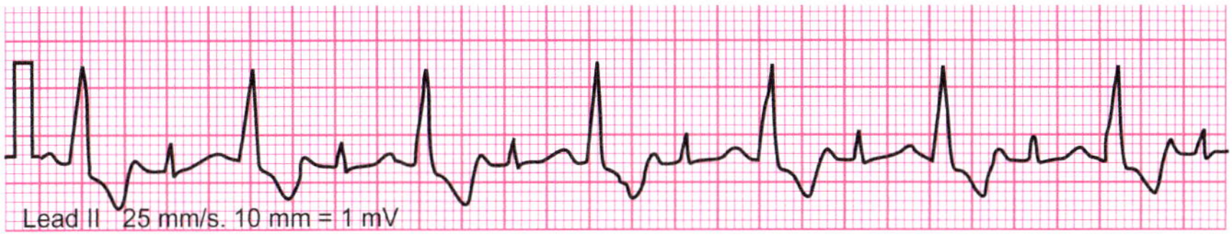


**Fig. 20.10** Ventricular bigeminy

**Box 20.2 Classification of Severity of Ventricular Extrasystoles**

| | |
|---|---|
| Class 0 | No ectopy |
| Class 1 | Less than 30 extrasystoles/h |
| Class 2 | More than 30 extrasystoles/h |
| Class 3 | Multiform complexes |
| Class 4A | Couplets |
| Class 4B | Runs of three or more |
| Class 5 | R on T phenomenon |

**Tips and Tricks**

- Ventricular extrasystoles are common findings in normal individuals and do not require active treatment in most of the cases.
- Precipitating factors and underlying causes should be treated.
- Beta-blockers and calcium channel blockers are required in some cases.

## *20.2.2 Ventricular Tachycardia*

Ventricular tachycardia (VT) occurs due to rapid discharge from an ectopic ventricular focus. When three or more ventricular extrasystoles occur in rapid succession at a rate of more than 100 bpm, it is known as ventricular tachycardia. It is associated with severe myocardial disease and the commonest cause is ischaemic heart disease. It is also frequently seen in digitalis toxicity. VT is practically always an indicator of serious heart disease. It is very rarely seen in patients without any heart disease. It is a very serious arrhythmia and the underlying cause should be detected quickly and the arrhythmia should be treated on emergency basis. VT may lead to ventricular fibrillation. The causes of ventricular tachycardia are enumerated in Box 20.3.

**Box 20.3 Causes of Ventricular Tachycardia**
Acute myocardial infarction
Digitalis toxicity
Rheumatic heart disease
Acid base imbalance
Electrolyte imbalance
Catecholamines

VT is often preceded by frequent ventricular extrasystoles. VT may be sustained (more than 30 s) or nonsustained (less than 30 s). The atrial rate is not discernible, ventricular rate is 100 to 250 bpm. P waves may be present or absent. If P waves are visible, then it bears no relation with QRS complex. The QRS complex is wide (greater than 0.12 s) and bizarre. The ventricular rate is usually regular. In VT, the QRS complexes in a single lead are similar in morphology and direction (concordance pattern) (Figs. 20.11, 20.12 and 20.13). Often it becomes difficult to

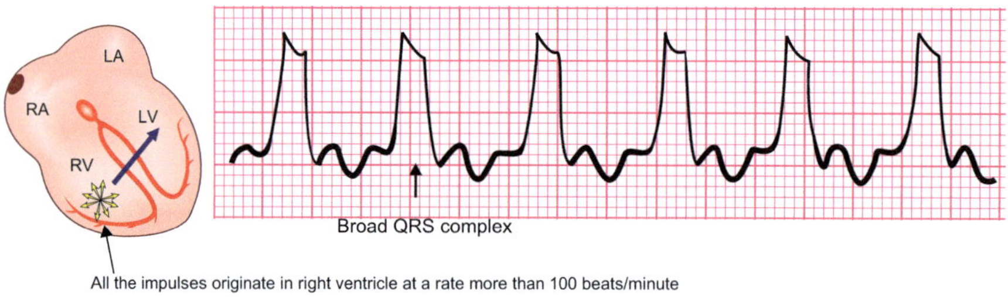


**Fig. 20.11** Illustration of genesis of ventricular tachycardia. Note that the impulse is originating from a focus in right ventricle at a rate of more than 100 bpm. The impulses are not traveling via the normal conducting system resulting in broad complexes with bizarre shape

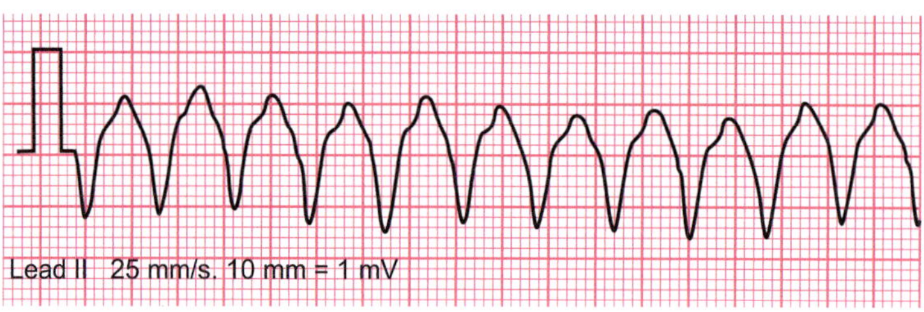


**Fig. 20.12** Ventricular tachycardia. The VPCs are occurring at a rate of more than 100 bpm

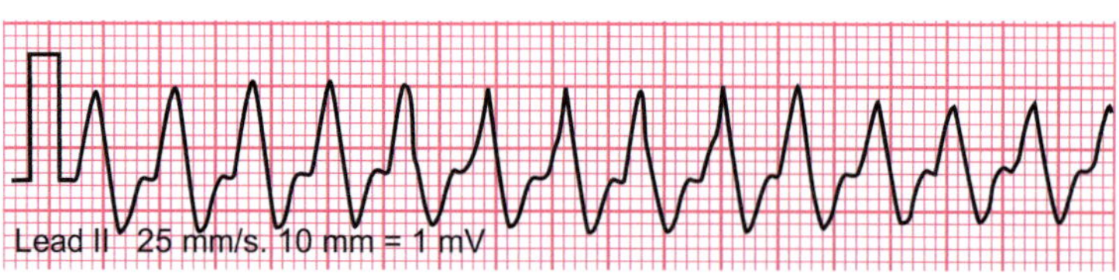


**Fig. 20.13** Ventricular tachycardia. Note the wide QRS complexes occurring at a rate of more than 100 bpm

differentiate between VT and SVT with intraventricular conduction defect. In this situation, the rhythm should be treated as VT until and unless proved otherwise.

The following characteristics suggest ventricular origin of the arrhythmia:

- QRS duration > 0.14 s.
- AV dissociation with or without fusion and captured beat.
- Superior QRS axis in presence of RBBB.
- Concordance of QRS pattern in all precordial leads, i.e. all positive or all negative waves.

The sinus beat and the ventricular beat are usually dissociated and they bear no relation with each other. The sinus impulse and the ventricular impulse meet with each other in the AV node and interfere with each other, thus P waves bear no relation with QRS complex. This is called 'atrioventricular dissociation' (AV dissociation). Sometimes the atria may be retrogradely activated by ventricular impulse and then the QRS complex will be followed by a P′ wave. This P′ wave may be inverted in leads II, III and aVF.

#### 20.2.2.1 Capture Beat and Fusion Beat

Sometimes it may happen that a sinus impulse is able to travel into the ventricle via the AV node during its non-refractory phase. This impulse has the power to activate the ventricles in a normal fashion resulting in a normal QRS complex and this QRS complex is preceded by a normal P wave. This normal PQRS complex can be identified if prior sinus rhythm is recorded in ECG. This beat in the presence of VT is called capture beat and is a reliable indicator of ventricular origin of the arrhythmia. Usually, one capture beat is seen only, between two ventricular extrasystoles during VT (Fig. 20.14).

Sometimes the capture beat may enter into the ventricles concomitantly with the ectopic ventricular impulse and the resulting beat will have feature of both capture beat and ventricular extrasystole, i.e. in between pure sinus beat and pure ventricular extrasystole. This beat is called 'fusion beat' (Fig. 20.14). It is the most reliable indicator of ventricular origin of the arrhythmia.

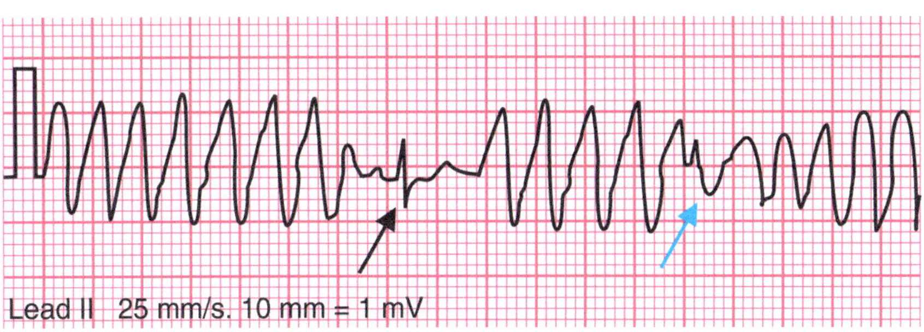


**Fig. 20.14** Capture beat and fusion beat. The capture beat is shown with a black arrow. It is a normal PQRS complex among the ongoing VT. The fusion beat is shown with a blue arrow. It has a morphology of capture beat and ventricular extrasystole

**Tips and Tricks**

- Fusion beat and capture beat confirm VT.
- Suspect VT if there is wide complex tachycardia with absent P waves.
- Suspect VT if there is wide complex tachycardia with all complexes either positive or negative (concordance pattern).
- DC cardioversion with high energy is required when pulse is absent.
- Lignocaine (1–1.5 mg/kg IV bolus) and procainamide are most effective drugs in acute therapy, especially when there is no haemodynamic compromise.
- Implanted cardioverter/defibrillator is often required in recurrent VT.

### *20.2.3 Torsades de Pointes*

This is a type of ventricular tachycardia or ventricular flutter. The QRS complexes are of multiform type. It is also called polymorphic VT. Torsades de pointes means twisting or torsion of points. The QRS complexes have beat-to-beat variation or change in amplitude and direction. This gives an appearance of rotation of QRS complexes around an isoelectric line (Figs. 20.15 and 20.16). It is usually associated with an underlying prolongation of Q-T interval, which favours ventricular tachycardia. It can complicate advanced and complete heart block. Due to prolongation of Q-T interval, there is also a likelihood of development of R on T phenomenon.

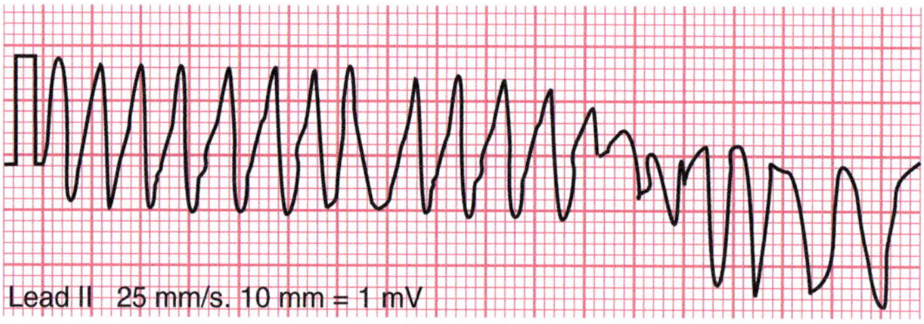


**Fig. 20.15** Torsades de pointes. Note the twisting of the points. The wide QRS complexes are positive at the beginning and then they become negative, i.e. twisting of the QRS complexes along the isoelectric line

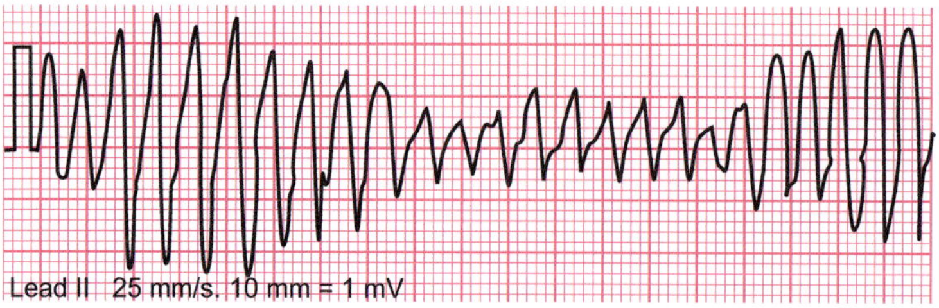


**Fig. 20.16** Torsades de pointes. Note the change in amplitude of the complexes

**Tips and Tricks**

- Look out for Q-T prolongation if normal beats are recorded before onset of tachycardia to diagnose Torsades de pointes.
- Intravenous magnesium, beta-blocker and phenytoin (shortens Q-T interval) are the mainstay of therapy.
- Metabolic abnormalities and drugs causing Torsades de pointes should be removed.

## 20.2.4 Ventricular Flutter and Fibrillation

Ventricular flutter occurs due to rapid and regular discharge from an ectopic ventricular focus. The QRS and T wave deflections are very broad, bizarre and often it is difficult to separate the QRS complex, S-T segment and the T wave. This is because of intraventricular conduction disturbance. The complexes are usually large in amplitude (Fig. 20.17).

Ventricular fibrillation (VF) occurs due to rapid and irregular discharge from an ectopic ventricular focus. This results in irregular, chaotic, deformed deflections of varying height and width (Figs. 20.18 and 20.19). ECG shows an undulating baseline with irregular waveforms that vary in morphology. Ventricular fibrillation with low amplitude waves (less than 3 mm) is called fine ventricular fibrillation, whereas waves, which are more than 3 mm, are often called coarse ventricular fibrillation.

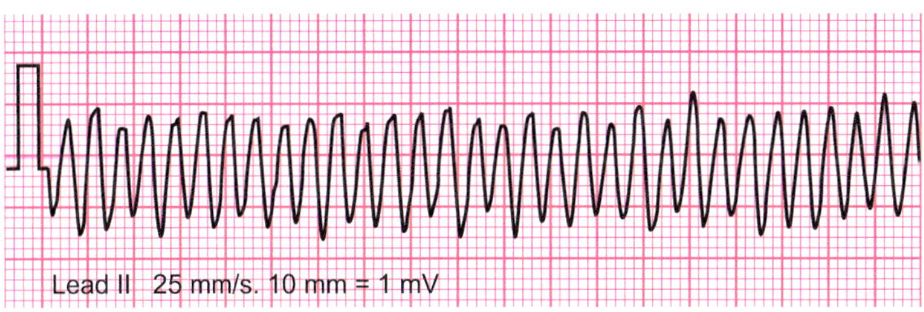


**Fig. 20.17** Ventricular flutter

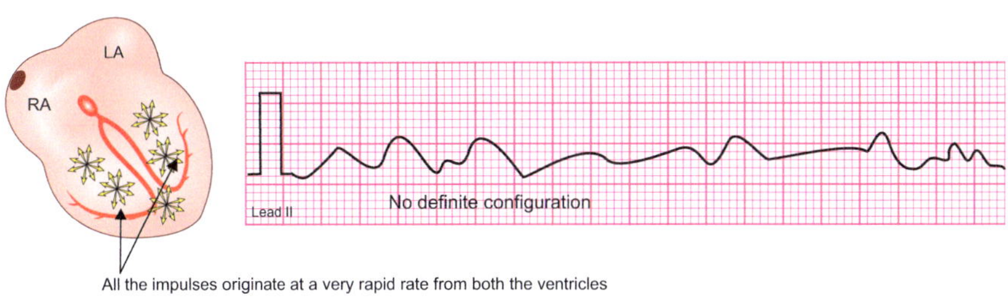


**Fig. 20.18** Illustration of genesis of ventricular fibrillation. The impulses are originating at a very rapid rate from the ventricles resulting in chaotic, deformed deflections of various sizes and shapes

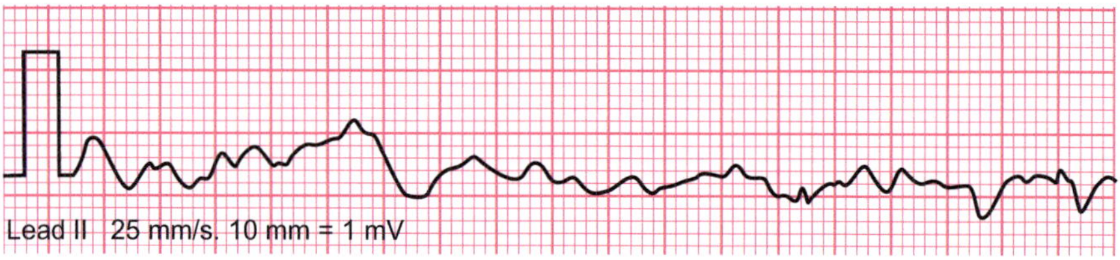


**Fig. 20.19** Ventricular fibrillation. Note that the complexes have no definite configuration. They are totally chaotic in nature

The ventricular activation is chaotic and they are not able to respond properly to each stimulus. The coordinated muscle contraction is lost and thus, the patient loses the pulse and blood pressure.

Ventricular fibrillation is a very serious life threatening arrhythmia. It is seen in almost all the conditions that are associated with VT. The commonest cause is myocardial infarction and it is the commonest cause of death within first hour of infarction. Cardiac surgery, electric shock and hypothermia may also cause VF. It should be immediately treated with DC shock. The various causes of ventricular fibrillation are summarized in Box 20.4.

**Box 20.4 Causes of Ventricular Fibrillation**
Coronary artery disease
Digitalis and quinidine toxicity
Hypothermia
Cardiac surgery
Electric shock
Electrolyte imbalance
Acid base disturbance
Untreated ventricular tachycardia

**Tips and Tricks**
- You will get only a few seconds to make a diagnosis of VF.
- Treatment is immediate defibrillation.
- Patient will require implanted cardioverter/defibrillator if recurrent VF is seen.

### *20.2.5 Idioventricular Rhythm*

Idioventricular rhythm (IVR) is a type of ectopic rhythm that originates from an ectopic pacemaker located in the ventricular myocardium. The inherent ventricular rate is roughly 20–40 bpm. It is considered to be an escape rhythm as it occurs when the rate of formation of impulse from SA node or the AV node becomes less than the pacemaker in the ventricles.

The QRS complexes are wide and bizarre, regular or may be slightly irregular and have no relation with atrial activity (Fig. 20.20).

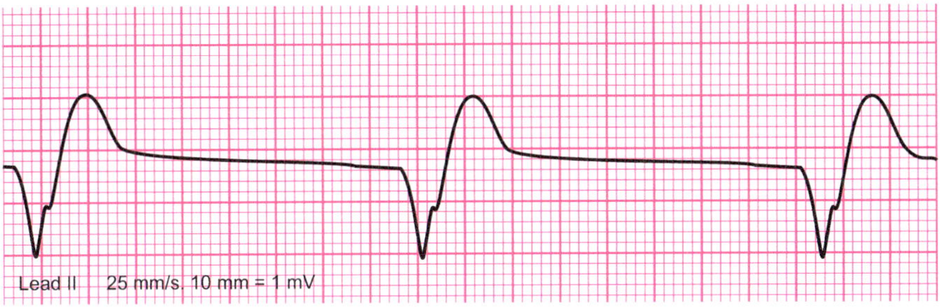


**Fig. 20.20** Idioventricular rhythm. Note the slow rate of extrasystoles at less than 40 bpm

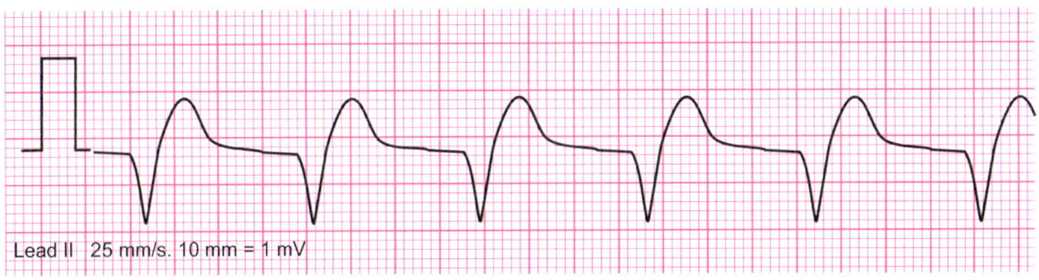


**Fig. 20.21** Accelerated idioventricular rhythm. The wide QRS complexes are of ventricular origin and the rate is 79 bpm

### *20.2.6 Accelerated Idioventricular Rhythm*

Accelerated idioventricular rhythm (AIVR) also originates from an ectopic pacemaker located in the ventricle like IVR but the rate of generation of impulse is 50–100 bpm. The term accelerated means the rate is more than IVR but less than that of VT. It is also called slow VT. ECG is just like that of IVR, only the rate is more (Fig. 20.21).

AIVR is commonly seen after myocardial infarction and reperfusion therapy, digitalis toxicity, myocarditis, etc. AIVR can be treated by increasing the sinus rate with atropine, but it is usually not required.

### *20.2.7 Ventricular Asystole*

Ventricular asystole is also called ventricular standstill. There is no electrical activity in the ventricles. Most often in ECG, it is manifested by a straight line (Fig. 20.22). It usually occurs after ventricular fibrillation. The chance of revival is very low. CPR must be started at the earliest.

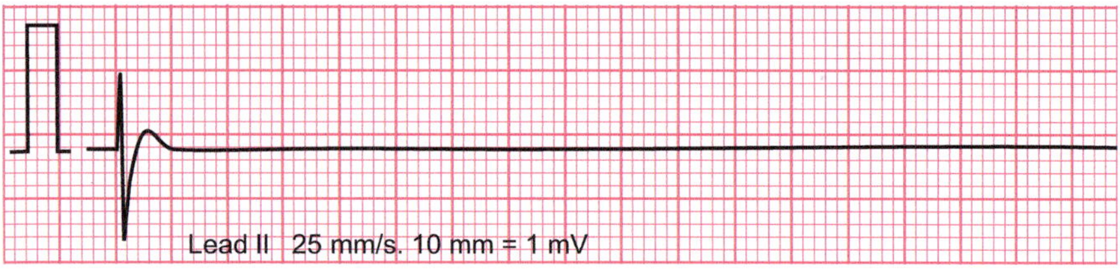


**Fig. 20.22** Ventricular asystole. After one complex there is ventricular asystole

**Self-Assessment Questions**

1. Ventricular premature beats typically appear as wide QRS complexes on the ECG. True or false?
2. Ventricular fibrillation is characterized by chaotic, irregular electrical activity on the ECG. True or false?
3. In ventricular extrasystoles, the compensatory pause following the premature beat is usually incomplete. True or false?
4. Ventricular tachycardia is commonly associated with narrow QRS complexes on the ECG. True or false?
5. In IVR, the heart rate is typically between 80 and 120 bpm. True or false?
6. **Ventricular premature beats are characterized by:**

   a. Wide QRS complexes b. Narrow QRS complexes c. Absent QRS complexes d. Prolonged P-R intervals

7. **A fusion beat occurs when:**

   a. Two or more atrial contractions occur at the same time b. Two or more ventricular contractions occur at the same time c. A combination of normal sinus rhythm and ventricular ectopic beats occurs d. The atria and ventricles contract at the same time

8. **In VF, the ECG shows:**

   a. Regular P waves b. Narrow of QRS complexes c. Wide QRS complexes d. Undulating baseline with ill-defined complexes

9. **IVR is defined as:**

   a. A regular ventricular rhythm with narrow QRS complexes b. A regular ventricular rhythm with wide QRS complexes c. An irregular ventricular rhythm with wide QRS complexes d. An irregular ventricular rhythm with narrow QRS complexes

10. **Torsades de pointes is characterized by:**

    a. Regular ventricular rhythm b. Narrow QRS complex c. Regular P waves d. Wide QRS complexes

**Case Studies**

1. A 30-year-old lady came for routine check-up. She had no symptoms. There was no past history of hypertension, diabetes or any chronic illness. Her blood pressure was 110/70 mmHg, pulse was irregular, chest was clear. Her rhythm strip is given in Fig. 20.23. What is the diagnosis?
2. A 75-year-old gentleman was admitted for inguinal hernia repair. On third post-operative day, he complained of chest discomfort for last one hour. Physical examination revealed a faint pulse and blood pressure was 70/40 mmHg. He was drowsy and breathless. Chest examination revealed widespread crepitations bilaterally more at the bases. His rhythm strip is given in Fig. 20.24. What does the ECG show? How will you manage this patient?
3. A 70-year-old gentleman suddenly collapsed in the emergency department. He had past history of CAD, hypertension and dyslipidaemia. Immediately ECG was done. Rhythm strip is given in Fig. 20.25. What is your diagnosis? How will you manage this patient?
4. A 65-year-old patient was admitted in ICU suffering from pneumonia with sepsis. His rhythm strip from cardiac monitor is given in Fig. 20.26. Identify the rhythm.
5. This rhythm strip (Fig. 20.27) was given for spot identification in final year MBBS examination. Identify the abnormality and give two reasons in favour of your diagnosis.
6. You are on duty in CCU. The duty nurse called you to examine this 67-year-old patient who suddenly complained of palpitation, dizziness and uneasy feeling. His pulse is feeble and blood pressure is 106/70 mmHg. The rhythm strip (Fig. 20.28) from bedside cardiac monitor reveals abnormal rhythm. Can you identify the rhythm?

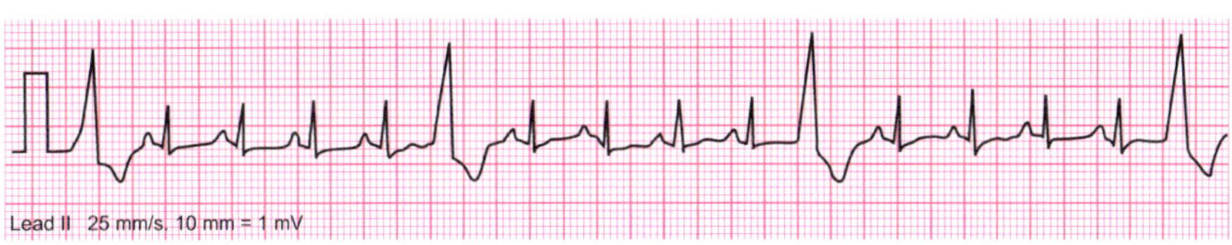


**Fig. 20.23** Analyse the rhythm strip

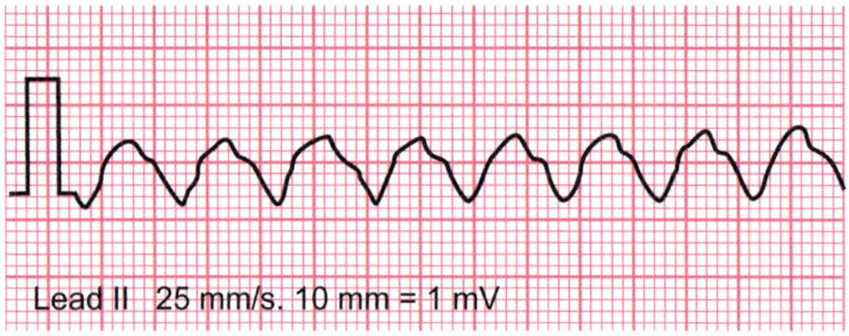


**Fig. 20.24** Analyse the rhythm strip

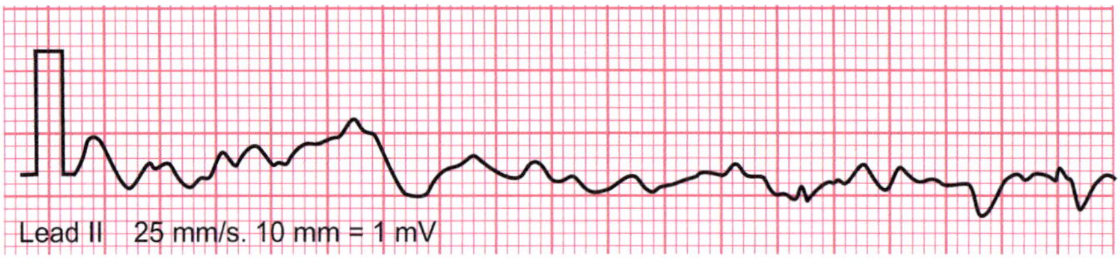


**Fig. 20.25** Analyse the rhythm strip

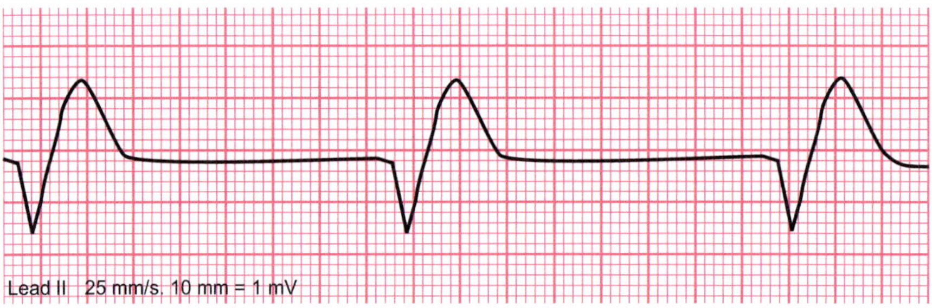


**Fig. 20.26** Analyse the rhythm strip

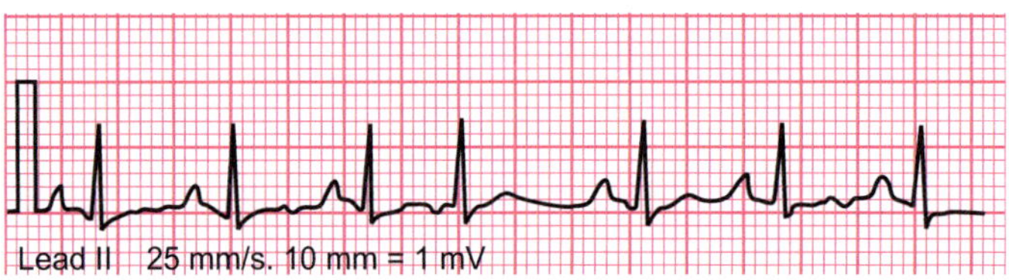


**Fig. 20.27** Analyse the rhythm strip

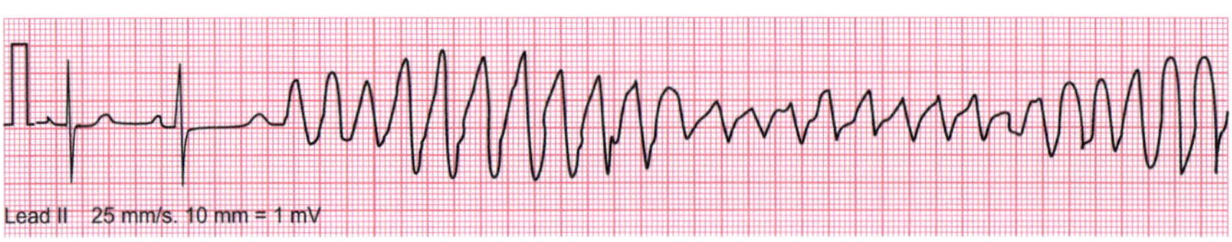


**Fig. 20.28** Analyse the rhythm strip

7. Identify the rhythm strip (Fig. 20.29). Give two points in favour of your diagnosis.
8. A 55-year-old patient had anterior wall myocardial infarction. While undergoing reperfusion therapy, the following abnormality appeared in the bedside cardiac monitor. Can you identify the rhythm strip given in Fig. 20.30.
9. Identify the rhythm (Fig. 20.31). What is your diagnosis?
10. You were on duty in CCU. Suddenly the cardiac monitor sounded the alarm. The rhythm strip from the monitor is given in Fig. 20.32. Identify the abnormality. What will you do to manage this patient?

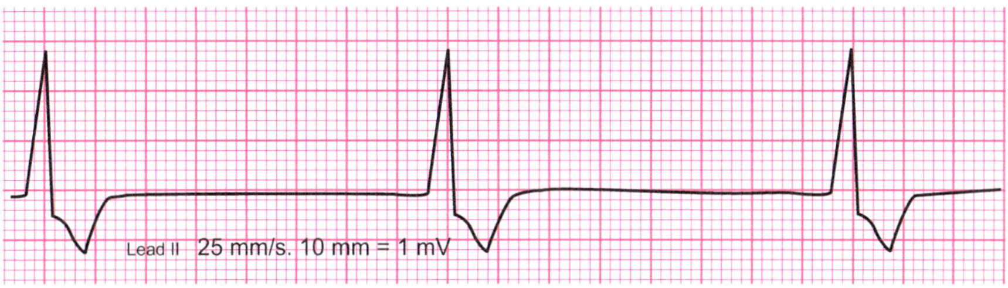


**Fig. 20.29** Analyse the rhythm strip

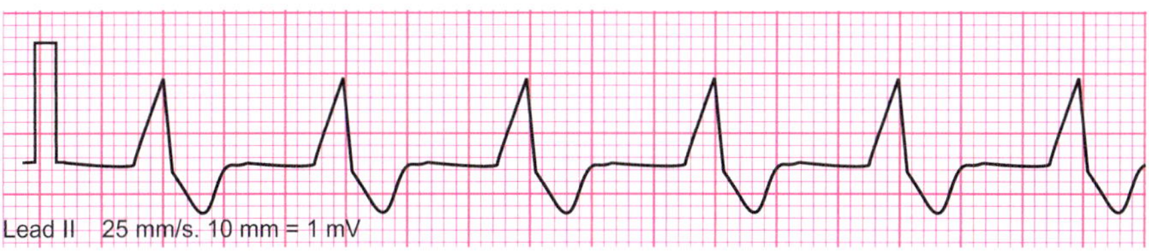


**Fig. 20.30** Analyse the rhythm strip

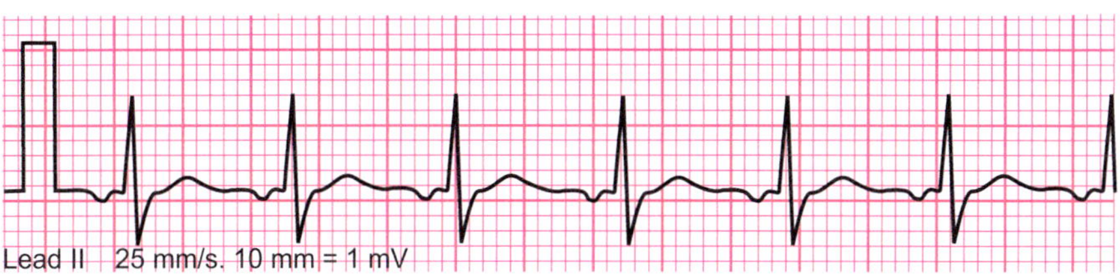


**Fig. 20.31** Analyse the rhythm strip

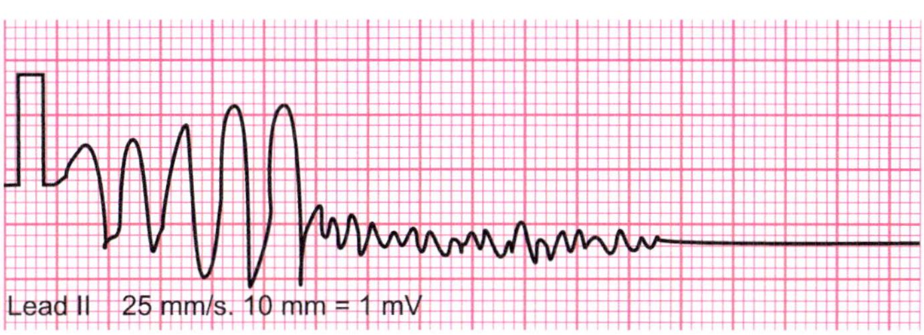


**Fig. 20.32** Analyse the rhythm strip

**Answers**

1. True 2. True 3. False 4. False 5. False 6. a 7. c 8. d 9. b 10. d

**Case Studies**

1. The rhythm strip (Fig. 20.23) shows ventricular extrasystoles occurring after every four normal PQRS complexes. The extrasystoles have wide QRS complex and amplitude and morphology is entirely different from normal PQRS complexes.

   The patient has irregular pulse which means the extrasystoles are occurring at random without maintaining any rhythm even if the rhythm strip shows them at a regular pattern occurring after every four normal complexes.

   Ventricular extrasystoles are commonly seen in daily clinical practice. In this patient, investigations should be carried out to rule out any underlying heart disease. If no underlying heart disease is detected, it indicates good prognosis and nothing more needs to be done. However, she should be advised to reduce intake of caffeine. If she becomes symptomatic, she may need beta-blockers to control the symptoms.
2. The diagnosis is VT (Fig. 20.24). There is wide QRS complex with duration more than 0.14 s and ventricular rate is about 166 bpm.

   Treatment of VT depends upon haemodynamic status. In this drowsy patient, there is hypotension and pulmonary oedema. This is a medical emergency. Immediate DC cardioversion should be done. After resuscitation, he should be evaluated for postoperative myocardial ischaemia or infarction.

   In patients with structural heart disease and hemodynamically stable ventricular tachycardia, intravenous procainamide, amiodarone, lidocaine and sotalol (depending on availability) are recommended for the acute treatment of ventricular tachycardia.
3. The diagnosis is VF (Fig. 20.25). There is undulating baseline with no identifiable PQRS complex.

   This is a life threatening emergency. Immediately guideline-directed management as per Advanced Cardiac Life Support (ACLS) protocol should be initiated. He should be shocked immediately with 120–200 J on a biphasic defibrillator or 360 J using a monophasic defibrillator. Administer epinephrine and amiodarone as per ACLS protocol in patients sustaining VF rhythm regardless of receiving three shocks. Amiodarone significantly improves survival to hospital admission without affecting survival to hospital discharge. Identifying and addressing the cause of inciting event is equally important.
4. The rhythm strip shows IVR (Fig. 20.26). There is no P wave, and the QRS complexes are wide, more than 0.14 s. The ventricular rate is 37 bpm. This is also called slow VT.

   Usually, IVR is a benign rhythm which settles down of its own. Sometimes, a patient may be symptomatic and may not tolerate idioventricular rhythm secondary to atrioventricular dyssynchrony, fast ventricular rate or degenerated ventricular fibrillation of idioventricular rhythm. Atropine may be trialled in such cases to increase sinus rate.

5. The rhythm strip in Fig. 20.27 shows premature junctional complex. The fourth PQRS complex is premature in timing and it is followed by compensatory pause. The P wave is inverted. Rest all the PQRST complexes are normal.
6. The rhythm strip (Fig. 20.28) shows Torsades de pointes, polymorphic VT. The first PQRS complex is normal. The second PQRS complex has prolonged Q-T interval. It is 0.68 s. It is followed by VT with big amplitude complexes at the beginning followed by small amplitude complexes. At the end of the strip again big amplitude complexes are seen. Hence it is Torsades de pointes precipitated by long Q-T interval.

   Intravenous magnesium is the first-line pharmacologic therapy in Torsades de Pointes. The patient has a feeble pulse and blood pressure is normal. Hence magnesium should be given. The recommended initial dose of magnesium is a slow 2 g IV push. An infusion of 1–4 g/h. should be started to keep the magnesium levels greater than 2 mmol/L. Magnesium has been shown to stabilize the cardiac membrane. If the patient becomes unstable haemodynamically, synchronized cardioversion should be performed (100 J monophasic, 50 J biphasic). Pulseless torsades should be defibrillated.
7. The rhythm is IVR (Fig. 20.29). Two points in favour of diagnosis are wide QRS complex, absent P waves and ventricular rate of about 40 bpm.
8. The diagnosis is AIVR (Fig. 20.30). There are no P waves, wide QRS complex at a rate of 100 bpm. This is also called slow VT.

   AIVR is usually a benign and well-tolerated arrhythmia. Most of the cases will require no treatment. It is frequently seen during reperfusion therapy and it signifies complete reperfusion although many disagree with it. Atropine may be required sometimes to increase the sinus rate to suppress the arrhythmia.
9. The diagnosis is junctional tachycardia (Fig. 20.31). The QRS complex is narrow. The ventricular rate is 125 bpm. The P waves are all inverted. Inverted P wave signifies that the rhythm is originating from AV junction. Hence, it is junctional tachycardia also called junctional ectopic tachycardia.

   Junctional tachycardia is more common in infants and children as compared to adults. It is often seen after cardiac surgery for congenital heart disease in infants. Beta-blockers, diltiazem and verapamil are recommended for treatment. Amiodarone is often effective in non-postoperative junctional tachycardia. Catheter ablation may be reasonable in patients with junctional tachycardia when medical therapy is not effective.
10. The diagnosis is VT degenerating into VF ultimately progressing to ventricular asystole (Fig. 20.32). Broad QRS tachycardia indicates VT at the beginning. There are no P waves. After this suddenly it degenerates into ill-formed complexes, which is VF and the following straight line indicates asystole.

    Immediate resuscitation should be started according to current ACLS guidelines. High-quality CPR is the mainstay of treatment. Asystole is a non-shockable rhythm. Therefore, if asystole is noted on the cardiac monitor, no attempt at defibrillation should be made. High-quality CPR should be continued with minimal (less than 5 s) interruption. CPR should not be stopped to allow for endotracheal intubation. Epinephrine (1 mg via intravenous or intraosseous line) should be delivered every 3–5 min. Cardioversion should be done the moment VT is diagnosed or else it may be too late.

# Chapter 21
# Approach to Arrhythmias

**Learning Objectives**
After studying this chapter, the reader will learn about:

- Analysis of arrhythmias by analysing rate and rhythm
- Analysis of arrhythmias by studying P wave

## 21.1 Approach to Arrhythmia

There are various ways of approaching arrhythmia. The choice of course depends upon the knowledge and the level of understanding of the reader. The easy method is to analyse by starting with the rate and regularity and then narrow down to the various possibilities. While analysing by this method, the following questions should be asked while inspecting the rhythm strip.

(a) Is the rate normal, fast or slow?
(b) Is the rhythm regular?
(c) If the rhythm is irregular, whether there is pattern of regularity to the rhythm that is regularly irregular or it is absolutely irregular that is irregularly irregular?
(d) If there are only a few beats interrupting the regularity, then it needs to be seen whether these are ectopic beats or whether these beats are followed by compensatory pause?

Now let us see the interpretation of these questions.



T. K. Koley, *Rapid Review of ECG*,
https://doi.org/10.1007/978-981-99-9116-7_21

### *21.1.1 Consider the Following Possibilities When the Rhythm Is Regular*

#### 21.1.1.1 Normal Rate

(a) Sinus rhythm (regular P waves present)
(b) Sinus rhythm absent (regular P waves absent)

  (i) Ectopic atrial pacemaker (P′ wave present)
  (ii) Accelerated AV nodal rhythm
  (iii) Implanted pacemaker (ventricular)

#### 21.1.1.2 Tachycardia

(a) Sinus tachycardia (P waves present, narrow QRS complex)
(b) PSVT/PAT (P waves usually not seen, narrow QRS complex)
(c) Ventricular tachycardia (P waves usually not seen, wide QRS complex)

#### 21.1.1.3 Bradycardia

(a) Sinus bradycardia
(b) Idioventricular rhythm with SA block or complete AV block
(c) AV nodal rhythm with SA block or complete AV block

### *21.1.2 Consider the Following Possibilities When the Rhythm Is Irregular*

#### 21.1.2.1 Regularly Irregular Arrhythmias

(a) Sinus arrhythmia
(b) Mobitz type I block (Wenckebach block)
(c) Bigeminy or trigeminy of atrial, AV nodal or ventricular origin

#### 21.1.2.2 Irregularly Irregular Arrhythmias

(a) Atrial flutter with variable AV block
(b) Atrial fibrillation
(c) Ventricular fibrillation

#### 21.1.2.3 Infrequent Irregularity

(a) Atrial, AV nodal or ventricular premature beats
(b) Mobitz type II AV block

### 21.1.3 *Consider the Following When There Are Pauses*

#### 21.1.3.1 Long Pause

(a) Sinus pause
(b) Complete AV block with failure of escape beat

#### 21.1.3.2 Short Pause

(a) Ventricular ectopic (complete pause)
(b) Atrial ectopic (incomplete pause)

Another method of analysing arrhythmias is by the study of the P wave and its relation with the QRS complexes. Here initially it has to be seen whether sinus rhythm is present or not. If the sinus rhythm is absent, then the number and the morphology of the P waves are to be studied and then the irregularities of the P waves are to be correlated with the QRS complexes. It is always better to mark out all the P waves in the rhythm strip at the beginning. The duration of the QRS complex should also be measured because a wide QRS complex points towards the ventricular origin of the arrhythmia. Let us consider the following:

#### 21.1.3.3 Sinus Rhythm

(a) Regular sinus rhythm
(b) Sinus bradycardia
(c) Sinus tachycardia
(d) Sinus arrhythmia

#### 21.1.3.4 Absent Sinus Rhythm

(a) Absent P waves

- (i) Infrequent absence
  - Ventricular ectopic
  - Premature beat of nodal origin

(ii) Constant absence of P wave (or P wave buried in T wave)

- Atrial fibrillation
- Ventricular tachycardia
- Nodal rhythm
- Accelerated nodal rhythm
- PSVT/PAT

(b) Abnormal shape of P wave (P′ wave)

(i) Atrial ectopic beat
(ii) Wandering atrial pacemaker
(iii) Incorrect placement of arm electrodes
(iv) Nodal rhythm with retrograde conduction of P waves

(c) More than one P wave for each QRS complex

(i) Complete AV block
(ii) 2:1 or higher AV block (Mobitz type I and II)
(iii) Atrial flutter or fibrillation with second degree AV block (very difficult to identify P wave in these cases)

One can use either of these methods alone or together to analyse arrhythmia, but it is easier said than done because analysis of arrhythmia is one of the most difficult aspects of ECG. This comes not by reading book only, but by constant daily practice.

# Part VI
# Miscellaneous ECG

# Chapter 22
# ECG in Electrolyte Imbalance

**Learning Objectives**
After studying this chapter, the reader will learn about:

- Hyperkalaemia
- Hypokalaemia
- Hypercalcaemia
- Hypocalcaemia
- Magnesium effect

Resting membrane potential of a cardiac cell is dependent upon the maintenance of a normal ionic balance across the cell membranes. Potassium, sodium and calcium influence the resting membrane potential as well as generation of action potential. Potassium is the most important contributor to the resting membrane potential. The normal ECG depends upon the concentration of these ions across the cardiac cell membranes. Imbalance in the level of potassium and calcium has profound effect on the ECG. Electrolyte abnormality is frequently encountered in our day-to-day practice in patients suffering from renal failure, patients on IV fluids and severely ill patients in ICU.

## 22.1 ECG in Potassium Imbalance

Electrophysiology of cardiac cell is profoundly affected by increase or decrease in level of potassium ions, thereby affecting the electrical stability of heart. Potassium ions play a key role in repolarization of cardiac cells. Severe hyperkalaemia and hypokalaemia can be life threatening and require urgent treatment.



T. K. Koley, *Rapid Review of ECG*,
https://doi.org/10.1007/978-981-99-9116-7_22

### 22.1.1 *Hyperkalaemia*

The normal range of serum potassium is between 3.5 and 5.5 mEq/L. A departure from this narrow range can have significant changes in ECG. Hyperkalaemia (serum potassium more than 5.5 mEq/L) increases cell membrane excitability. The ECG changes are frequently seen when the serum potassium level is more than 6 mEq/L. The typical progressive ECG changes of hyperkalaemia are:

- Peaked, tall and tented T wave
- Gradual decrease and disappearance of P wave
- Widening of QRS complex
- Virtual disappearance of S-T segment
- Atrioventricular conduction defect
- Cardiac arrhythmias

#### 22.1.1.1 Peaked, Tall and Tented T Waves

The earliest ECG manifestation of hyperkalaemia is peaked, tall and tented T wave best seen in the chest leads. At first the T wave becomes tall and then becomes slightly wide. This is called 'tented' T wave. This is seen when serum potassium is between 6 and 7 mEq/L. Similar picture may also be seen in normal individuals and posterior wall infarction. The proximal limb is usually steep but the distal limb of the T wave has more gradual descent (Figs. 22.1, 22.2, 22.3, 22.4, 22.5, 22.6 and 22.7).

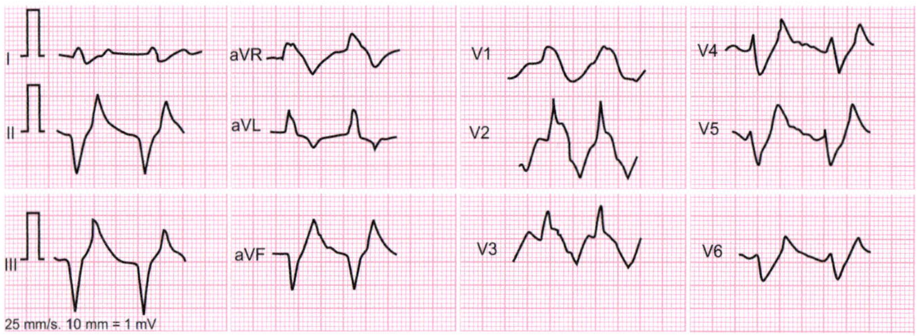


**Fig. 22.1** ECG showing hyperkalaemia. This is ECG of a 50-year-old gentleman suffering from Addison's disease who presented with hyperkalaemia. This is the ECG at the time of presentation. Note the wide QRS complexes and disappearance of P wave

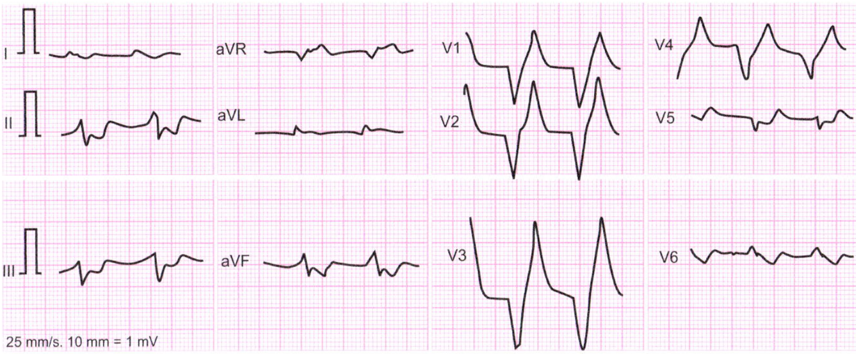


**Fig. 22.2** ECG showing hyperkalaemia. This is the ECG of the same patient after 10 min. Note the wide QRS complexes and tall T waves. At this time, the serum potassium was 9.1 mEq/L. Injection calcium gluconate was administered and insulin glucose drip was started

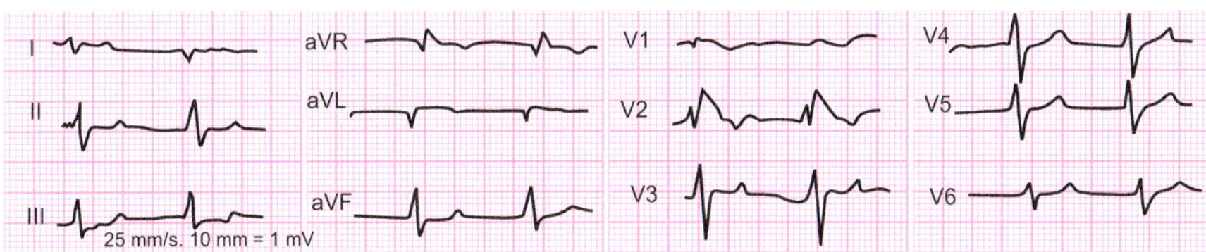


**Fig. 22.3** ECG showing hyperkalaemia. This is the ECG of the same patient after calcium and insulin glucose therapy. Note the narrowing of the complexes with treatment. Also note the bundle branch block appearance in lead V2

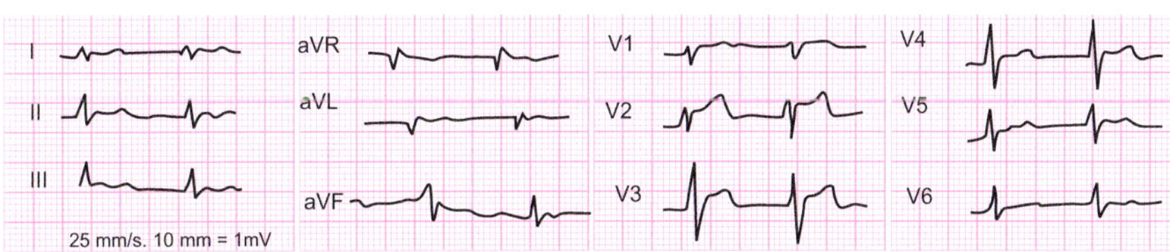


**Fig. 22.4** ECG of the same patient after correction of serum potassium

**Fig. 22.5** Hyperkalaemia showing sine wave configuration of QRS complex

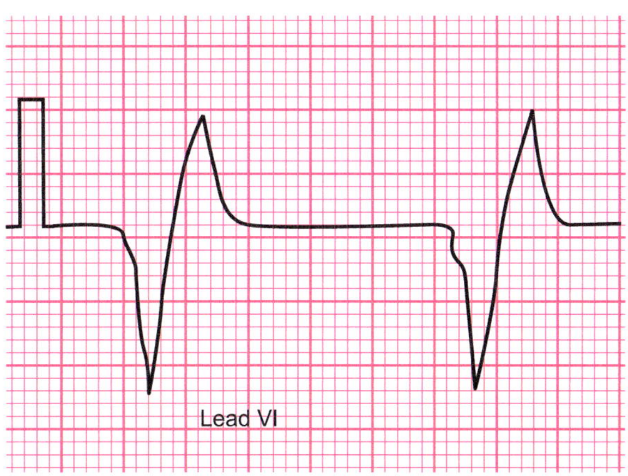

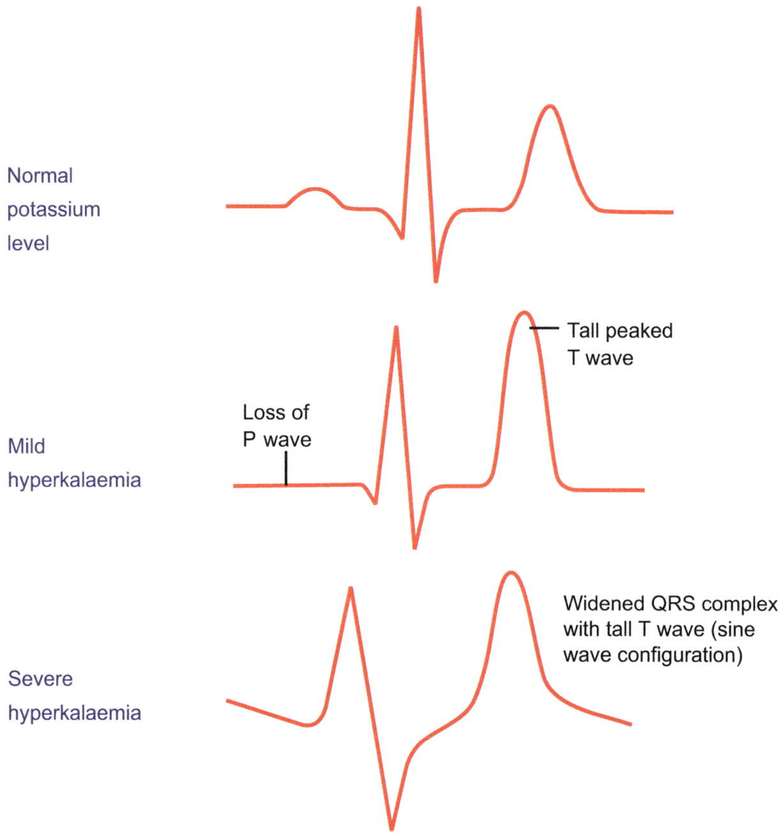


**Fig. 22.6** Diagram showing progressive hyperkalaemia

**Fig. 22.7** Diagram showing progressive hyperkalaemia. (**a**) Normal complex. (**b**) Raised serum potassium. Note the tall and peaked T wave with blunting of the P wave. (**c**) With further rise in serum potassium, there is widening of the QRS complex with peaked T wave and disappearance of the P wave

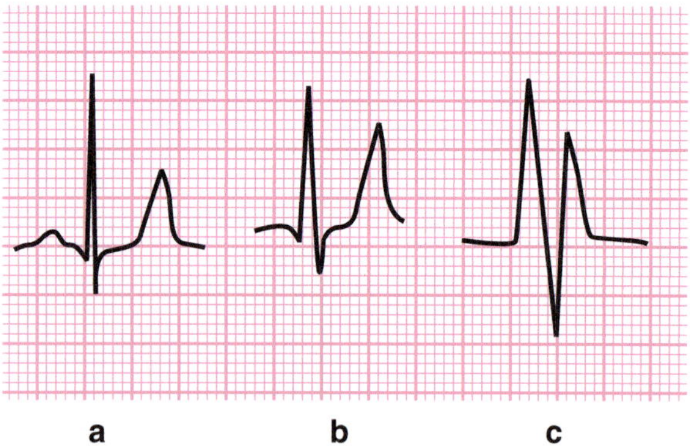

#### 22.1.1.2 Gradual Decrease and Then Disappearance of P Wave

With further rise in serum potassium level (7–8 mEq/L), there is further increase in height on T wave. The P wave first decreases in amplitude and then disappears. The prolongation of P-R interval may precede the disappearance of P wave.

#### 22.1.1.3 Widening of QRS Complex

The QRS complex becomes wide and bizarre in shape when the serum potassium lies between 8 and 9 mEq/L. This mainly affects the terminal deflection. This conduction disturbance resembles bundle branch block. There is further peaking of T waves. S-T segment depression starts.

#### 22.1.1.4 Virtual Disappearance of S-T Segment

With rise in serum potassium level (more than 9 mEq/L), the S-T segment virtually disappears as if the proximal limb is incorporated in the ascending limb of T wave. The QRS complex continues to widen and eventually blends with the T wave, producing the classic sine-wave ECG.

#### 22.1.1.5 Atrioventricular Conduction Defect

Atrioventricular conduction defects are observed in patients suffering from severe hyperkalaemia. In the initial phase, P-R interval prolongation and QRS widening are seen but later the sequential changes include atrioventricular junctional delay, followed by acceleration of junctional pacemakers, conduction delays in the His-Purkinje system and delays in ventricular muscle. Fascicular blocks and bundle branch blocks are also seen.

#### 22.1.1.6 Cardiac Arrhythmias

Sinus tachycardia and bradycardia, idioventricular rhythm, ventricular tachycardia, ventricular fibrillation have all been observed in ECG of patients suffering from hyperkalemia. Asystole may develop if urgent steps are not taken to manage life threatening hyperkalaemia.

### *22.1.2 Hypokalaemia*

Hypokalaemia (serum potassium less than 3.5 mEq/L) is commonly seen in patients receiving diuretics, prolonged intravenous fluid therapy, vomiting and diarrhoea. It causes delayed ventricular repolarization shortened refractory period and increased automaticity. The gradual fall in serum potassium level is reflected electrocardiographically by the following features:

#### 22.1.2.1 Gradual Decrease and Then Disappearance of T Wave

The earliest ECG change of hypokalaemia is decrease in the amplitude of T wave. The T wave gradually becomes flat and then disappears. Later it may be seen as a small hump on the S-T segment.

#### 22.1.2.2 Presence of Prominent U Waves, Best Seen in Leads V2–V4

With fall in serum potassium, the U wave becomes prominent. When the height of U wave is more than that of T wave, the serum potassium level is below 3 mEq/L. When the T wave has disappeared, the U wave may give a false impression of T wave. Thus, it may also lead to an appearance of pseudo-prolonged Q-T interval, which is basically Q-U interval. The U wave maintains its round shape (Figs. 22.8, 22.9 and 22.10).

#### 22.1.2.3 Slight Depression of S-T Segment

There may be S-T segment depression in all the leads.

#### 22.1.2.4 Increase in P-R Interval

The P-R interval gradually increases along with increase in amplitude of P wave and the P wave falls almost on the preceding U wave. Wenckebach type of second-degree block is usually seen with very low level of serum potassium.

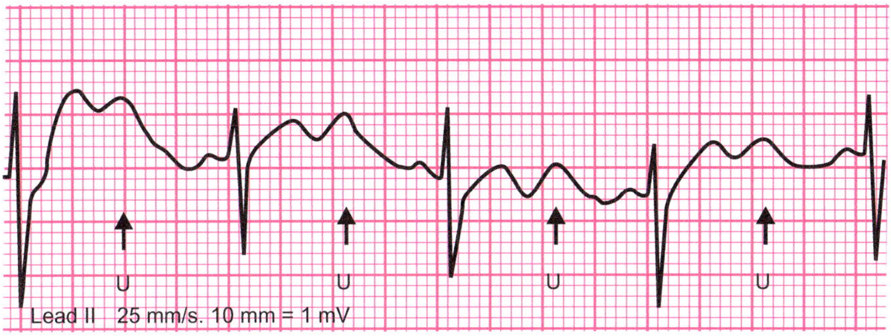


**Fig. 22.8** Hypokalaemia

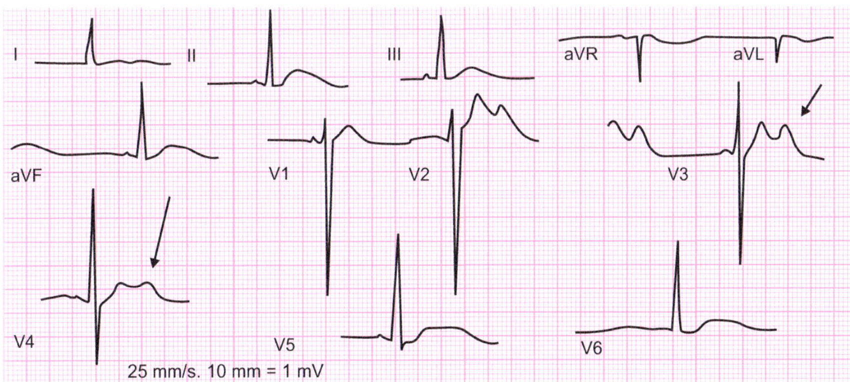


**Fig. 22.9** Hypokalaemia. This ECG was taken from a patient suffering from hypokalaemic periodic paralysis. Note the prominent U waves (arrows) in leads V2, V3 and V4

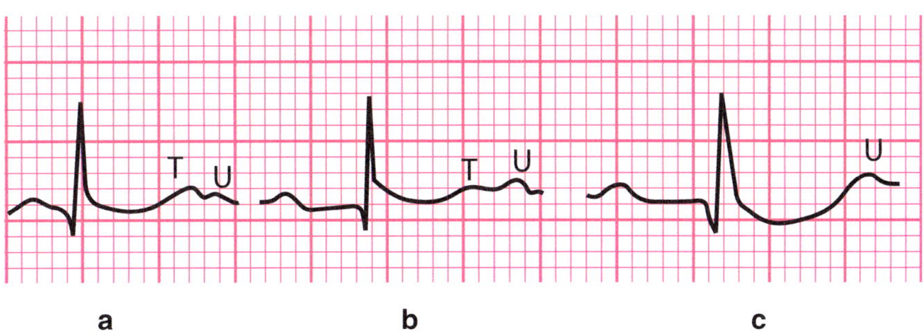


**Fig. 22.10** Diagram showing progressive changes in hypokalaemia. (**a**) Normal complex. (**b**) Hypokalaemia. Note the prominence of U wave, which is taller than the T wave. The P-R interval is prolonged. (**c**) With further fall in serum potassium, the U wave becomes very prominent with disappearance of the T wave. Note the further prolongation of the P-R interval

#### 22.1.2.5 Arrhythmias

Severe hypokalaemia can cause arrhythmias including ventricular tachycardia and Torsades de Pointes. It also may cause ventricular fibrillation and sudden cardiac death.

**Tips and Tricks**

- Look for tall and tented T waves to diagnose hyperkalaemia.
- Look for U waves which are preferably taller than T waves to diagnose hypokalaemia.
- Always remember that tall T waves and prominent U waves are seen in normal persons as well.
- If you find tall T waves, keep in mind the possibility of hyperacute myocardial infarction.

## 22.2 ECG in Calcium Imbalance

Calcium imbalance is seen in patients suffering from renal failure, disorder of parathyroid glands, pancreatitis and malignancy. Calcium ion is mainly responsible for phase 2 of action potential when calcium ions enter into the cardiac cells. Calcium imbalance mainly produces changes in the duration of S-T segment with practically no changes in QRS complex or T waves.

### *22.2.1 Hypercalcaemia*

The normal serum calcium level is 9–10.5 mg/dL. The ECG changes usually appear when the serum calcium level is more than 12 mg/dL. The most characteristic ECG change is shortening of Q-T interval and the shortening is due to shortening of the S-T segment. This occurs due to the shortening of the phase 2 of action potential. The S-T segment virtually disappears and gets incorporated in the T wave as if it forms the proximal limb of T wave (Figs. 22.11 and 22.12). There may be P-R

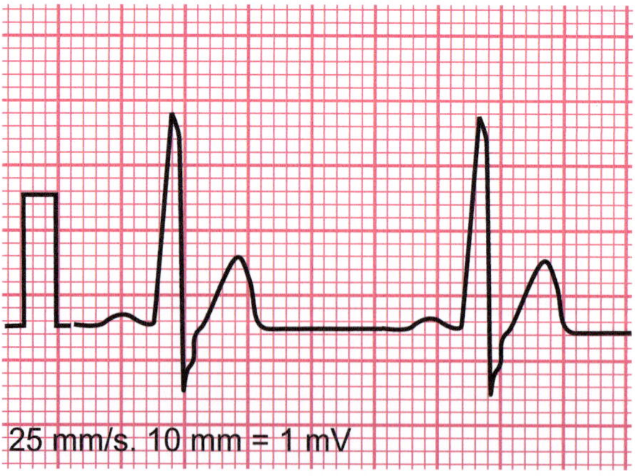


**Fig. 22.11** Hypercalcaemia

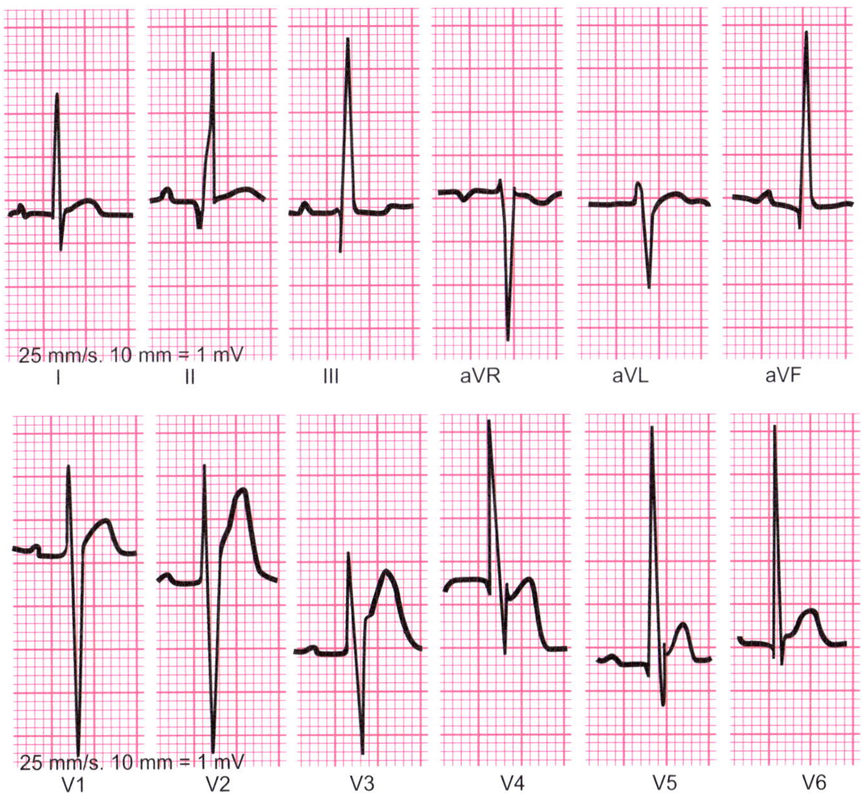


**Fig. 22.12** Hypercalcaemia. Note the shortened Q-T interval

interval prolongation and increased duration of QRS interval also. J point elevation has also been observed in hypercalcaemia.

Additional ECG manifestations in severe hypercalcaemia include S-T segment elevation, biphasic T waves and prominent U waves.

### *22.2.2 Hypocalcaemia*

Hypocalcaemia occurs when the serum level of calcium is below the lower limit of normal. The most characteristic ECG change is prolongation of Q-T interval. The increase in Q-T interval is due to increase in the S-T segment, which is due to prolongation of phase 2 of action potential. The prolongation of Q-T interval is proportional to degree of hypocalcaemia. However the S-T segment is not displaced. The Q-T interval may be in the region of 0.5–0.6 s (Fig. 22.13).

**Fig. 22.13** Hypocalcaemia

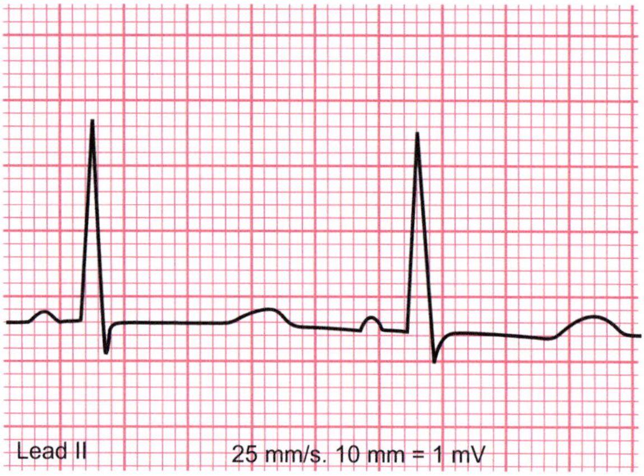


Rarely, there may be decreased T wave amplitude, T wave flattening, terminal T wave inversion or deep T wave inversion in severe hypocalcaemia. In certain patients, S-T segment elevation mimicking acute myocardial infarction has also been observed.

**Tips and Tricks**

- To diagnose hypercalcaemia, look for shortened Q-T interval.
- To diagnose hypocalcaemia, look for prolonged Q-T interval.
- If Q-T interval is prolonged beyond 0.48 s, keep in mind the possibility of development of Torsades de pointes.

## 22.3 Magnesium Effect

Usually, the serum potassium and magnesium go hand in hand and the ECG changes are also similar. The ECG changes of hypomagnesaemia resemble that of hypokalaemia. The U wave increases in amplitude, and the T wave becomes flattened. The S-T segment may be depressed.

The ECG changes of hypermagnesaemia resemble that of hyperkalaemia. There may be widening of QRS complex and increase of P-R interval.

**Self-Assessment Questions**

1. Hyperkalaemia can cause a flat or absent P wave on the ECG. True or false?
2. Hyperkalaemia can cause a wide QRS complex and peaked T waves on the ECG. True or false?
3. Hypercalcaemia can cause a shortened Q-T interval on the ECG. True or false?
4. S-T segment is isoelectric in hypercalcaemia. True or false?
5. ECG changes of hypomagnesaemia resemble that of hyperkalaemia. True or false?

6. **Electrolyte disturbances can cause major changes in the:**

   a. QRS complex  b. P-R interval  c. T wave  d. All of the above

7. **Hypokalaemia is associated with:**

   a. Prominent U waves  b. Peaked T waves  c. Tall R waves  d. Deep S waves

8. **Severe hypercalacaemia is sometimes associated with:**

   a. Prolonged Q-T interval  b. S-T segment elevation  c. Peaked T waves  d. Widened QRS complex

9. **Which electrolyte disturbance can cause Torsades de Pointes on the ECG?**

   a. Hypokalaemia  b. Hypercalcaemia  c. Hypomagnesaemia  d. Hyponatraemia

10. **Hypomagnesaemia can cause:**

    a. Prominent U waves  b. Peaked T waves  c. Shortened Q-T interval  d. S-T segment depression

**Case Studies**

1. A 55-year-old gentleman presented to emergency with history of uneasy feeling for last six hours. He gave history of suffering from hypertension, diabetes and dyslipidaemia. He was taking Enalapril and Telmisartan for control of blood pressure. He was on metformin and glimepiride for control of diabetes. His pulse rate was 80 bpm, regular and blood pressure was 130/90 mmHg. His 12-lead ECG is given in Fig. 22.14. Identify the abnormality. What is the treatment?

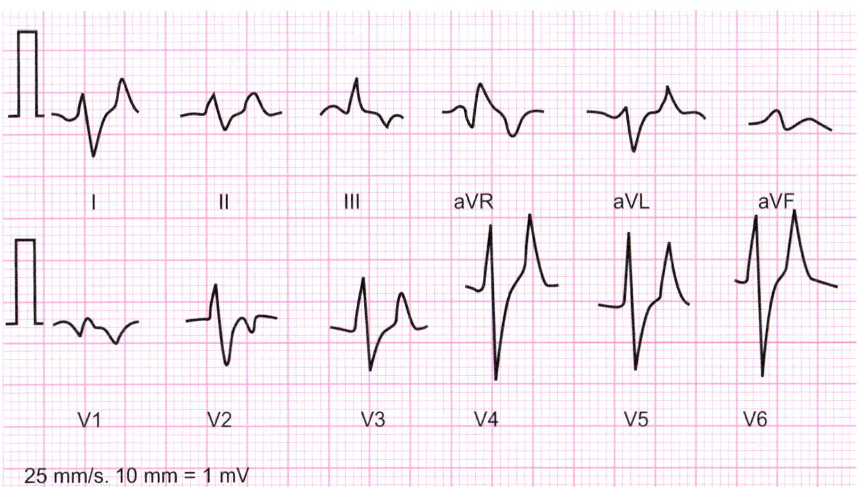


**Fig. 22.14** Identify the ECG abnormality

2. A 60-year-old lady presented with history of numbness and tingling in perioral area, fingers and toes for last five days. She also complained of backache. On examination, she did not seem to be in any apparent distress. Her blood pressure was 110/84 mmHg, pulse rate was 72 bpm, afebrile, heart sounds were normal and chest was clear. Her rhythm strip is given in Fig. 22.15. Identify the abnormality.
3. A 26-year-old lady presented with history of several bouts of watery diarrhoea and vomiting for past twenty four hours. On examination, her blood pressure was 100/60 mmHg, pulse rate was 100 bpm. Her rhythm strip is given in Fig. 22.16. Identify the abnormality.
4. A 57-year-old gentleman suffering from renal cell carcinoma presented with history of episodic abdominal pain, nausea and vomiting for last 3 months, backache and left knee pain, increased thirst, fatigue and lethargy. His rhythm strip is given in Fig. 22.17. What does the ECG show?
5. The rhythm strip in Fig. 22.18 is given for spot diagnosis in final year MBBS examination. What is your diagnosis?

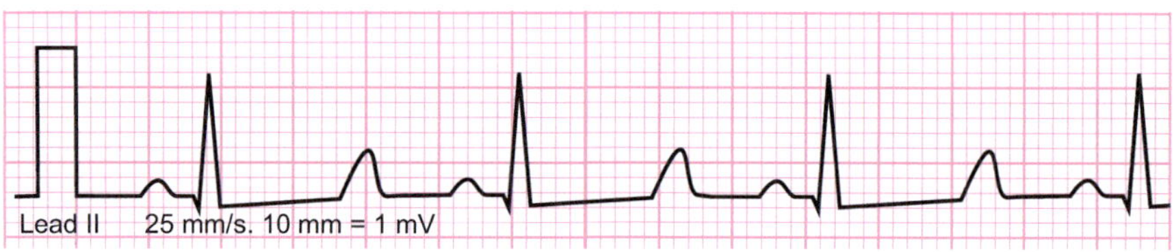


**Fig. 22.15** Identify the ECG abnormality

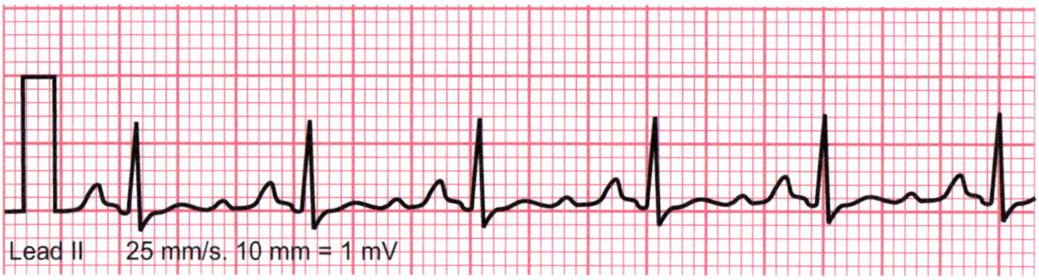


**Fig. 22.16** Identify the ECG abnormality

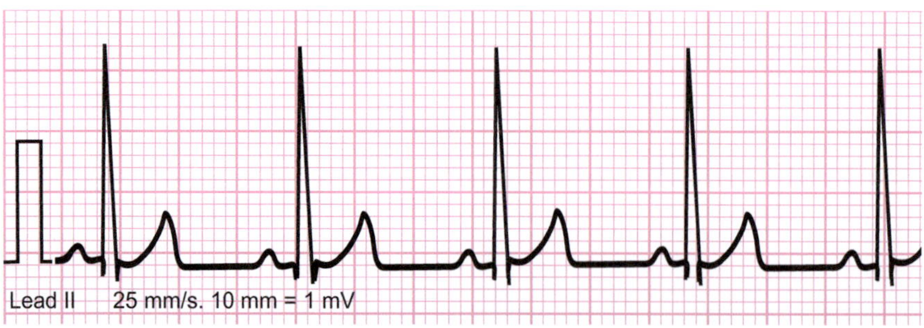


**Fig. 22.17** Analyse the rhythm strip

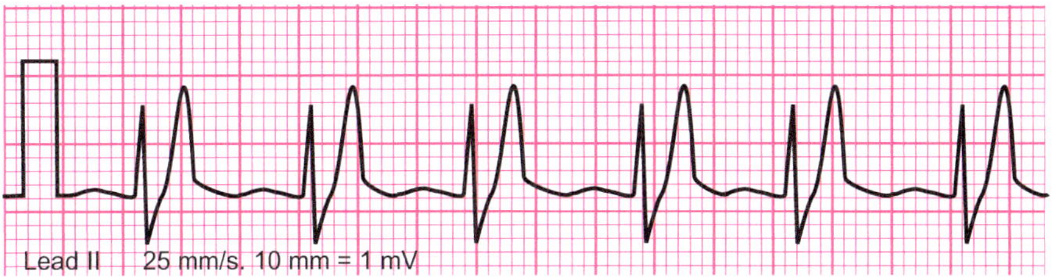


**Fig. 22.18** Analyse the rhythm strip

**Answers**

1. True 2. True 3. True 4. True 5. False 6. d 7. a 8. b 9. c 10. a

**Case Studies**

1. The ECG (Fig. 22.14) shows hyperkalaemia. There are tall and tented T waves in leads V4, V5 and V6. There is also widening of QRS complexes. If untreated, the P waves will disappear; there will be further widening of QRS complex and there may be sine wave appearance. Ventricular fibrillation and asystole may follow.

   This patient should be urgently given intravenous calcium to negate the cardiac toxicity. Glucose plus insulin intravenous drip should be started without delay to increase intracellular uptake of potassium, thereby reducing serum potassium. Cation exchange resin like sodium polystyrene sulfonate should be started later on. The combination of ACE inhibitor and ARB may cause hyperkalaemia, especially in presence of kidney dysfunction. Hence, kidney function should be assessed and this combination of antihypertensives should be stopped at the earliest.
2. The rhythm strip (Fig. 22.15) shows hypocalcaemia. There is Q-T interval prolongation. It is 0.52 s.

   Hypocalcaemia is commonly due to inadequate levels of vitamin D or parathyroid hormone or resistance to these hormones. Treatment is with oral calcium and vitamin D supplements. It is important to correct coexisting magnesium deficiency if any.

   In acute hypocalcaemia, intravenous calcium gluconate is given.
3. The ECG (Fig. 22.16) shows hypokalaemia. There is U wave which is bigger in amplitude as compared to the T wave. This signifies that these are not the normal U waves which are often seen in healthy people. The patient is suffering from acute gastroenteritis. There is loss of potassium in watery loose stool and vomiting.

   The patient should be started intravenous potassium infusion at a rate of 10–20 mEq every hour. If potassium level does not correct, look out for coexisting hypomagnesaemia. Treat acute gastroenteritis with IV fluids and antiemetics. Appropriate antibiotics may be started as early as possible if required.

4. The ECG (Fig. 22.17) shows hypercalcaemia. The Q-T interval is shortened. It is 0.28 s.

   Hypercalcaemia in an adult patient is usually due to either hyperparathyroidism or malignancy. This patient is suffering from hypercalcaemia most likely due to renal cell cancer. The treatment options for hypercalcaemia include IV hydration, calcitonin, bisphosphonates, denosumab, gallium nitrate, prednisone and haemodialysis.
5. The ECG (Fig. 22.18) shows hyperkalaemia. There are tall tented T waves that are diagnostic of hyperkalaemia.

# Chapter 23
# Digitalis Effect and Toxicity

**Learning Objectives**
After studying this chapter, the reader will learn about:

- Digitalis effect
- Digitalis toxicity

## 23.1 Digitalis Effect

Digitalis (digoxin) is one of the commonest drugs to produce changes in ECG. Digitalis is water soluble and is highly concentrated in the myocardium. It influences the repolarization of myocardium. The serum level of digitalis, at a standard dose, in which no toxicity is seen is 1.0–1.5 ng/mL. The ECG change produced at this level is called digitalis effect. The ECG changes are:

- S-T segment depression
- Decrease in magnitude of T wave
- Decrease in Q-T interval
- Prolongation of P-R interval

### *23.1.1 S-T Segment Depression*

The S-T segment is depressed. The J point remains at isoelectric level. After that the S-T segment slopes downwards with a sharp terminal rise and blends with the T wave. This produces the mirror image of a correction mark or reverse check sign (Figs. 23.1, 23.2, 23.3 and 23.4). The depression of S-T segment has also been



T. K. Koley, *Rapid Review of ECG*,
https://doi.org/10.1007/978-981-99-9116-7_23

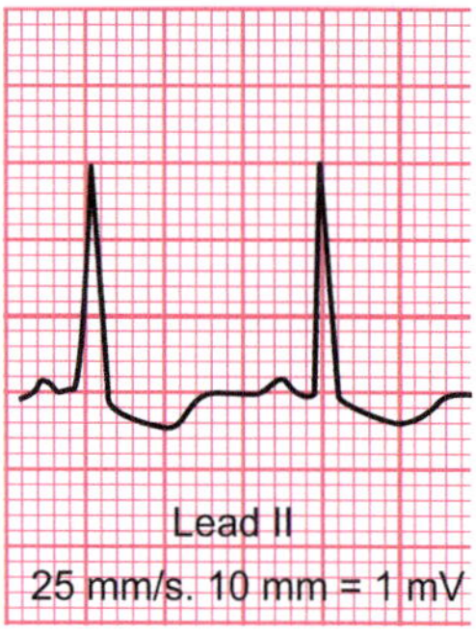


**Fig. 23.1** Digitalis effect

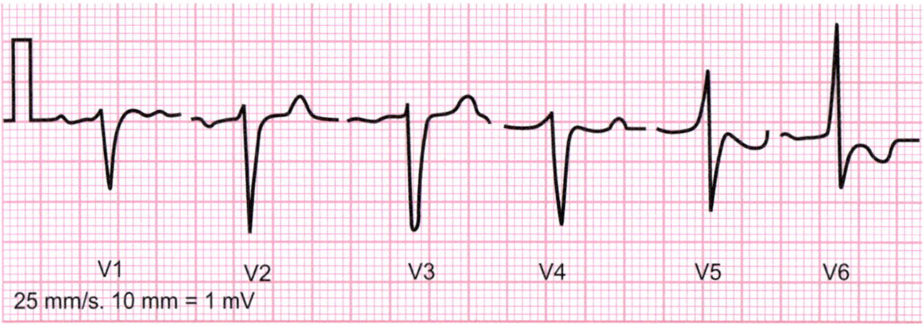


**Fig. 23.2** Digitalis effect. Note the reverse check sign in leads V5 and V6

described as a scooped S-T segment depression. The S-T segment often has a scooped configuration also. If the J point is also depressed, it indicates digitalis toxicity. This change is mainly seen in the leads with the tall R waves, i.e. the epicardial leads. If this change is also seen in leads with dominantly negative QRS complex, then it may be a sign of digitalis toxicity.

### 23.1.2 Decrease in Magnitude of T Wave

In digitalis effect, the T wave is slightly diminished in magnitude but the direction remains unchanged. Along with a depressed S-T segment often the T wave seems to be dragged down. In digitalis toxicity, the amplitude of T wave is decreased and often it is inverted. However, it should be kept in mind that the T wave may be inverted due to preexisting coronary artery disease. In digitalis effect, the T wave is depressed and rises above the baseline before becoming isoelectric, but in digitalis toxicity, the T wave does not rise above the baseline. See Fig. 23.4. Sometimes digitalis may cause slight increase in amplitude of U wave.

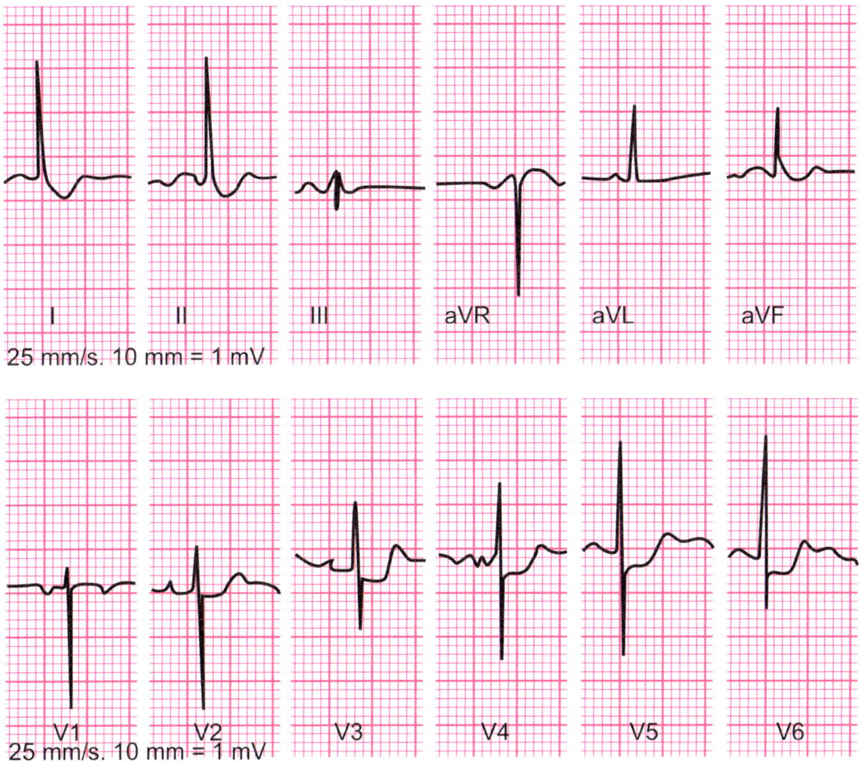


**Fig. 23.3** Digitalis effect. Note the reverse check sign best seen in leads I, II and note the terminal positivity of the inverted T wave in leads II, V3 to V6

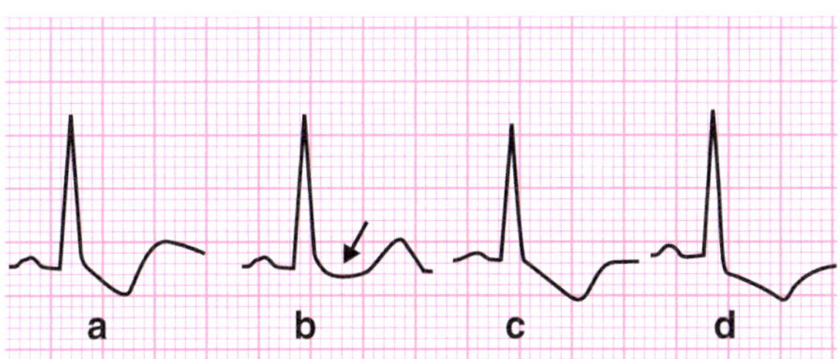


**Fig. 23.4** Diagrams of digitalis toxicity and digitalis effect. (A) Reverse check sign. Note the terminal positivity of the T wave. (B) Scooped S-T segment. The depressed S-T segment is shown with an arrow. (C) Digitalis toxicity. Note that the terminal part of the T wave does not rise above the baseline. (D) Digitalis toxicity. Note that the terminal part of the T wave does not rise above the baseline. The J point is also depressed. It can also be due to primary T wave abnormality due to coronary artery disease

### *23.1.3 Decrease in Q-T Interval*

Digitalis decreases the duration of electrical systole. The Q-T interval is shortened in digitalis effect because the refractory period of ventricular myocardium is shortened. This change is seen early during digitalization and does not represent digitalis toxicity. The refractory period of atrial myocardium is also shortened, but it is difficult to measure directly. It is however important to remember that digitalis increases the refractory period of SA and AV node.

### *23.1.4 Prolongation of P-R Interval*

Digitalis causes vagal stimulation which reduces AV conduction. As a result, the P-R interval is prolonged within the range of 0.02–0.30 s. It also slows down the ventricular rate.

**Tips and Tricks**

- Look for reverse check sign and scooped S-T segment to diagnose digitalis effect.

## 23.2 Digitalis Toxicity

The serum level of digitalis is usually more than 2–3 ng/mL when the features of digitalis toxicity appear in the ECG. Hypokalaemia due to diuretic therapy is one of the most common factors that precipitates digitalis toxicity. The various ECG changes are:

### *23.2.1 S-T Segment Depression*

There is downsloping S-T segment depression like digitalis effect, but along with it there is depression of the J point also and there is no terminal positivity of the inverted T wave (Fig. 23.5). The T wave does not rise above the baseline.

### *23.2.2 Cardiac Arrhythmia*

Almost any type of cardiac arrhythmia is seen in digitalis toxicity. The arrhythmias commonly seen are sinus bradycardia, first-degree AV block, ventricular extrasystoles (uniform and multiform) and ventricular bigeminy. Wenckebach type of block may be seen. Complete heart block, SA block, AV dissociation, AV junctional

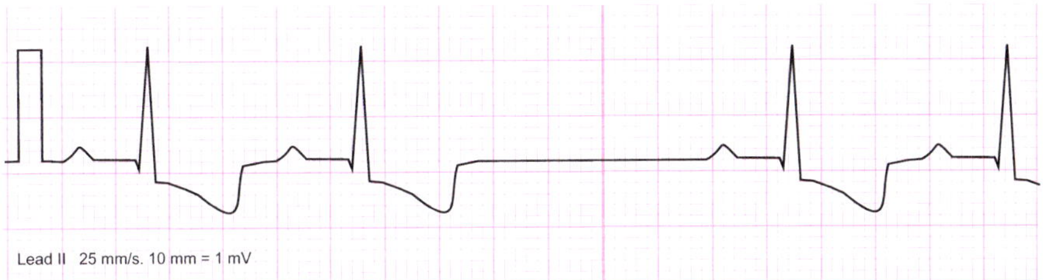


**Fig. 23.5** Digitalis toxicity. There is S-T segment depression with reverse check sign. The J point is depressed with T wave inversion. The terminal part of T wave does not rise above the baseline. There is pronged P-R interval (0.28 s) and the third PQRST complex is missing indicating SA block

rhythm and ventricular fibrillation may be observed sometimes. Nonparoxysmal atrial tachycardia with variable AV block is characteristic of digitalis toxicity. Atrial flutter, atrial fibrillation and Mobitz type II second degree AV block are the least likely of all the arrhythmias to be caused by digoxin toxicity. The various ECG changes in digitalis toxicity are summarized in Box 23.1.

**Box 23.1 Changes in Digitalis Toxicity**

S-T segment depression (including J point depression)
T wave inversion
Sinus bradycardia
Uniform or multiform ventricular extrasystoles
Ventricular tachycardia, flutter and fibrillation
Paroxysmal atrial tachycardia
SA block
Bundle branch block
First, second and third degree AV block
Atrial flutter and fibrillation

Digitalis toxicity is manifested by anorexia, nausea, vomiting, yellow vision, etc. The toxicity commonly occurs because of a narrow therapeutic window. Toxicity is seen when serum level exceeds 2 ng/mL. Coadministration of quinidine, verapamil, amiodarone and propafenone predisposes to toxicity.

### Tips and Tricks

- If you find S-T segment downsloping depression with depression of J point and T wave inversion think of digitalis toxicity.
- If you find S-T segment depression with T wave inversion always rule out myocardial ischaemia before considering it a case of digitalis toxicity.

### Self-Assessment Questions

1. Digitalis toxicity can result in a characteristic scooped S-T segment depression in the ECG. True or false?

2. Digitalis effect is commonly associated with an increased risk of atrial fibrillation in the ECG. True or false?
3. Digoxin toxicity may cause ventricular tachycardia on the ECG. True or false?
4. Digitalis toxicity is precipitated by hyperkalaemia. True or false?
5. **Which of the following ECG findings is typically associated with chronic digitalis use?**

   a. Bradycardia b. S-T segment depression c. Presence of J waves d. Atrioventricular block

6. **Which of the following is seen in an ECG in patients with digitalis effect?**

   a. Prolonged Q-T interval b. Mild prolongation of P-R interval c. Increased QRS complex duration d. Elevated S-T segment

7. **Which ECG abnormality is commonly observed in patients with digoxin toxicity?**

   a. Sinus bradycardia b. Sinus tachycardia c. Ventricular fibrillation d. Normal sinus rhythm

8. **The ECG finding of digitalis toxicity can mimic which cardiac condition?**

   a. Ventricular septal defect b. Brugada syndrome c. Wolff-Parkinson-White syndrome d. Acute myocardial ischaemia

9. **Digoxin effect can result in the appearance of "reversed tick" or "Salvador Dali" sign, which is characterized by:**

   a. Biphasic T waves b. Peaked T waves c. S-T segment depression d. Absent T waves

10. **Digoxin intoxication may lead to:**

    a. Ventricular bigeminy b. AV junctional rhythm c. Sinus node depression d. All of the above

**Case Studies**

1. A 63-year-old gentleman was prescribed some medicine and was taking it for past five years. Previously, he was taking it once daily but for last six months he had been taking it twice daily by mistake. Now he complains of nausea, vomiting and yellow vision. He had two rhythm strips with him. One strip was recorded 2 years back (Fig. 23.6) and another was recorded 5 days back (Fig. 23.7). Examine both the rhythm strips and make your diagnosis.
2. Examine the rhythm strip given in Fig. 23.8. Identify it.

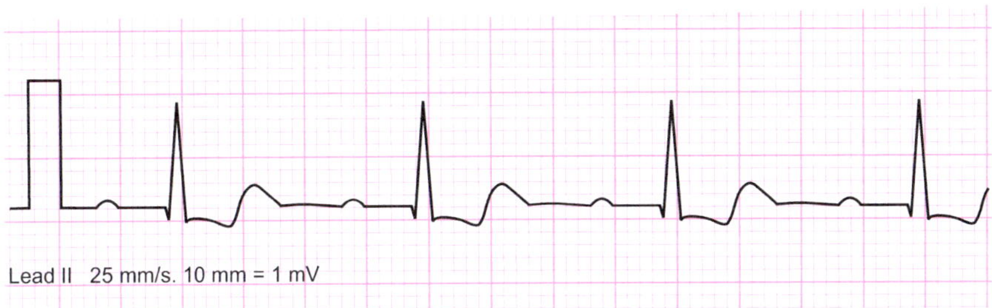


**Fig. 23.6** Rhythm strip recorded 2 years back

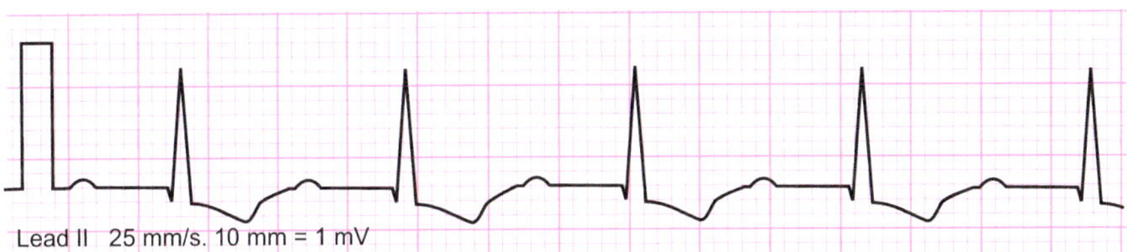


**Fig. 23.7** Rhythm strip recorded 5 days back

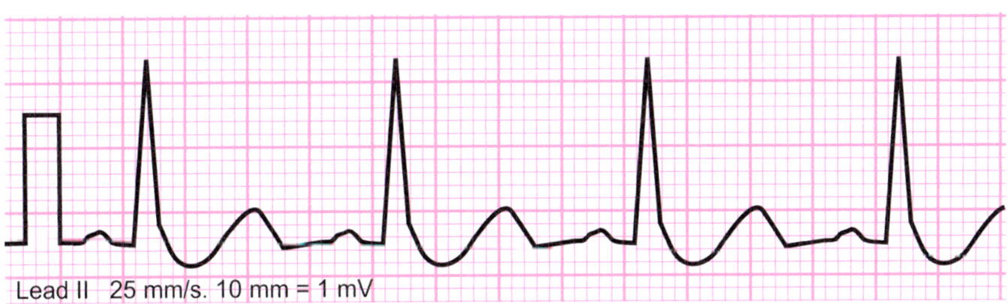


**Fig. 23.8** Analyse the rhythm strip

**Answers**

1. True 2. False 3. True 4. False 5. b 6. b 7. a 8. d 9. c 10. d

**Case Studies**

1. The patient has complained of nausea, vomiting and yellow vision. This indicates that most likely the patient was taking digitalis. The rhythm strip in Fig. 23.6 shows digitalis effect. There is reverse check sign of downsloping S-T segment depression. The T wave rises above the baseline. The P-R interval is 0.22 s.

The rhythm strip of the same patient in Fig. 23.7 shows digitalis toxicity. The J point is depressed below the baseline. The S-T segment is depressed like a reverse check sign but the T wave does not rise above the base line. Besides this the P-R interval is 0.28 s.

This patient was taking digitalis in appropriate dose which is reflected in the first rhythm strip. However, he took double dose of digitalis that led to digitalis toxicity. This patient was probably also taking loop diuretics due to heart failure. Loop diuretics cause hypokalaemia and hypokalaemia precipitates digitalis toxicity. Hence, hypokalaemia should be ruled out in this patient and if detected should be corrected. However, one must remember that the major electrolyte disturbance in acute digoxin toxicity is hyperkalaemia.

Treatment with digoxin immune Fab is considered first-line therapy for dysrhythmias including AV block and ventricular tachycardia caused by suspected digoxin toxicity.

2. The rhythm strip (Fig. 23.8) shows scooping S-T segment depression and the T wave rises above the baseline. Most likely it is due to digitalis effect.

# Chapter 24
# ECG in Miscellaneous Heart Diseases

**Learning Objectives**
After studying this chapter, the reader will learn about:

- Valvular heart disease
- Acute rheumatic carditis
- Pericardial disease
- Congenital heart disease
- Miscellaneous conditions

## 24.1 Valvular Heart Disease

Rheumatic heart disease is still common in many parts of the world. Rheumatic carditis and resultant valvular heart disease can both lead to notable changes in an ECG, aiding in their diagnosis and management. Rheumatic carditis, a consequence of rheumatic fever, may present with prolonged P-R intervals, S-T, T wave abnormalities and atrial fibrillation. Valvular heart disease, such as aortic stenosis or regurgitation, mitral stenosis or regurgitation and tricuspid regurgitation can exhibit distinct ECG findings. Valvular diseases can cause both structural and functional changes in the heart. These include left ventricular hypertrophy, left or right atrial enlargement, repolarization abnormalities and various P wave abnormalities. Accurate interpretation of ECG changes in rheumatic carditis and valvular heart disease plays a pivotal role in identifying these conditions, guiding treatment decisions and monitoring patient progress.


T. K. Koley, *Rapid Review of ECG*,
https://doi.org/10.1007/978-981-99-9116-7_24

### 24.1.1 Mitral Stenosis

Mitral stenosis is usually of rheumatic origin. There is left atrial and right ventricular hypertrophy (Figs. 24.1 and 24.2). In long standing cases, there is right atrial enlargement. Pulmonary hypertension is commonly observed in these patients. They often suffer from atrial fibrillation. The various ECG manifestations of mitral stenosis are:

- P mitrale in lead II and biphasic P wave in lead V1
- P pulmonale is present in mitral stenosis with pulmonary artery hypertension
- Features of RVH (R:S ratio > 1 in lead V1 with S-T segment, T wave change)
- Right axis deviation
- Presence of atrial fibrillation (absence of P wave with varying R-R interval)

### 24.1.2 Mitral Regurgitation

Mitral regurgitation is due to several causes like rheumatic heart disease, dilated cardiomyopathy, mitral valve prolapse, etc. There is left ventricular and left atrial hypertrophy. Pulmonary hypertension is usually absent. Atrial fibrillation may be seen. The ECG manifestations are:

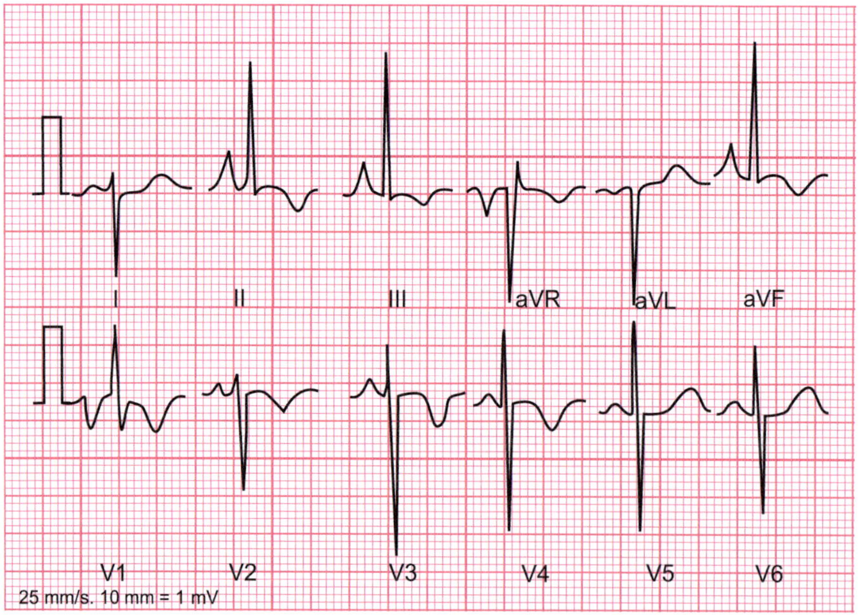


**Fig. 24.1** Mitral stenosis

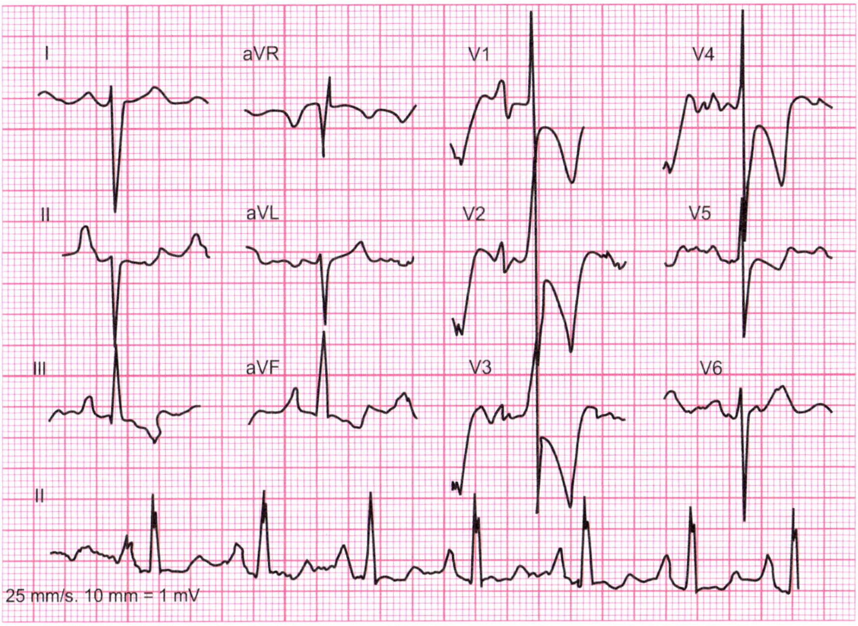


**Fig. 24.2** Mitral stenosis. This ECG is recorded from a 17-year-old boy suffering from pure mitral stenosis. Note the tall R waves in lead V1 with small S waves and S-T segment, T wave changes suggestive of gross RVH. Note the biphasic P wave in leads V1 and V2 and tall P wave in lead II. Also note the widening of P wave in lead I

- Left atrial enlargement (deep and prominent negative component of biphasic P wave in lead V1)
- Left ventricular hypertrophy due to diastolic overload (S in lead V1 plus R in lead V5 or V6 is >35 mm, with S-T segment, T wave change in lead V5 or V6)
- Normal QRS axis
- Atrial fibrillation (absence of P wave with varying R-R interval)

### *24.1.3 Aortic Stenosis*

In aortic stenosis, there is concentric hypertrophy of left ventricle. There is systolic overload of the left ventricle. The ECG features are:

- Left ventricular hypertrophy (S in lead V1 plus R in lead V5 or V6 is >35 mm, with S-T segment, T wave change in lead V5 or V6)
- Normal QRS axis
- Incomplete left bundle branch block (rSr' complex in lead V5 or V6 with QRS duration <0.12 s)
- Left atrial enlargement
- Inversion of U wave

### *24.1.4 Aortic Regurgitation*

Aortic regurgitation is often of rheumatic origin. There is volume overload of the left ventricle. There is gross hypertrophy of the left ventricle. The left atrium is also enlarged. The ECG manifestations are:

- Left ventricular hypertrophy (diastolic overload pattern)
- Left atrial enlargement
- Usually normal QRS axis, sometimes left anterior hemiblock may be seen
- Sometimes inversion of U wave is seen

### *24.1.5 Acute Rheumatic Carditis*

Acute rheumatic carditis occurs during acute rheumatic fever. Myocardium, pericardium and the endocardium are involved. The ECG manifestations of acute rheumatic carditis are:

- Prolonged P-R interval
- Sinus tachycardia
- Features of acute pericarditis
- Features of acute myocarditis

  (a) Depression or elevation of S-T segment
  (b) Notching or slurring of QRS complex
  (c) Non-specific T wave changes
  (d) Prolonged Q-Tc interval

## 24.2 Pericardial Diseases

Pericardial diseases can give rise to characteristic ECG changes that aid in their diagnosis and management. Pericarditis and pericardial effusion are common clinical condition where ECG plays a major role in making a diagnosis.

### *24.2.1 Pericarditis*

Pericarditis may be of viral or bacterial origin. Tuberculous pericarditis is also very common. It is often associated with pericardial effusion. Uraemia is also an important cause of pericarditis. Acute pericarditis is diagnosed by the following ECG features:

- Sinus tachycardia
- S-T segment elevation with upward concavity in leads oriented towards the affected surface (Fig. 24.3)
- T wave inversion (this occurs after S-T segment becomes isoelectric)
- Sometimes depression of P-R segment is seen

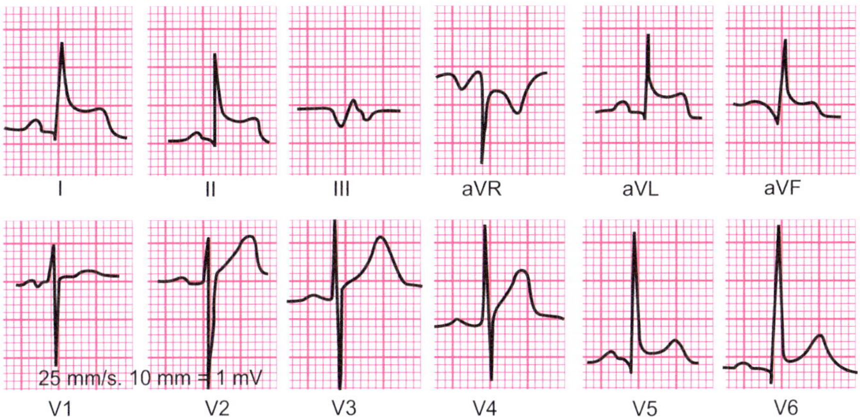


**Fig. 24.3** Acute pericarditis

### *24.2.2 Pericardial Effusion*

There are several causes of pericardial effusion. Tuberculosis, uraemia, viral pericarditis are some of the common causes. There is collection of fluid in the pericardial sac that compresses the heart often leading to cardiac tamponade. The ECG features of pericardial effusion are:

- Low voltage complex, i.e. less than 5 mm amplitude in standard leads and less than 10 mm amplitude in chest leads (Figs. 24.4 and 24.5)
- T wave inversion in most of the leads except aVR
- Electrical alternans (alternating low and normal voltage QRS complexes)

## 24.3 Congenital Heart Disease

Congenital heart disease (CHD) encompasses a broad range of structural abnormalities in the heart present at birth. ECG changes can provide valuable insights into the presence and severity of CHD. ASD, VSD and Fallot's tetralogy are some of the common CHDs that we come across in day-to-day clinical practice. The structural deformities and the functional changes due to CHDs produce numerous changes in the ECG including abnormalities in P wave, QRS complex and QRS axis. These ECG findings, combined with clinical evaluation, aid in diagnosing and managing individuals with CHD, facilitating timely intervention when necessary.

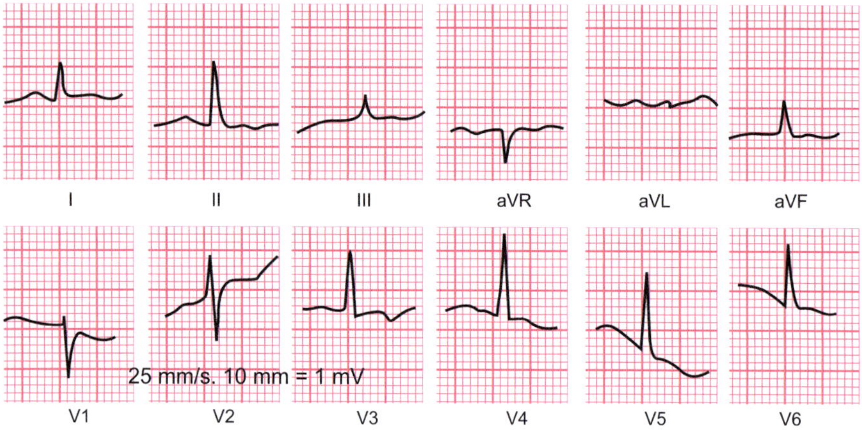


**Fig. 24.4** Pericardial effusion

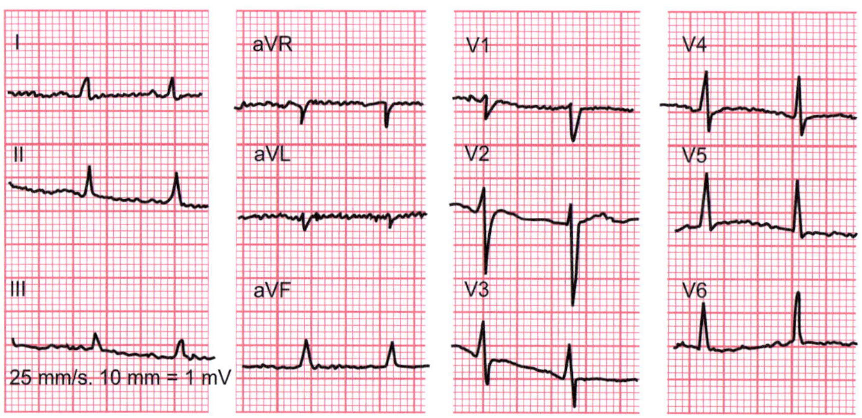


**Fig. 24.5** Pericardial effusion. This ECG is recorded from a 45-year-old gentleman suffering from tubercular pleural effusion. Note the low voltage complexes with sinus tachycardia

## *24.3.1 Atrial Septal Defect*

Atrial septal defect (ASD) is of two types: ostium secundum type and ostium primum type. Ostium secundum defect is not associated with any malformation of the AV canal. In this defect, there is volume overload of right atrium and right ventricle (Figs. 24.6 and 24.7). The ECG features of ostium secundum type of ASD are the following:

- rsR' complex in lead V1 with biphasic P wave
- Right axis deviation
- Right atrial enlargement
- Decrease in amplitude of R wave in leads V5 and V6
- Atrial fibrillation and atrial flutter may be observed
- Clockwise electric rotation: The transition zone is shifted to lead V5 or V6

Ostium primum defect is often associated malformation of atrioventricular canal. The ECG features of ostium primum type of ASD are:

- rsR' complex in lead V1
- Left axis deviation

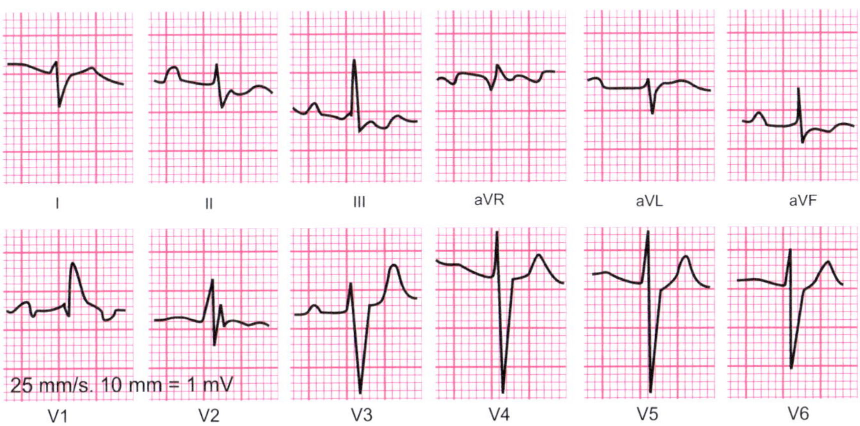


**Fig. 24.6** Atrial septal defect

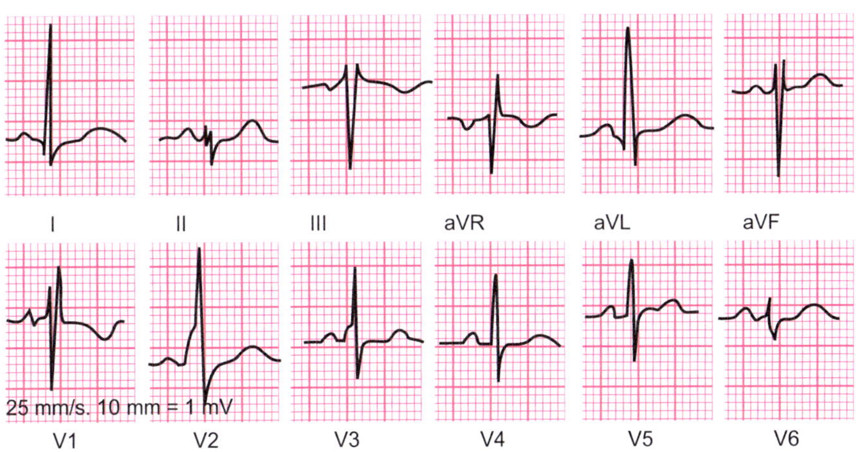


**Fig. 24.7** Atrial septal defect

- First degree AV block
- Atrial arrhythmias

### 24.3.2 *Ventricular Septal Defect*

The ventricular septum is made up of a membranous part and a muscular part. Most of the defects lie in the membranous part of the interventricular septum. The muscular part is rarely affected. There is left to right shunt. There is volume overloading of the left atrium and the left ventricle. Due to gradual increase in the pulmonary resistance, there is increase in right ventricular pressure, i.e. systolic overload. In later stage, there may be reversal of shunt resulting in Eisenmenger complex. The ECG features of VSD are the following:

- Features of left ventricular hypertrophy or combined left and right ventricular hypertrophy
- Large amplitude equiphasic QRS deflections in leads V2, V3 and V4 (Fig. 24.8)
- Prominent q waves in leads II, III and aVF
- QRS axis is normal but with development of pulmonary hypertension there may be right axis deviation

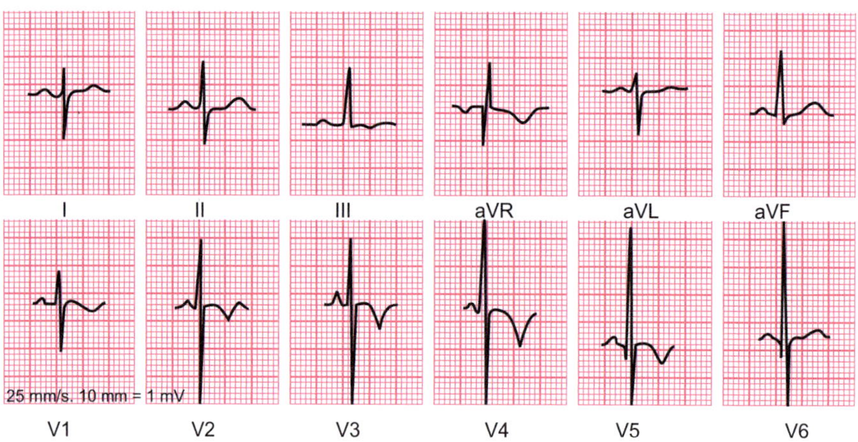


**Fig. 24.8** Ventricular septal defect

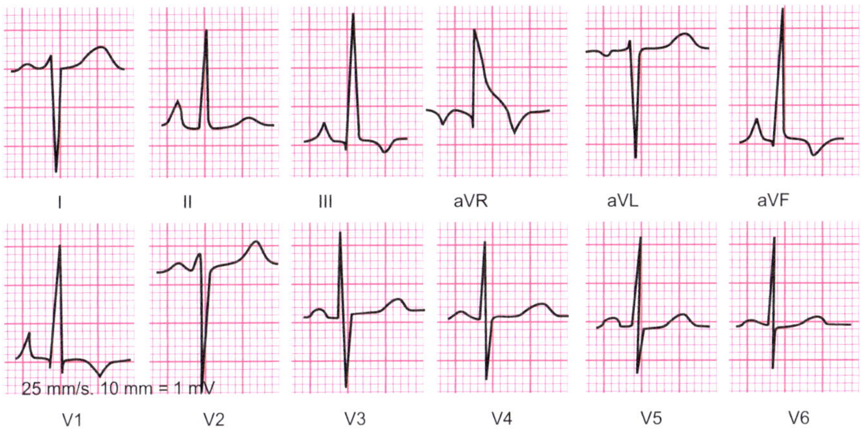


**Fig. 24.9** Fallot's tetralogy

### *24.3.3 Fallot's Tetralogy*

Fallot's tetralogy is the commonest congenital cyanotic heart disease in the adults. The four defects in the heart are a) infundibular pulmonary stenosis, b) dextroposition of aorta, c) ventricular septal defect, d) right ventricular hypertrophy. The ECG features of Fallot's tetralogy are:

- Right ventricular hypertrophy due to systolic overload (Fig. 24.9)
- Tall and peaked P waves in lead II due to right atrial enlargement

### *24.3.4 Pentalogy of Fallot*

In this rare condition, there are all the features of tetralogy along with ostium secundum ASD. There is volume overloading of left atrium and left ventricle. Thus, there is enlargement of all the cardiac chambers. The ECG features consist of right atrial enlargement with right ventricular hypertrophy (systolic overload) and mild left ventricular hypertrophy (diastolic overload).

### *24.3.5 Trilogy of Fallot*

Trilogy of Fallot is pulmonary stenosis (valvular) with any of the following types of interatrial septal defect: (a) patent foramen ovale, (b) ostium secundum ASD, (c) ostium primum ASD. The ECG features are:

- Right atrial hypertrophy
- Right ventricular hypertrophy due to systolic overload
- Possible left atrial and left ventricular hypertrophy

## 24.4 Miscellaneous Conditions

### *24.4.1 Preexcitation Syndrome (WPW Syndrome)*

Wolff–Parkinson–White syndrome (WPW) is the prototype of preexcitation syndrome. This electrocardiographic syndrome is mainly due to an anomalous atrioventricular pathway or the accessory pathway (Fig. 24.10). This pathway is of congenital origin and bypasses the AV node. This accessory pathway is known as Bundle of Kent. WPW syndrome is commonly associated with Ebstein's anomaly and hypertrophic cardiomyopathy.

The ECG of WPW syndrome has the following features:

- Short P-R interval (< 0.12 s)
- Widened QRS complex (> 0.12 s)
- Delta wave: This is the slurred upstroke of QRS complex (Figs. 24.11 and 24.12)
- Secondary S-T segment, T wave change

Depending upon the location of the accessory pathway in relation to the SA node and the relative transmission characteristics of the accessory pathway and the AV node, the morphology of the ECG may vary from a classic presentation to near normal.

The treatment of preexcitation is mainly removal of the accessory pathway. The pathway is detected precisely by electrophysiological studies and then it is removed by radio frequency catheter ablation (Fig. 24.13).

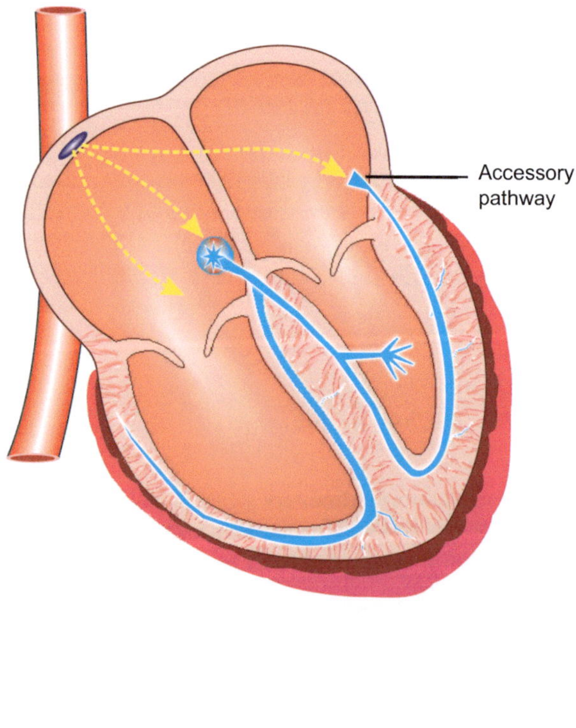


**Fig. 24.10** The accessory pathway

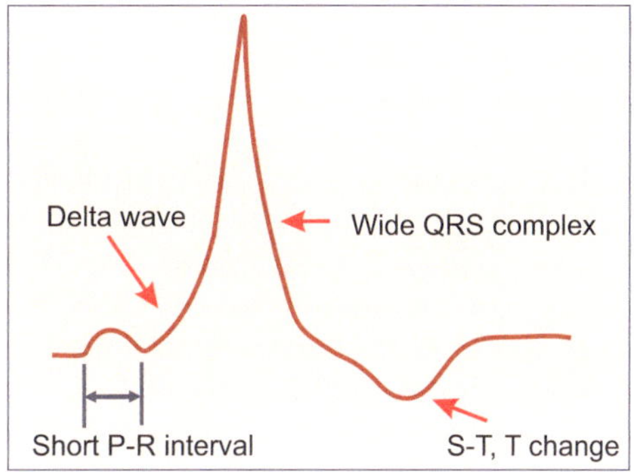


**Fig. 24.11** WPW syndrome. Note the delta wave, short P-R interval, wide QRS complex and the accompanying S-T segment, T wave change

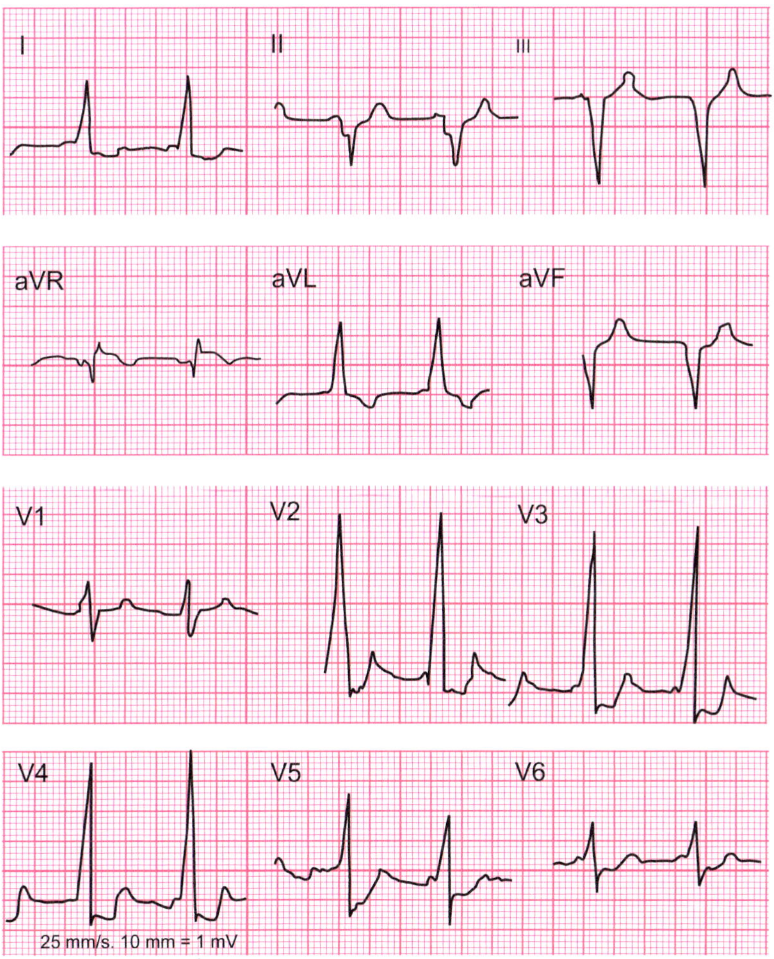


**Fig. 24.12** WPW syndrome. This ECG is taken from a 40-year-old gentleman who presented with PSVT. After termination of PSVT, the ECG revealed WPW syndrome. Note the wide QRS complexes with delta waves and short P-R interval

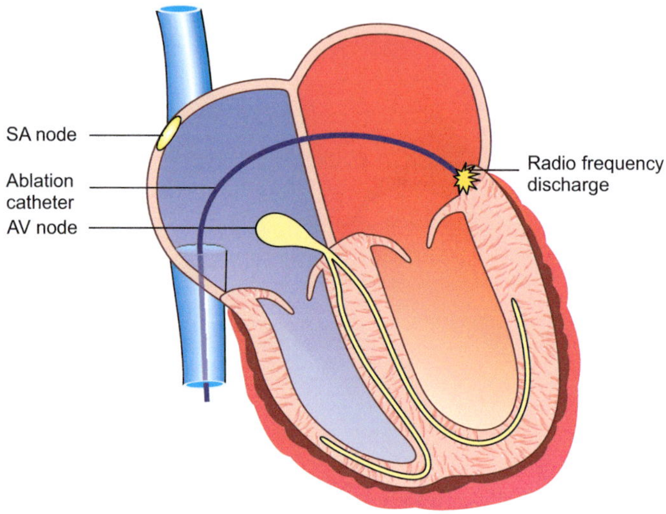


**Fig. 24.13** Radiofrequency catheter ablation of bypass tract

### *24.4.2 Myocarditis*

Myocarditis is acute infection of the myocardium. Almost any acute infectious disease may involve the myocardium. Myocarditis may be due to viral or bacterial origin. It is very frequently a part of rheumatic fever. The ECG features are:

- S-T segment, T wave changes in chest leads
- First-degree heart block or defective intraventricular conduction
- Prolongation of Q-Tc interval
- Various types of arrhythmias
- QRS abnormalities that may mimic myocardial infarction

### *24.4.3 Cardiac Trauma*

ECG changes may be seen in both penetrating and non-penetrating cardiac trauma. The ECG abnormalities may be the following:

- Various types of arrhythmias
- Non-specific S-T segment, T wave changes
- Features similar to pericarditis
- Changes of myocardial infarction

### 24.4.4 Cardiac Malignancy

Primary cardiac malignancy is rare but metastasis to heart is not uncommon. Cardiac malignancy is often not diagnosed in life. The ECG features of cardiac malignancy are the following:

- Atrial or ventricular arrhythmias
- Features similar to pericarditis
- Features similar to myocardial infarction

### 24.4.5 Hypertrophic Cardiomyopathy

Hypertrophic cardiomyopathy (HOCM) is characterized by asymmetric hypertrophy of the left ventricle. The interventricular septum is markedly hypertrophied. The ECG features are the following:

- Features of LVH and rarely of RVH. Due to septal hypertrophy, there are deep and narrow Q waves in left and inferior oriented leads (Fig. 24.14).
- Intraventricular conduction defects in the form of bundle branch block or LAHB.
- Enlargement of left and/or right atrium.
- Prolongation of P-R and Q-Tc interval.
- Cardiac arrhythmias.

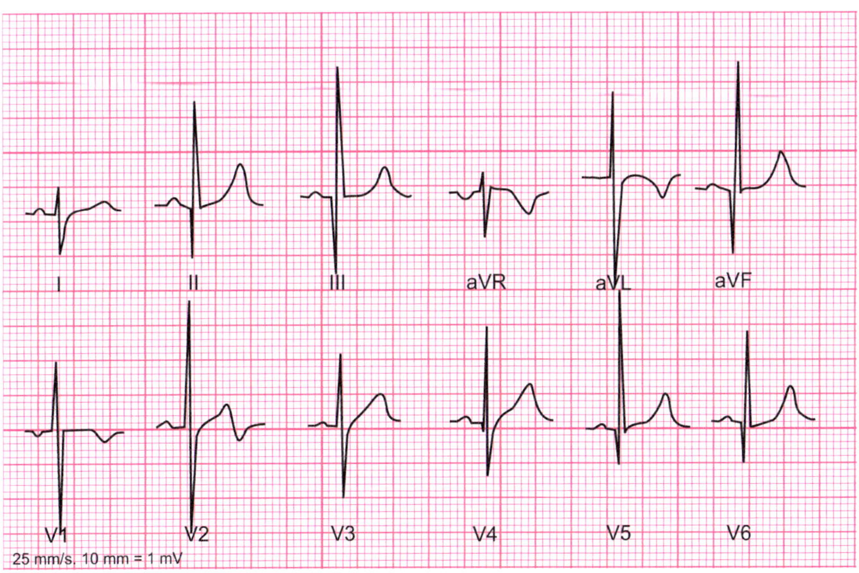


**Fig. 24.14** HOCM. The ECG shows evidence of LVH in precordial as well as limb leads. There are deep dagger shaped narrow Q waves in leads II, III, aVF and leads V5 and lead V6

### 24.4.6 Parasystole

Parasystole is a type of dual rhythm where two pacemakers together but independent of each other govern the rhythm of the heart. In normal condition, the sinus pacemaker that is the SA node controls the heart rhythm. The sinus pacemaker prematurely discharges all the other slower and subsidiary pacemakers. Thus, it can be said that the sinus pacemaker dominates over the other potential pacemakers. However, in some cases the subsidiary pacemakers develop the property to protect themselves from the effect of the sinus or other dominant pacemaker and they are not affected by the dominant pacemaker. In those conditions, the two pacemakers together but independent of each other govern the rhythm of the heart and this is known as parasystole. The commonest parasystole is ventricular parasystole. The ECG features are:

- Varying coupling interval. It is the interval between the ventricular ectopic beat and the preceding sinus beat. In simple ventricular extrasystoles, the coupling intervals are constant, but in parasystole they vary.
- The intervals between ectopic beats are in multiples of shortest interectopic interval.
- Fusion beats.

### 24.4.7 Dextrocardia

Dextrocardia is congenital malposition of heart. The left ventricle and left atrium are present in the right side of right ventricle and right atrium. The right atrium is on the left side and the aortic knob is on the right side. The ECG features of dextrocardia are the following:

- Inverted P waves in leads I and aVL.
- QRS complexes are upright in leads II, III and aVF.
- QRS complexes are negative in leads I and aVL.
- The P, QRS and T waves in aVL resemble that of aVR and vice versa (Fig. 24.15).
- R wave is prominent in lead V1 and the height of R wave gradually diminishes in lead V6, because the lead V1 overlies left ventricle and lead V6 overlies right ventricle.
- The P, QRS and T waves in leads V4R and V5R resemble that of leads V4 and V5.
- The QRS axis is the mirror image of the normal QRS axis (+60°), i.e. +120°.

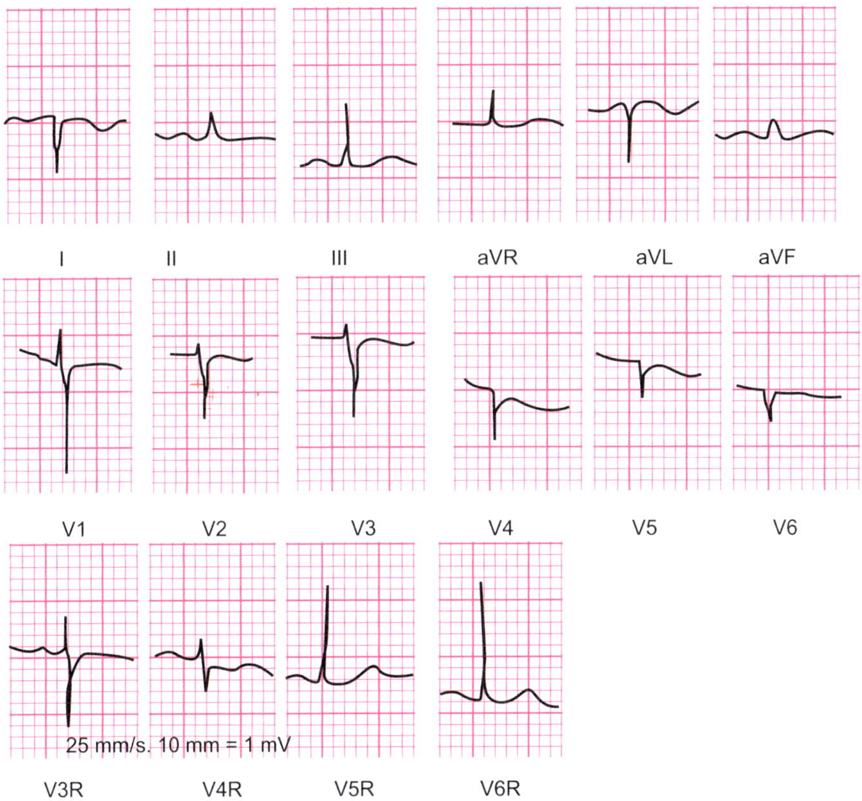


**Fig. 24.15** Dextrocardia. Note the negative complexes in lead aVL and positive complexes in lead aVR

## *24.4.8 Dextroversion*

Dextroversion is congenital malposition of heart. The heart is displaced to right and the ventricles are rotated in counterclockwise direction. The ventricles and the atria are not transposed. The aorta is in normal position. QRS vector is directed more anteriorly because of counterclockwise rotation of heart. The T wave is inverted in lead I (Fig. 24.16).

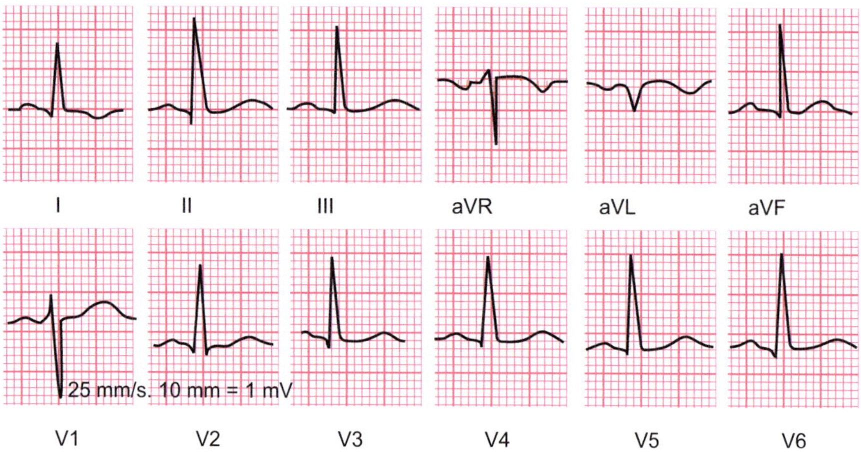


**Fig. 24.16** Dextroversion

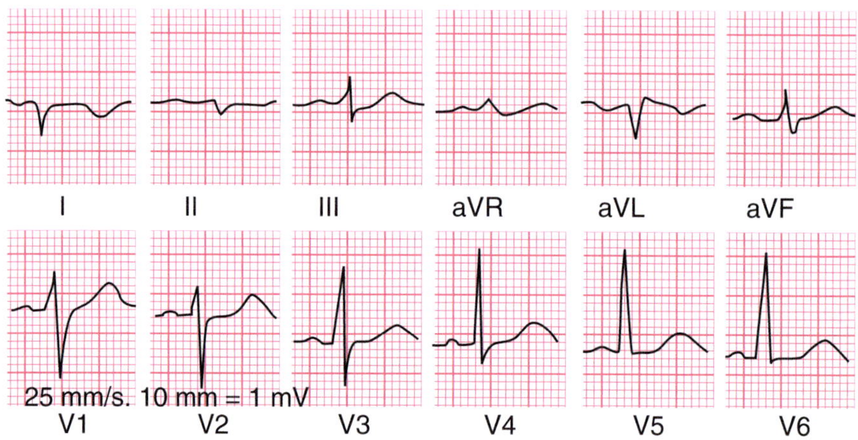


**Fig. 24.17** Technical dextrocardia

### *24.4.9 Technical Dextrocardia*

Technical dextrocardia is the term used when ECG is recorded by mistake in which the right and the left arm electrodes are interchanged with each other. There are features of dextrocardia in limb leads (Fig. 24.17). The recordings in chest leads are normal.

### 24.4.10 *Brugada Syndrome*

Brugada syndrome is an inherited, rare, life threatening disease that predisposes to fatal cardiac arrhythmias. It is more common in males than females. It is often responsible for sudden cardiac death. The main ECG features are:

- Right bundle branch block
- S-T segment elevation in leads V1–V3

Three different ECG patterns have been described in Brugada syndrome patients:

- Type 1: Coved S-T segment elevations greater than 2 mm accompanied with an inverted T wave (Fig. 24.18)
- Type 2: Saddleback-shaped S-T segment elevation greater than 2 mm
- Type 3: Saddle-back shaped S-T segment elevations less than 2 mm

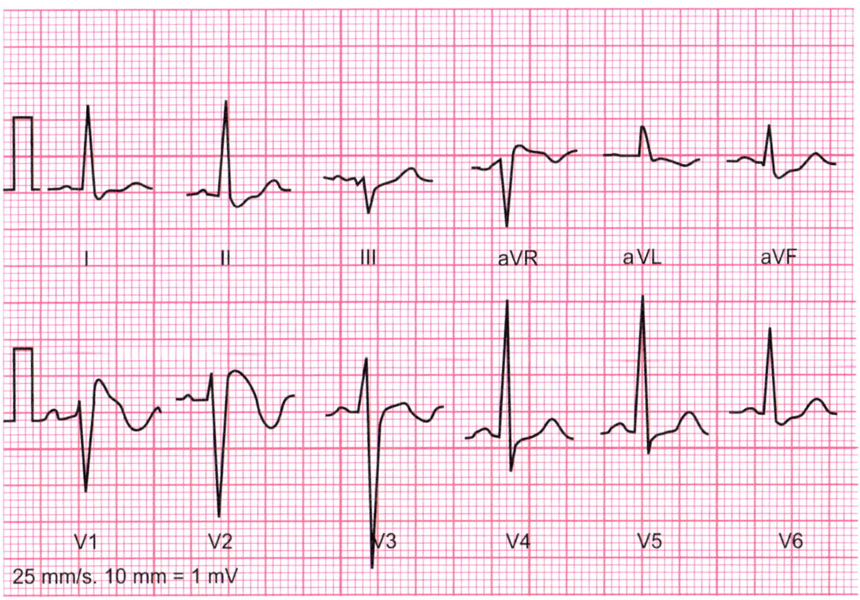


**Fig. 24.18** Brugada syndrome. Coved S-T segment elevation >2 mm in leads V1–V3 followed by a negative T wave

**Tips and Tricks**

- If you find P mitrale, suspect mitral stenosis.
- If you find concave upwards S-T segment elevation, think of acute pericarditis.
- If you find electric alternans, think of pericardial effusion.
- If you find rSR' complex in lead V1 with right axis deviation, think of ostium secundum ASD.
- If you detect short P-R interval, think of WPW syndrome. Next you should look for presence of delta wave.
- If you find QRS complex negative in aVL and positive in lead aVF, think of dextrocardia.
- If you find coved S-T segment elevation in leads V1–V3 with T wave inversion, think of the possibility of Brugada syndrome.

**Self-Assessment Questions**

1. Mitral stenosis is typically associated with a wide and notched P wave on the ECG. True or false?
2. Pericardial effusion can lead to low voltage QRS complexes on the ECG. True or false?
3. Rheumatic heart disease can cause a prolonged P-R interval and sinus tachycardia on the ECG. True or false?
4. P-R interval is more than 0.2 s in WPW syndrome. True or false?
5. Features of RVH in ECG are seen in Fallot's tetralogy. True or false?
6. **Dextrocardia is most commonly associated with:**

   a. Atrial fibrillation b. Negative complexes in lead aVL c. Sinus bradycardia d. Complete heart block

7. **WPW syndrome is characterized by:**

   a. Prolonged P-R interval b. Delta waves c. Tall R waves in V1 d. Absent P waves

8. **ECG findings in ostium secundum ASD may include:**

   a. Right axis deviation b. Left bundle branch block c. Peaked T waves in precordial leads d. Deep S waves in lead V1

9. **VSD can lead to which ECG abnormality?**

   a. Left ventricular hypertrophy b. Prolonged P-R interval c. Tall R waves in V1 d. Upsloping S-T segment depression

10. **In pericarditis ECG shows:**

    a. S-T segment elevation with concavity upwards b. S-T segment is isoelectric c. S-T segment elevation with convexity upwards d. Tall T waves

**Case Studies**

1. A 35-year-old gentleman presented with history of fever for five days followed by retrosternal, sharp chest pain which increases on lying down. The pain improves upon sitting up and bending forward. On auscultation, a superficial scratchy sound is audible over the precordium. Pulse rate was 110 bpm and blood pressure was 110/70 mmHg and temperature was 100.2°F. His ECG is given in Fig. 24.19. What is your diagnosis?
2. A 6-year-old male child suffering from cough and cold for two days was examined by a paediatrician. A soft ejection systolic murmur was audible over the pulmonary area and a wide fixed splitting of second heart sound was detected. His ECG is given in Fig. 24.20. What is your diagnosis?
3. A 30-year-old gentleman presented with history of three episodes of palpitation over last one year. Each episode lasted for about two minutes and stopped of its own. He has no history of hypertension, diabetes or dyslipidaemia. Physical examination was unremarkable. His ECG is given in Fig. 24.21. What is your diagnosis?
4. A 45-year-old gentleman suffering from pulmonary tuberculosis presented with history of fatigue, swelling of feet, chest pain and breathlessness that improves on sitting up. Examination revealed muffled heart sound, blood pressure of 96/70 mmHg and pulse rate 114 bpm, temperature 99°F. Chest X-ray showed nonhomogeneous opacities in left apex and water bottle shaped cardiac shadow. His rhythm strip is given in Fig. 24.22. Identify the rhythm and name the condition in which you will get it.

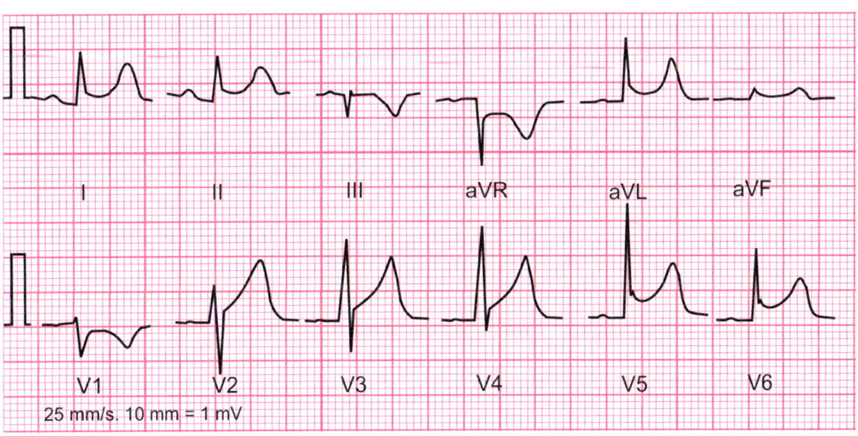


**Fig. 24.19** Interpret the ECG

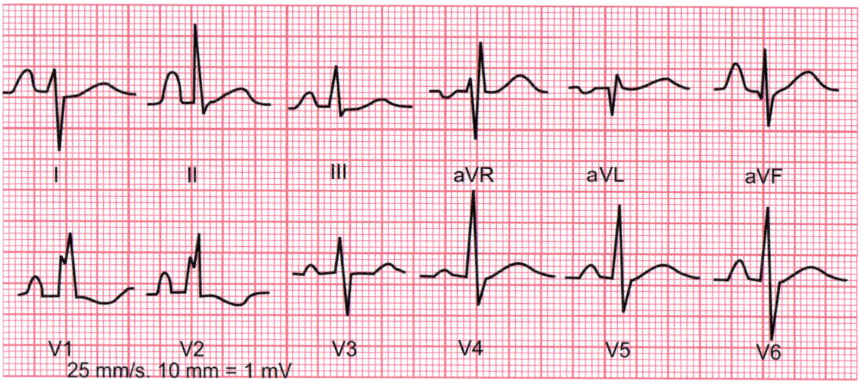


**Fig. 24.20** Interpret the ECG

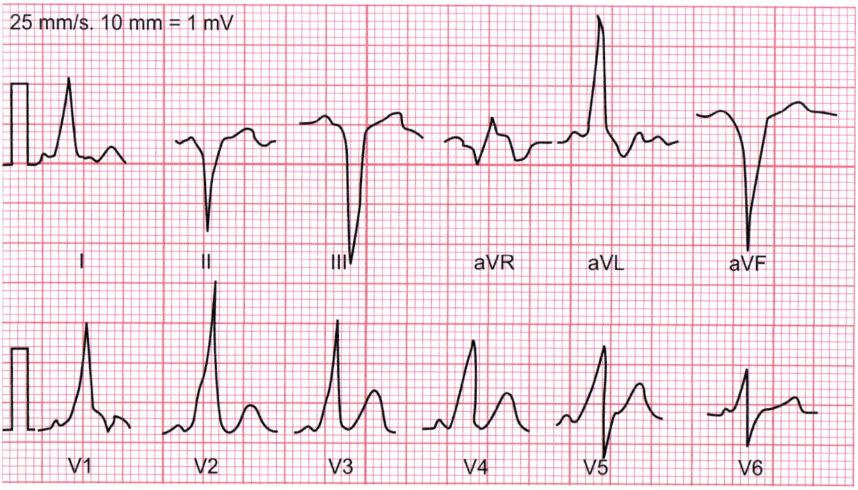


**Fig. 24.21** Interpret the ECG

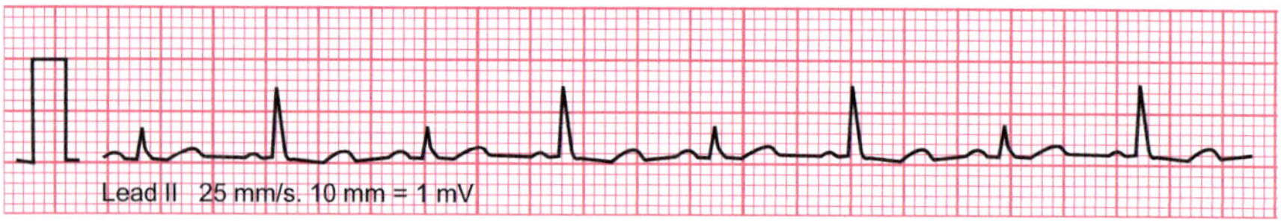


**Fig. 24.22** Analyse the rhythm strip

**Answers**

1. True 2. True 3. True 4. False 5. True 6. b 7. b 8. a 9. a 10. a

**Case Studies**

1. The ECG (Fig. 24.19) shows S-T segment elevation with concavity upwards in leads I, II, aVL and V2–V6. The T waves are not inverted and there are no Q waves. In light of the clinical features, the ECG is diagnostic of acute pericarditis. Most likely pericarditis is of viral origin.

   Echocardiography should be performed to rule out pericardial effusion. CRP is usually high in acute pericarditis. Pericarditis is treated empirically with NSAIDs. Colchicine may be used to treat recurrent pericarditis or that does not respond to conventional treatment.
2. The ECG (Fig. 24.20) shows P pulmonale, right bundle branch block, deep S waves in lead V5 and lead V6 and right axis deviation. Correlating with the clinical features, it is a case of ostium secundum ASD. If there was left axis deviation, a diagnosis of ostium primum ASD would be made.

   Echocardiography is the gold standard for diagnosis of ASD. Defects that are greater than 1 cm will most likely require medical/surgical intervention to close the defect. If an ASD requires closure, options include percutaneous and surgical intervention. Percutaneous transcatheter closure may be considered in this patient.
3. The ECG (Fig. 24.21) shows short P-R interval (< 0.12 s), delta wave and wide QRS complex (> 0.12 s). Delta waves are clearly visible in leads I, aVL, V1–V6. This ECG is diagnostic of WPW syndrome.

   In general, asymptomatic, young, healthy patients without comorbid conditions who have the WPW pattern on ECG and without a history of suspected tachyarrhythmia will require cardiology follow-up. However, patients who have suffered tachyarrhythmias should be referred for close cardiology follow-up for risk stratification testing and/or electrophysiologic study with accessory pathway mapping and possible ablation. Accessory tract ablation is commonly done by radiofrequency current ablation, but cryoablation can also be utilized.
4. The ECG (Fig. 24.22) shows electrical alternans. One large QRS complex is alternating with a QRS complex of smaller amplitude. Electrical alternans is seen in pericardial effusion.

   Most likely this patient is suffering from pulmonary tuberculosis with pericardial effusion. Echocardiography will confirm the presence of fluid in the pericardial sac. Small effusions usually do not require any treatment. The patient should receive anti-tubercular treatment and should be asked for follow-up on a regular basis.

   Large effusions may need a diagnostic and therapeutic pericardiocentesis to evaluate the aetiology and drained to provide symptomatic relief if the patient has associated symptoms such as dyspnoea, chest discomfort, pulmonary oedema or lower extremity oedema.

# Chapter 25
# ECG in Miscellaneous Clinical Conditions

**Learning Objectives**
After studying this chapter, the reader will learn about:

- Myxoedema
- Hyperthyroidism
- Pulmonary embolism
- COPD
- Hypothermia
- Neuromuscular disease
- SI, SII, SIII syndrome

In this chapter, ECG changes of some common diseases will be discussed. It is very important to understand the changes, as ECG is often the first investigation for these diseases that help us in making a diagnosis and start appropriate treatment.

## 25.1 Myxoedema

In myxoedema, body metabolism is decreased. There may be pericardial effusion. The ECG features of myxoedema are the following:

- Low voltage complex (Fig. 25.1)
- Sinus bradycardia
- Shallow or inverted T waves
- Prolonged P-R interval



T. K. Koley, *Rapid Review of ECG*,
https://doi.org/10.1007/978-981-99-9116-7_25

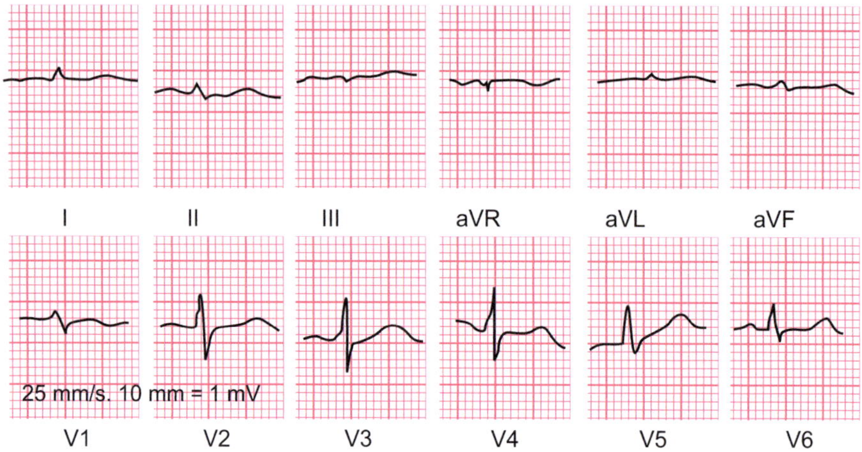


**Fig. 25.1** Myxoedema

## 25.2 Hyperthyroidism

Hyperthyroidism is due to effect of excess circulating thyroid hormones. The body metabolism is increased and hence there is tachycardia, which is a cardinal feature of hyperthyroidism. The ECG features are:

- Sinus tachycardia
- S-T segment, T wave change in left ventricular chest leads
- Atrial and ventricular extrasystoles
- Atrial fibrillation

## 25.3 Pulmonary Embolism

Acute pulmonary embolism is characterized by sudden onset of chest pain and dyspnoea. There is sudden right ventricular strain. Often these patients suffer from various types of cardiac arrhythmias. Sinus tachycardia is the commonest ECG finding. It is diagnosed electrocardiographically by the following criteria:

- SI, QIII, TIII pattern, i.e. prominent S wave in lead I, Q wave in lead III and T wave inversion in lead III (Figs. 25.2 and 25.3)
- Right axis deviation
- S-T segment depression in leads I and II
- Tall peaked P waves may appear in lead II
- T inversion in leads V1–V3 due to right ventricular ischaemia
- Low voltage complexes
- RBBB
- Atrial arrhythmias

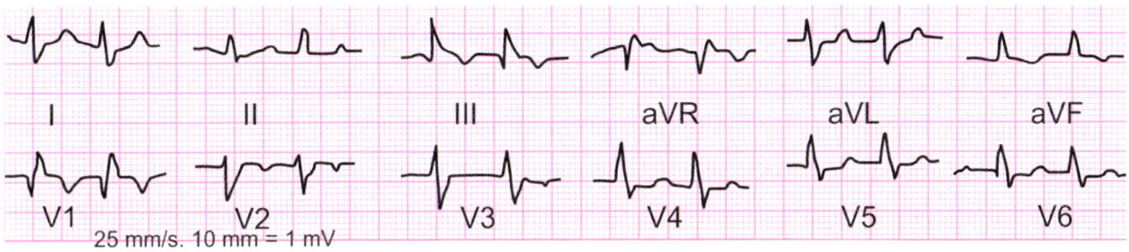


**Fig. 25.2** Pulmonary embolism. There is sinus tachycardia with T wave inversion in leads V1 and V2. Note the SI, QIII and TIII pattern

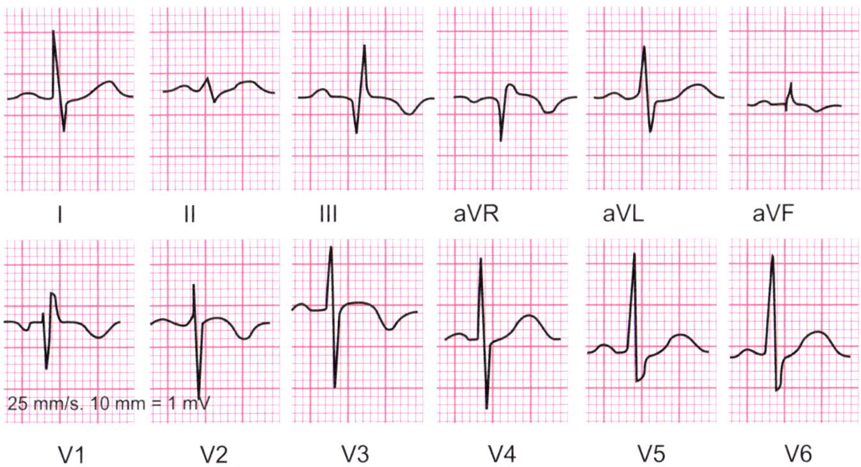


**Fig. 25.3** Acute pulmonary embolism. Note the SI, QIII and TIII pattern

## 25.4 Chronic Obstructive Pulmonary Disease

Chronic obstructive pulmonary disease (COPD) is a very common disease. Patients often present with acute exacerbation. In long standing cases, there is right ventricular hypertrophy with pulmonary hypertension. There is right atrial enlargement as well. These patients often suffer from rhythm disturbances and conduction disturbances.

The ECG manifestations are:

- P-pulmonale (height of P wave > 2.5 mm), best seen in leads II, III and aVF (Figs. 25.4 and 25.5)
- Clockwise rotation
- Right axis deviation
- Right ventricular hypertrophy (R:S ratio > 1 in lead V1)
- Decreased amplitude of QRS complexes
- Incomplete or complete right bundle branch block (rSR' complex in lead V1 with S-T segment, T wave change and QRS duration > 0.12 s)

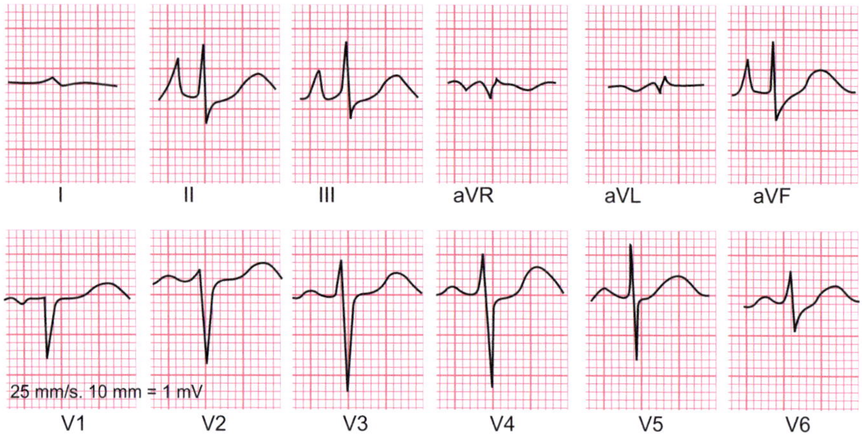


**Fig. 25.4** Chronic obstructive pulmonary disease

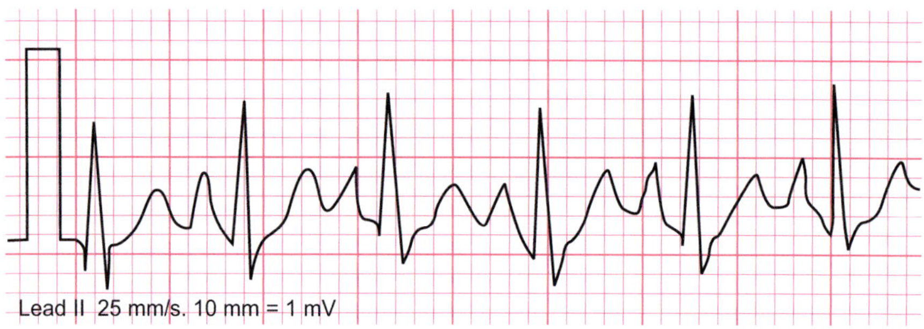


**Fig. 25.5** Note the tall and peaked P wave of COPD (p pulmonale)

## 25.5 Hypothermia

Hypothermia is mainly due to exposure to cold air or water for a long time. Osborne wave or J wave is the characteristic finding of hypothermia. Ventricular fibrillation may be seen when the core temperature falls below 28°C. The ECG features of hypothermia are the following:

- Presence of J waves (Fig. 25.6)
- Prolongation of P-R, QRS and Q-T intervals
- Atrial fibrillation
- Sinus bradycardia
- AV junctional rhythm
- Ventricular fibrillation may occur

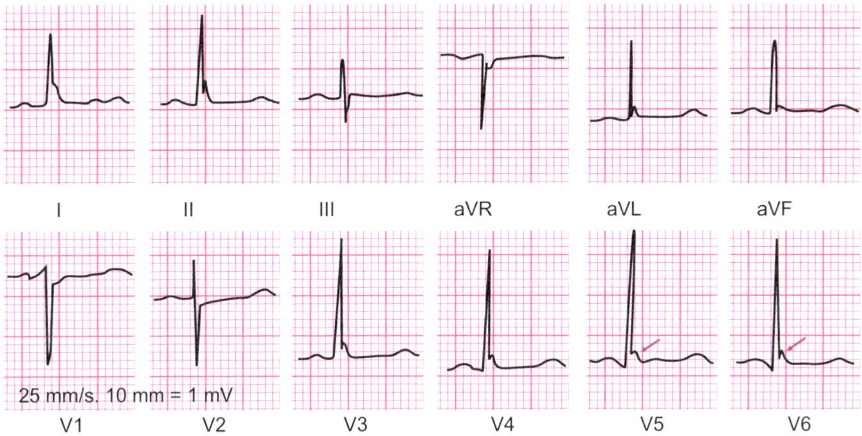


**Fig. 25.6** Hypothermia. The J waves are shown with arrow

## 25.6 Neuromuscular Diseases

ECG changes are often seen in neuromuscular diseases. These diseases are Friedreich's ataxia, progressive muscular dystrophy, etc. The ECG changes are the following:

- First-degree heart block
- Various types of arrhythmias
- Non-specific S-T segment, T wave changes

## 25.7 SI, SII, SIII Syndrome

SI, SII, SIII syndrome means there are S waves in all the three standard leads. There are several causes of this syndrome. It can be seen in normal healthy adults who do not have any heart disease. It is often considered a normal variant. It may be the persistence of physiological dominance of the right ventricular outflow tract, which is present during infancy. It can also be seen in those congenital heart diseases, which have right ventricular dominance like Fallot's tetralogy, pulmonary atresia, Fallot's trilogy, endocardial cushion defect, VSD with pulmonary hypertension, etc. Besides this, it can also be seen in apical myocardial infarction and straight back syndrome. The ECG changes are:

- S waves in leads I, II and III. The depth of S wave is maximum in lead II. The depth of S wave should be greater than the preceding R wave in at least one of the three leads. (Remember in LAHB, the maximum depth of S wave is in lead III.)
- The QRS axis is in northwest region. It is usually within $-90°$ to $-150°$.

**Tips and Tricks**

- Sinus tachycardia is the commonest ECG manifestation of acute pulmonary embolism.
- SI, QIII, TIII is specific ECG change in acute pulmonary embolism.
- P pulmonale is typically seen in COPD with pulmonary hypertension.
- If you find J wave, it may be due to hypothermia.
- If you find northwest axis, look for SI, SII, SIII syndrome. However, it is extremely rare. Remember: Rare diagnosis is rarely correct.

**Self-Assessment Questions**

1. Sinus tachycardia is common in ECG of patient suffering from hyperthyroidism. True or false?
2. ECG may show atrial fibrillation in thyroid storm. True or false?
3. COPD is associated with high amplitude QRS complexes in ECG. True or false?
4. J waves are seen in hypothermia. True or false?
5. SI, QIII, TIII pattern is seen in ECG of acute pulmonary embolism. True or false?
6. **Which ECG finding is commonly seen in hyperthyroidism?**

   a. Prolonged P-R interval b. Sinus tachycardia c. Right axis deviation d. Sinus bradycardia

7. **Which ECG finding is commonly observed in COPD?**

   a. Left axis deviation b. Prolonged P-R interval c. Peaked P waves d. Prominent R waves in precordial leads

8. **ECG of patient suffering from hypothermia is likely to show:**

   a. J waves b. Prolonged P-R interval c. Sinus bradycardia d. All of the above

9. **ECG of patient suffering from myxoedema is likely to show:**

   a. Low voltage complex b. Prolonged P-R interval c. Sinus bradycardia d. All of the above

10. **Northwest QRS axis is seen in:**

    a. COPD b. SI, SII, SIII syndrome c. Hypothermia d. CVA

**Case Studies**

1. A 55-year-old lady was admitted with fracture shaft femur of left leg. She was operated. On third postoperative day, she suddenly complained of chest pain and became breathless. After about five minutes she had a bout of haemoptysis. On examination, her pulse rate was 128 bpm, blood pressure was 86/60 mmHg. There was loud P2. There were bilateral crepitations with decreased breath sounds. There was tenderness in left calf muscle. Her ECG is given in Fig. 25.7. What is your diagnosis?

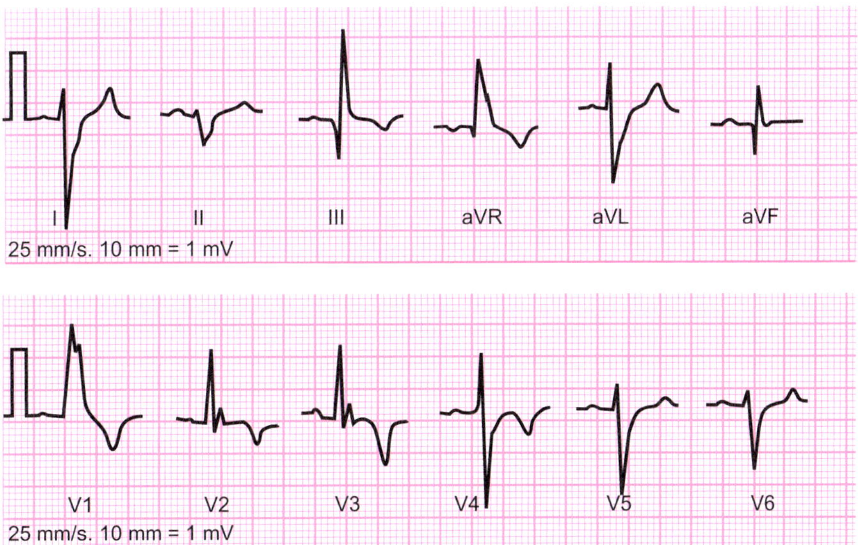


**Fig. 25.7** Interpret the ECG

2. A 50-year-old gentleman presented in emergency department with severe breathlessness and cough for last six hours. He is a chronic smoker. He has history of hypertension and dyslipidaemia. He is on irregular treatment. Patient had dyspnoea. His pulse rate was 110 bpm, blood pressure was 150/90 mmHg, afebrile. Chest examination revealed bilateral wheeze and crepitations with decreased breath sound. The chest was barrel shaped. Heart sounds were normal except for loud P2. Examine his ECG given in Fig. 25.8 and make your diagnosis.
3. A 70-year-old gentleman was brought to the emergency department in a drowsy state by his relatives at around 6 AM on a very cold day. He was partially responding to verbal commands. His pulse was irregularly irregular and rate was about 50 bpm and blood pressure was 84/66 mmHg. His ECG is given in Fig. 25.9. What is your diagnosis?

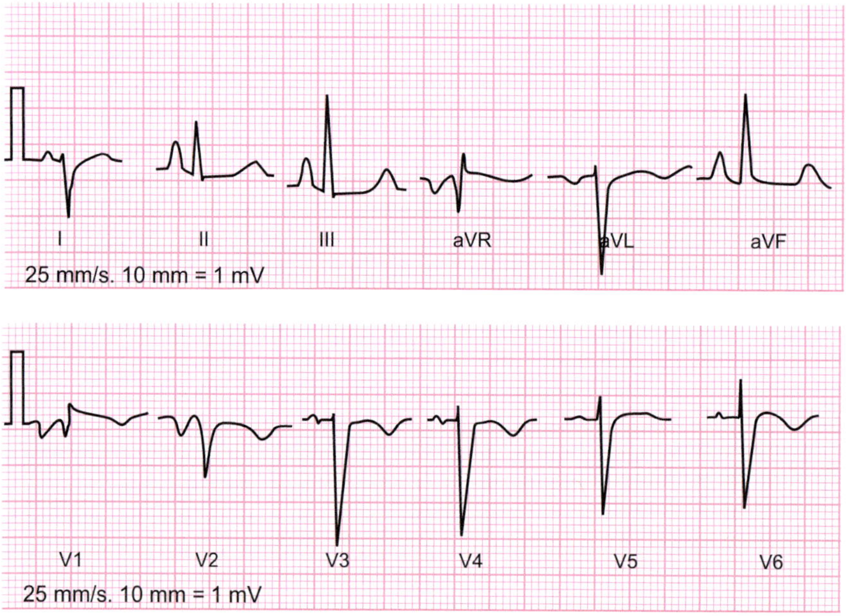


**Fig. 25.8** Interpret the ECG

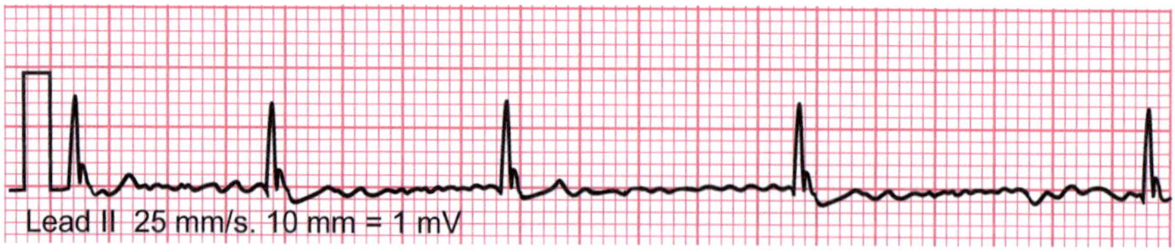


**Fig. 25.9** Interpret the ECG

**Answers**

1. True 2. True 3. False 4. True 5. True 6. b 7. c 8. d 9. d 10. b

**Case Studies**

1. The ECG (Fig. 25.7) shows the following:

    - Right axis deviation
    - RBBB (RsR' pattern in lead V1)
    - SI, QIII, TIII pattern
    - T wave inversion in lead V1 to lead V4

    This is a case of acute pulmonary embolism.

    The clinical picture of the patient is typical of acute pulmonary embolism. Calf tenderness signifies development of postoperative deep vein thrombosis. This has resulted in pulmonary embolism. The patient needs urgent investigation to confirm the diagnosis. She needs supportive measures and anticoagulation is the mainstay of treatment. Primary reperfusion treatment, usually, thrombolysis, is the treatment of choice for patients with hemodynamically unstable acute pulmonary embolism.
2. The ECG (Fig. 25.8) shows P pulmonale, right axis deviation, and right ventricular hypertrophy. There is clockwise rotation. The deep S waves persisting in lead V4 to lead V6 is due to RVH. Correlating the clinical finding with the ECG, it can be diagnosed as a case of COPD.

    Oxygen saturation should be checked and if required oxygen should be started. Immediately nebulization with bronchodilator and corticosteroid should be done. If required, intravenous bronchodilator and corticosteroid may be required.
3. The ECG (Fig. 25.9) shows atrial fibrillation with slow ventricular rate. J wave is visible in every QRS complex. In light of clinical findings, it can be diagnosed to be a case of hypothermia.

    Rewarming of the patient should be started without delay along with other supportive care. There always remains a possibility of cardiac collapse from a fatal arrhythmia due to increased cardiac irritability. Comorbid medical conditions merit considerations and appropriate treatment.

# Chapter 26
# Basic Aspects of Pacemaker

**Learning Objectives**
After studying this chapter, the reader will learn about:

- Temporary pacing
- Permanent pacing
- Pacemaker code
- Pacemaker terminology
- Pacemaker malfunction

A pacemaker (or artificial pacemaker) is a battery powered medical device that uses electrical current, delivered by electrodes contacting the heart muscles, to regulate the beating of the heart. The primary purpose of a pacemaker is to maintain an adequate heart rate and rhythm, either because the heart's native pacemaker is not fast enough, or there is a block in the heart's electrical conduction system. They function by sensing intrinsic cardiac electric potentials and if these potentials are too infrequent or absent, electric impulses are transmitted to the heart, thereby stimulating myocardial contraction.

Modern pacemakers are externally programmable and allow the selection of optimum pacing modes for individual patients. Some combine a pacemaker and implantable defibrillator in a single implantable device for dual function of pacing and defibrillation.

Artificial pacemakers can be used in management of these conditions:

- Sinus node dysfunction—when the SA node does not fire properly to contract the heart, e.g. sinus arrest, sinus block, sick sinus syndrome, etc.
- Bifascicular block, trifascicular block or third degree AV block
- Stokes-Adams attack involving disruption of conduction between the sinoatrial node and the AV node leading to syncopal attack
- Atrial fibrillation with a slow ventricular response



T. K. Koley, *Rapid Review of ECG*,
https://doi.org/10.1007/978-981-99-9116-7_26

- Chronotropic incompetence (inability to increase the heart rate to match a level of exercise)
- Prolonged QT syndrome

Relative indications include the following:

- Cardiomyopathy (hypertrophic or dilated)
- Severe refractory neurocardiogenic syncope
- Paroxysmal atrial fibrillation

## 26.1 Types of Pacing

Pacing is mainly of two types: temporary and permanent.

### *26.1.1 Temporary Pacing*

Temporary pacing is of two types: transcutaneous and transvenous pacing.

#### 26.1.1.1 Transcutaneous Pacing

Transcutaneous pacing is also called external pacing. It is recommended for the initial stabilization of hemodynamically significant bradycardias of all types like symptomatic bradycardia, second degree Mobitz type II AV block and complete heart block, etc. It is not effective if meaningful contractile activity is absent like ventricular standstill or pulseless electrical activity.

The procedure is performed by placing two pacing pads on the patient's chest on anterior and posterior side. The pacing pads are attached to the pacing cable. ECG leads are also attached to the patient. The pacing rate is set and gradually the pacing current (measured in mA) is increased until electrical capture (characterized by a wide QRS complex with a tall, broad T wave on the ECG) is achieved, with a corresponding pulse. The myocardium is stimulated indirectly by electric current passed through the chest wall.

External pacing should not be relied upon for an extended period of time. It is an emergency procedure that acts as a bridge until transvenous pacing or other therapies can be applied. The large amount of current passed may cause chest wall pain and skin burns.

#### 26.1.1.2 Transvenous Pacing

Transvenous pacing or temporary internal pacing is an alternative to transcutaneous pacing. The pacemaker electrode is placed under sterile conditions via a central venous catheter via transvenous route (internal jugular vein, subclavian vein or femoral vein). The proximal tip of the electrode is placed into either the right atrium or right ventricle. The other end of the electrode is attached to the pulse generator, outside of the body. The endocardium is stimulated directly by electric current that is supplied by the pulse generator. Batteries are kept in the generator housing.

This type of pacing is useful for significant bradycardias like transcutaneous pacing and is not useful if meaningful contractile activity of heart is absent. Transvenous pacing is often used as a bridge to permanent pacemaker placement. Under certain conditions, a person may require temporary pacing but would not require permanent pacing like complete heart block due to viral or drug induced myocarditis. In this case, a temporary pacing wire may be the optimal treatment option.

### *26.1.2 Permanent Pacing*

Permanent pacing is done in cardiac catheterization laboratory under intravenous conscious sedation and local anaesthesia. Permanent pacing with an implantable pacemaker involves placement of one or more pacing electrodes within the chambers of the heart either right atrium or right ventricle or both in dual chamber pacing, via the cephalic vein or the subclavian vein (Fig. 26.1). One end of each electrode is attached to the muscle of the heart and the other end is attached into the pulse generator. Pulse generators contain, among other things, a battery, an output circuit, a sensing circuit and a timing circuit. The battery most commonly used in permanent pacers is a lithium-iodide type and has a life span of 5–8 years.

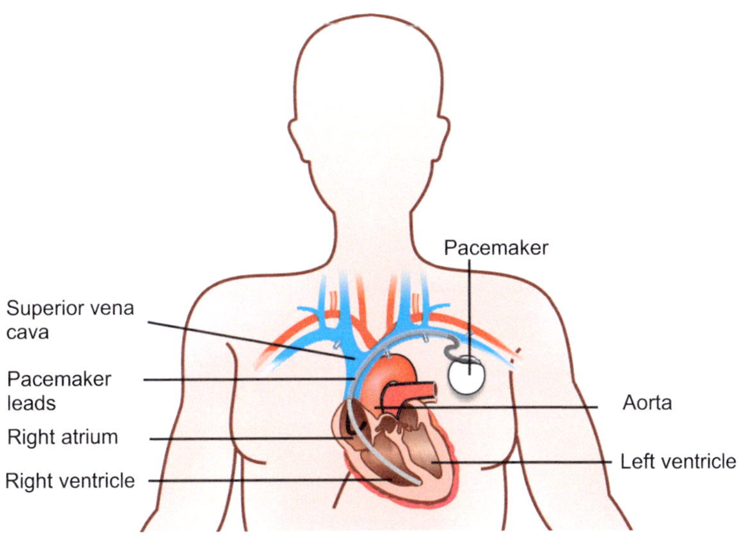


**Fig. 26.1** Permanent pacemaker

Most commonly, the pulse generator is placed below the subcutaneous fat of the chest wall, above the muscles and bones of the chest either in right or left pectoral area. However, the placement may vary on a case by case basis. The outer casing of pacemakers is so designed that it will rarely be rejected by the body's immune system. It is usually made of titanium, which is very inert inside the body.

Pulse generators can be set to a fixed-rate (asynchronous) or demand (synchronous) mode. In the fixed-rate mode, an impulse is produced at a set rate regardless to the patient's intrinsic cardiac activity. In this mode, there is a small but inherent danger of producing lethal arrhythmias should the impulse coincides with the vulnerable period of the T wave. This type of pacemaker is usually used when there is no intrinsic heart rate.

In the demand mode, the sensing circuit searches for an intrinsic depolarization potential. If this is absent, a pacing response is generated. When intrinsic activity is present, then the pacemaker is inhibited. This mode can closely mimic the intrinsic electric activity pattern of the heart.

Single chamber pacemakers sense and pace either the atrium or the ventricle. Dual chamber pacemakers are able to sense and pace both the atrium and the ventricles. Dual chamber pacing has the ability to stimulate the atria and the ventricles in sequence like normal cardiac cycle, thereby preserves the normal atrioventricular synchrony and the atrial kick that contributes to about 30% of ventricular filling.

## 26.2 Pacemaker Code

The North American Society of Pacing and Electrophysiology (NASPE) and the British Pacing and Electrophysiology Group (BPEG) have developed a code (Box 26.1) to describe the various pacing modes.

**Box 26.1 Pacemaker Code Used to Describe Various Pacing Modes**

| Chamber paced | Chamber sensed | Mode of response | Programmable functions | Special anti-tachyarrhythmia functions |
|---|---|---|---|---|
| V = Ventricle | V = Ventricle | T = Triggered | P = Programmable | P = Pacing (anti-tachyarrhythmia) |
| A = Atrium | A = Atrium | I = Inhibited (demand) | M = Multiprogrammable | S = Shock |
| D = Double (dual A + V) | D = Double (dual A + V) | D = Double (Dual function T + I) | O = None (permanent pacemaker only) | D = Double (P + S) |
| O = None | | O = None | C = Communicating | |
| | | R = Reverse | R = Rate modulation | |

The first three letters are used most commonly. A pacemaker in VVI mode means that it paces and senses the ventricle (right ventricle) and is inhibited by a sensed ventricular electrical activity. In absence of a sensed spontaneous activity, the pacemaker stimulates the right ventricle. AAI means pacemaker senses and paces the atrium only. Similarly, AAT mode represents pacing and sensing in the atrium and each sensed event triggers the generator to fire within the P wave.

The DDD mode denotes that both chambers are capable of being paced and sensed. This requires two functioning leads: one in the right atrium and the other in the right ventricle.

If pacemaker does not sense an atrial activity within a predetermined period, the atrial pacing lead will pace the atrium. A maximum P-R interval is predetermined. If a ventricular beat is not sensed, the ventricle will be paced as well. In the ECG, each QRS is preceded by two spikes: one indicating the atrial depolarization and the other indicating the initiation of the QRS complex. A left bundle-branch pattern may also be evident upon the ECG.

Pacemaker programming can be performed non-invasively. Because of the various types of pacemakers, patients should carry a card with them providing information about their particular model. Most pulse generators, however, have an X-ray code that can be seen on a standard chest X-ray. The markings, along with the shape of the generator, may assist with deciphering the manufacturer of the generator and pacemaker battery.

Placing a magnet over a permanent pacemaker causes sensing to be inhibited by closing an internal reed switch. This process only temporarily reprograms the pacer into the asynchronous mode, where pacing is initiated at a set rate. It does not turn the pacemaker off. Application of a magnet can determine if the pacer's battery needs to be replaced.

## 26.3 Pacemaker Terminology

Ability to sense, fire and capture are the basic functions of all pacemakers.

**Sensing:** It means the pulse generator is able to detect the intrinsic beat of the patient.

**Firing:** It means the pulse generator has delivered an electrical stimulus to the heart.

**Capture:** It means the heart has responded to the electrical stimulus (Figs. 26.2 and 26.3).

**Automatic interval:** It means the heart rate at which the pacemaker is set. The interval can be calculated by measuring the duration from one pacing spike to the next consecutive pacing spike (Fig. 26.4).

**Ventricular capture:** This means the ventricle has responded to a stimulus and this is reflected in ECG by a pacemaker spike followed by a wide QRS complex (Fig. 26.4).

**Intrinsic beat:** It is also called native beat (Figs. 26.4 and 26.5). This beat is produced by the patient's own heart and the pacemaker does not play any role.

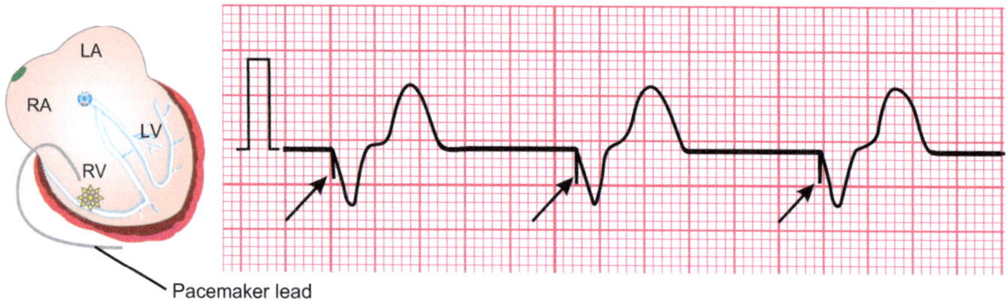


**Fig. 26.2** Illustration of pacemaker function. Note the pacing spikes (arrows) followed by broad QRS complex

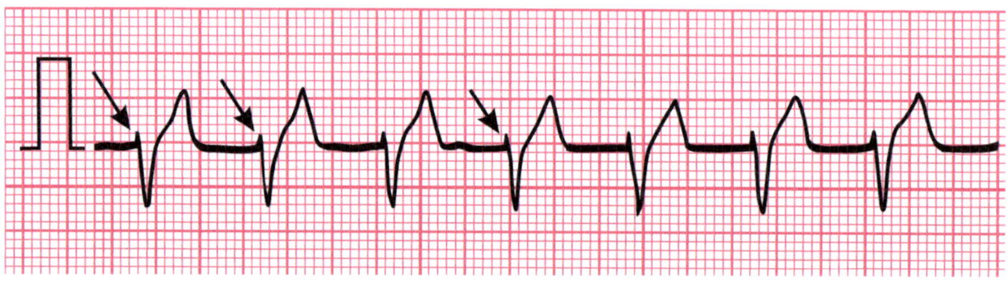

**Fig. 26.3** Normal pacemaker function. Note the pacing spikes (arrows) and the broad QRS complexes

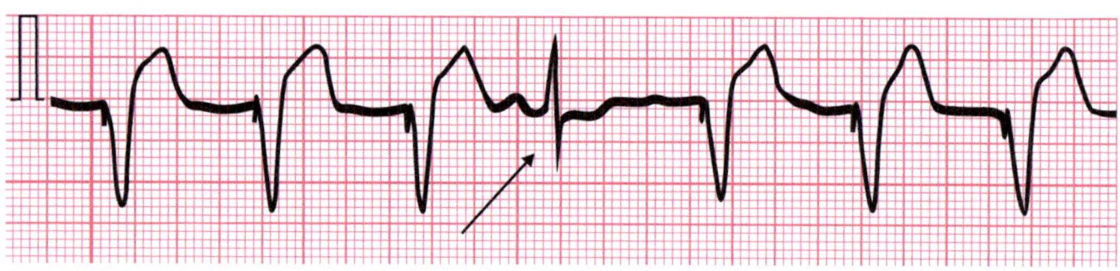

**Fig. 26.4** Ventricular capture. Note the pacing spikes. Also note the native beat (arrow). Automatic interval 83 bpm

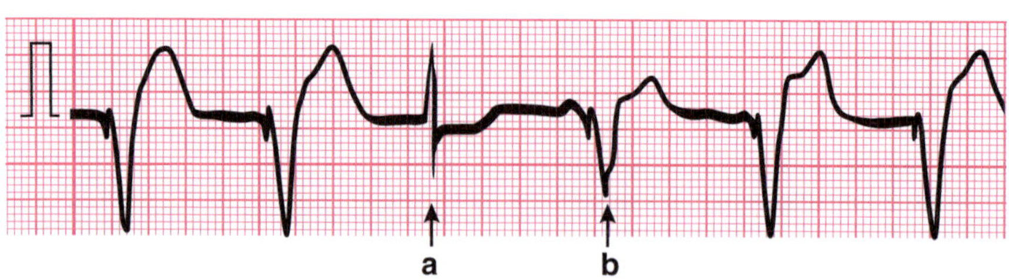


**Fig. 26.5** (**a**) Native beat, (**b**) fusion beat

**Fusion beat:** This is a beat produced by both the normal conduction system of the heart of its own electrical activity, as well as by the pacemaker. The two electrical activities together depolarize the ventricles (Fig. 26.5).

## 26.4 Pacemaker Malfunction

Major pacemaker malfunctions include failure to capture, failure to sense and failure to output, correctly.

### *26.4.1 Failure to Capture*

Failure to capture means when a pacing spike that occurs on time but is not followed by either an atrial or a ventricular complex (Fig. 26.6). This means that the atrium or the ventricle has failed to respond to the delivered electrical stimulus. This may be due to lead fracture, lead dislodgement, a break in lead insulation, an elevated pacing threshold, myocardial infarction at the lead tip, certain drugs (e.g. flecainide), metabolic abnormalities (e.g. hyperkalaemia, acidosis, alkalosis), cardiac perforation, poor lead connection at the takeoff from the generator and improper amplitude or pulse width settings.

By increasing the mA setting on pulse generator, the strength of the electric current delivered to the heart can be increased, and this will correct this problem. Chest X-ray may be required to determine the condition/position of the catheter and it may require repositioning.

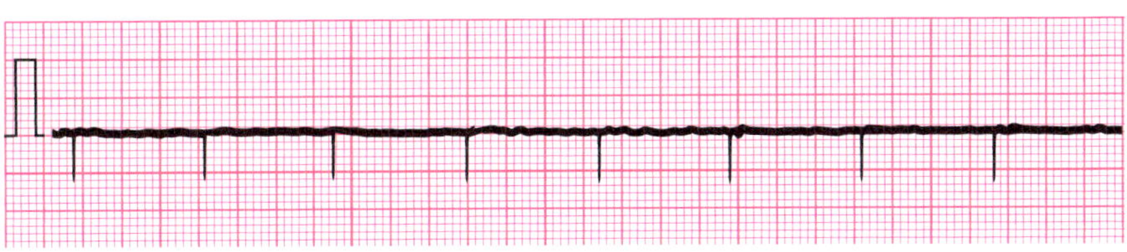

**Fig. 26.6** Complete failure to capture in ventricular asystole

### 26.4.2 Oversensing

Oversensing means when a pacer incorrectly senses noncardiac electrical activity and is inhibited from pacing correctly. The various causes are muscular activity, particularly oversensing of the diaphragm or pectoralis muscles, electromagnetic interference such as MRI or lead insulation breakage. In this condition, decrease the sensitivity of the pulse generator by turning the mV (millivolt) dial to a higher number.

### 26.4.3 Undersensing

Undersensing means when a pacer wrongly misses intrinsic depolarization and paces despite intrinsic activity of the heart (Fig. 26.7). The various causes are poor lead positioning, lead dislodgment, magnet application, low battery states and myocardial infarction. In this condition, increase the sensitivity of the pulse generator by turning the mV (millivolt) dial to a lower number. Chest X-ray may be required here also to determine the condition/position of the catheter and it may require repositioning.

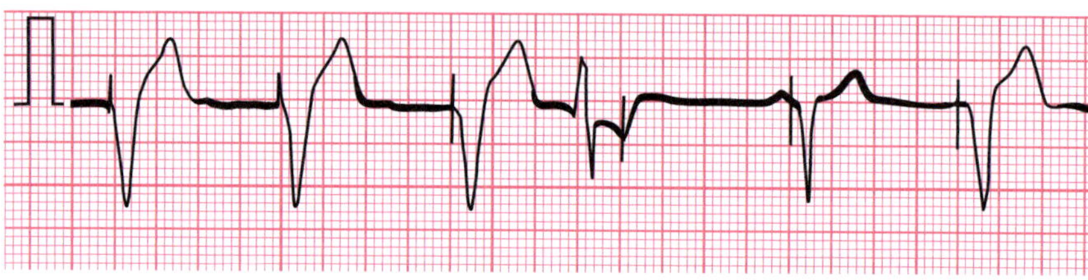

**Fig. 26.7** Failure to sense. The first three beats are paced beats. The fourth beat is a patient beat after which the spike occurs early. This is failure to sense. This is followed by a fusion beat. The last beat is again a paced beat

### 26.4.4 Failure to Output

Failure to output means when no pacing spike is present despite an indication to pace. The various causes are a break in lead insulation, oversensing, poor lead connection at the takeoff from the pacer, battery failure, lead fracture and cross-talk (a phenomenon seen when atrial output is sensed by a ventricular lead in a dual-chamber pacer).

Management of pacer output complications are medications to increase the intrinsic heart rate and placement of a temporary pacer. A chest X-ray is often required to check pacer leads especially to evaluate for possible lead fracture, which occurs most frequently at the clavicle/first rib location.

### 26.4.5 Operative Failures

Operative failure means malfunction due to mechanical factors, such as pericarditis, skin erosion, pneumothorax, haematoma, infection, lead dislodgment, venous thrombosis, etc. Treatment depends on the aetiology. Lead dislodgment usually occurs within two days following implantation of a permanent pacer and may be seen on chest X-ray.

**Tips and Tricks**

- If you find no pacing spikes but excellent own rhythm, consider good functional SA node.
- Any pause greater than the pacing interval should be considered as a cause of concern.
- If you find pacing spikes more than QRS complex, consider failure to capture.
- If you find no pacing spikes and no own rhythm, consider magnet application before inserting temporary pacemaker. It is a real emergency.
- If you find bradycardia, insert a temporary pacemaker. It is a real emergency because paced heart rate cannot fall below 70 bpm.
- In real emergency, temporary pacemaker insertion is often lifesaving.

**Self-Assessment Questions**

1. An ECG of a patient with a functioning cardiac pacemaker will show the presence of pacing spikes. True or false?
2. The location of the pacing spike in the ECG indicates the chamber being paced (atrium or ventricle). True or false?
3. The presence of pacing spikes indicates normal sinus rhythm in a patient with a cardiac pacemaker. True or false?
4. In an ECG of a patient with a pacemaker, the QRS complex following a pacing spike may be wider compared to a normal QRS complex. True or false?
5. Atrial pacing can be identified on the ECG by the presence of a pacing spike after P wave. True or false?
6. Pacemaker-mediated tachycardia can occur when the pacemaker fires too frequently and causes rapid ventricular rates. True or false?

7. Magnet application over a pacemaker can temporarily deactivate the pacing function and allow the patient's intrinsic rhythm to be recorded on the ECG. True or false?
8. Pacemaker syndrome refers to the presence of symptoms caused by improper pacing, such as palpitations and dizziness. True or false?
9. **Which component of an electrocardiogram (ECG) represents the electrical activity generated by a temporary cardiac pacemaker?**

   a. P wave b. QRS complex c. Pacing spike d. T wave

10. **In a temporary cardiac pacemaker, the pacing spike is typically followed by which waveform?**

    a. P wave b. T wave c. QRS complex d. U wave

11. **A pacing spike appearing before the P wave in an ECG indicates:**

    a. Atrial pacing b. Ventricular pacing c. Malfunction of the pacemaker d. Normal sinus rhythm

12. **A pacing spike appearing before the QRS complex in an ECG indicates:**

    a. Atrial pacing b. Ventricular pacing c. Normal sinus rhythm d. Malfunction of the pacemaker

13. **In a permanent cardiac pacemaker, the pacing spike is typically followed by:**

    a. P wave b. U wave c. T wave d. QRS complex

14. **A failure to capture malfunction in a pacemaker refers to:**

    a. Inability to detect intrinsic cardiac activity b. Inability to produce a T wave c. Inability to produce a QRS complex d. Inability to generate a pacing spike

15. **A failure to sense malfunction in a pacemaker refers to:**

    a. Inability to generate a pacing spike b. Inability to detect intrinsic cardiac activity c. Inability to produce a QRS complex d. Inability to produce a T wave

**Case Studies**

1. Analyse the rhythm strip given in Fig. 26.8.
2. Analyse the rhythm strip given in Fig. 26.9 and identify the problem.
3. Examine the rhythm strip given in Fig. 26.10 and identify the problem.
4. Examine the rhythm strip given in Fig. 26.11 and identify the problem.

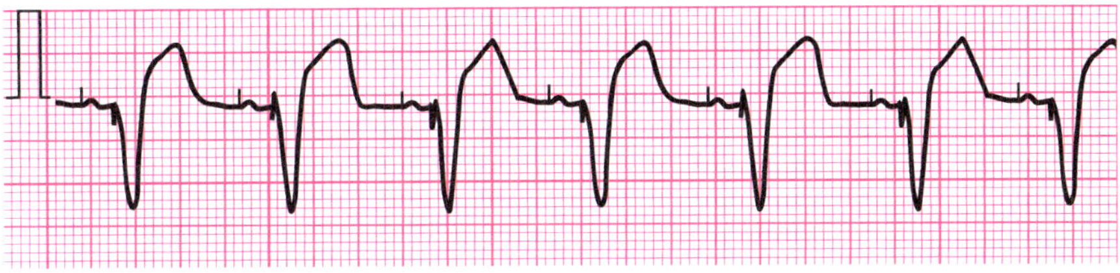

**Fig. 26.8** Analyse the rhythm strip

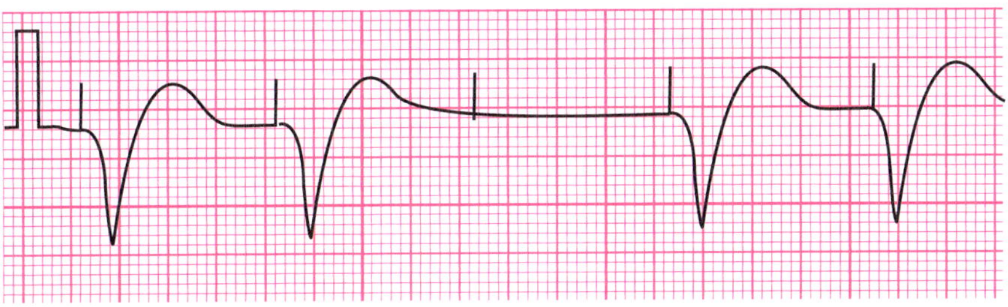

**Fig. 26.9** Analyse the rhythm strip

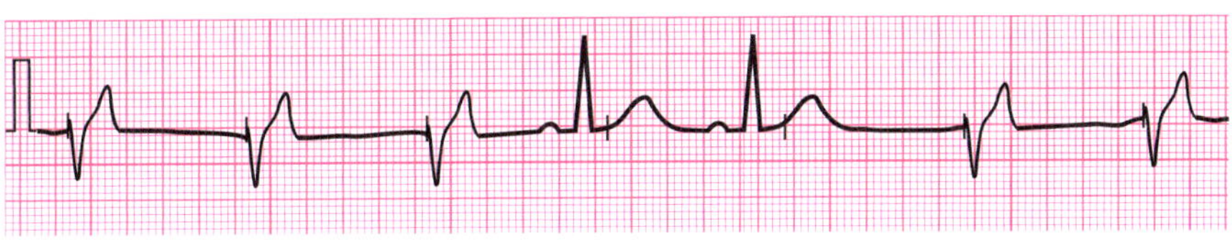

**Fig. 26.10** Analyse the rhythm strip

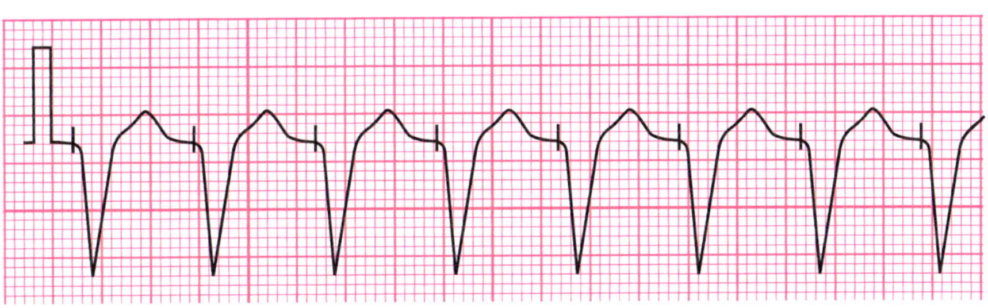

**Fig. 26.11** Analyse the rhythm strip

**Answers**

1. True 2. True 3. False 4. True 5. False 6. True 7. True 8. True 9. c 10. c 11. a 12. b 13. d 14. c 15. b

**Case Studies**

1. The rhythm strip (Fig. 26.8) shows pacing spike before every P wave and pacing spike before every QRS complex. Hence it is a dual chamber pacing. The QRS complex is wide. The ventricular rate is 88 bpm. There is no problem including failure to capture, failure to pace and failure to sense.
2. In ECG of Fig. 26.9, all the QRS complexes are preceded by pacing spike. Hence it is a single chamber pacing. However, after the third pacing spike QRS complex is absent. Hence, the diagnosis is failure to capture.
3. The rhythm strip (Fig. 26.10) shows ventricular pacing for the first three QRS complexes. After this, the fourth and the fifth beats are intrinsic beats of the patient having normal PQRS complexes. Here the pacemaker fails to sense the intrinsic beats. The pacemaker continues to pace throughout the intrinsic beats and ventricular pacing resumes for sixth and seventh beats. Hence, it is undersensing problem of the pacemaker.
4. The rhythm strip (Fig. 26.11) shows pacing spikes before each QRS complexes. The QRS complexes are paced at a rate of 125 bpm. Hence, it is a case of pacemaker mediated tachycardia.

# Part VII
# Recording and Monitoring of ECG

# Chapter 27
# Recording of ECG

**Learning Objectives**
After studying this chapter, the reader will learn about:

- Standardization of ECG
- Procedure of recording ECG

ECG should be recorded carefully and the technique of recording should be uniform from one recording to another. It is a safe, painless and quick procedure that can help detect various heart conditions such as arrhythmias, heart attacks and heart failure. A good quality ECG recording is essential to ensure accurate diagnosis and treatment of these conditions. A good quality recording is essential for correct interpretation. Any medical personnel who has received training on conducting an electrocardiogram can record an ECG, including a doctor, nurse and a qualified technician. Usually, it is performed by the technicians in clinics or hospitals and then interpreted by clinicians. Often, these findings are confirmed by a cardiologist in a hospital-based setting. Before recording ECG, it is essential to learn about standardization of ECG.

## 27.1 Standardization of ECG

Standardization of ECG is one of the most important but most often neglected aspects of recording of ECG. If standardization is not perfect, it may lead to wrong diagnosis.

Conventionally, ECG is standardized so that 1 mV is equal to 10 mm of upward deflection (Fig. 27.1).



T. K. Koley, *Rapid Review of ECG*,
https://doi.org/10.1007/978-981-99-9116-7_27

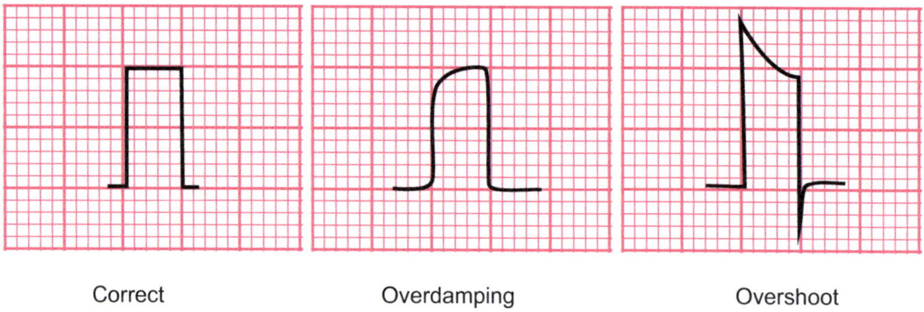


**Fig. 27.1** Diagram showing normal standardization, overdamping and overshoot

Overdamping: It is due to the stylus pressing too hard on paper and platform, resulting in rounded edges. It leads to widening of the complex.

Underdamping or overshoot: This happens when the stylus becomes too loose and causes spikes on the comer. The amplitude of the waves and complexes will increase as a result.

## 27.2 Procedure of Recording ECG

The procedure of recording a good quality of ECG is learnt by practice only. However, the theoretical aspect is essential for everyone involved in the process of recording ECG. A sound knowledge gets translated into an excellent ECG strip which in turn helps in making the exact diagnosis. The basic steps that need to be followed sequentially are discussed here.

### *27.2.1 Gather and Check All the Equipment*

The first step in recording a good quality ECG is to gather the proper equipment and check them thoroughly. Check the ECG machine and the leads properly before starting the procedure. Collect self-adhesive electrodes, razor and alcohol swipes which are essential to obtain a good ECG record.

### *27.2.2 Introduction and Consent*

The first step in recording a very good quality ECG is to prepare the patient for the procedure. Introduce yourself to the patient including your name and confirm the identity of the patient. A brief history regarding drugs and allergies to adhesive gel is necessary. Explain the patient the procedure of recording the ECG in a patient friendly language, preferably in the mother tongue of the patient including what to expect and how long it will take. They should be asked about any medical conditions, allergies, or medications they are taking that could affect the ECG results. The patient should know that certain electrodes are going to be attached to the chest and limbs and electrical activity of the heart will be recorded in the ECG machine. It must be explained that he will not feel any electric current. After this obtain a verbal consent. Female attendant should be present during recording of ECG in a female patient.

### 27.2.3 Preparation

At the very beginning, wash your hands cleanly with soap and running water and dry them properly. Patient must lie down comfortably and relax. The patient should be instructed to remove all clothing from the waist up and put on a gown or loose-fitting clothing. Any metallic object, like jewellery or a watch requires removal. The patient's skin should be clean, dry and free from any lotions, oils or powders that can affect the electrode's adhesion. Wipe the patient's skin with alcohol and allow it to dry. The patient should be advised not to move or talk during the recording, as this can cause interference.

### 27.2.4 Electrode Placement

The next step is to place the electrodes on the patient's body. The standard ECG uses ten electrodes that are attached to the patient's chest, arms and legs. The electrode placement is critical in recording a very good quality ECG. The electrodes must be placed correctly to ensure accurate results. Attach the four electrodes on the four limbs and the six chest electrodes on the designated areas on the anterior chest wall. The limb leads include I, II, III, aVL, aVR and aVF and the electrodes are named RA, LA, RL and LL. It is important to ensure each electrode has very good skin contact, which may involve cleaning or shaving the areas where you need to place electrodes. The need for shaving of chest hairs with razor should be explained to the patient properly and consent should be taken for it. If the skin is very oily, it should be cleaned with alcohol wipe properly and allowed to dry prior to electrode attachment. If the skin is visibly soiled, it should be cleaned, ideally with soap and water and dried properly prior to electrode application.

Properly check the colour codes of the limb leads and attach them to the electrodes. The limb lead and the chest lead cables should be properly attached to the ECG machine. There should not be any loose attachment.

### 27.2.5 *Recording the ECG*

Turn the ECG machine on and ensure ECG paper has been properly loaded into the machine. Next instruct the patient to remain still and not to talk or move during recording. It is essential to check the machine's calibration. The calibration ensures that the ECG machine is recording accurate results. The calibration should be checked regularly, preferably before each use, to ensure that the machine is functioning correctly. The paper speed should be set at 25 mm/s and standardization should be 10 mm = 1 mV. It is also essential to check that the machine is properly grounded and any electric equipment that may cause electrical interference should be removed.

Press the start button on the ECG machine to record the ECG trace. If the ECG trace is of poor quality, double-check the connections to ensure there is good skin contact. Once a good quality ECG is obtained, switch off the ECG machine and detach the ECG leads from the electrodes and then remove the electrodes carefully and discard them properly. Label the ECG with patient details like name, age, sex, date and time of ECG and hospital admission number.

In ECG, artifact is often recorded. The artifacts originate from sources other than electrical activity in the heart. The common causes are shivering, muscle tremor, loose electrodes, electrical equipment interference and improper grounding of ECG machine (Fig. 27.2).

**Tips and Tricks**

- Check calibration properly and standardization should be perfect for good recording.
- The ECG machine should be properly grounded.
- There should not be any loose connections and electrical interference.
- The colour codes should be checked properly.
- Patient should be absolutely comfortable.

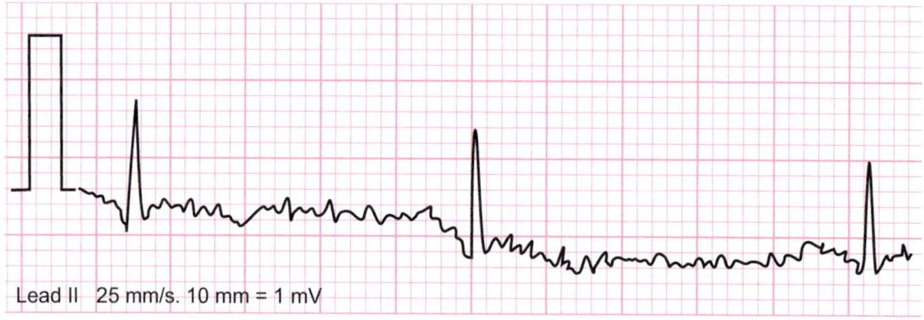


**Fig. 27.2** Shivering artifacts

# Chapter 28
# Bedside Cardiac Monitoring

**Learning Objectives**
After studying this chapter, the reader will learn about:

- Indications for cardiac monitoring
- Types of bedside cardiac monitoring
- Setting up of cardiac monitoring
- Monitor problems and their solutions

Bedside cardiac monitoring is an important aspect of management of a critical cardiac patient. Cardiac monitoring is a useful, noninvasive diagnostic tool to monitor the wide array of patient conditions. In this chapter, basic information will be provided for careful monitoring of sick patients. By this process, one can continuously monitor the electrical activity of the heart, which is useful for identification of arrhythmias and heart blocks, acute myocardial ischaemia, evaluate response of drugs and pacemaker function. Major improvements have occurred in cardiac monitoring systems, including computerized arrhythmia detection algorithms, S-T segment/ischaemia monitoring software, improved noise-reduction strategies, multilead monitoring and reduced lead sets for monitoring-derived 12-lead ECGs with a minimal number of electrodes. It is useful in coronary care unit, intensive care units, emergency departments, anaesthesia recovery rooms and operation theatres. Lead II is used more frequently for monitoring because most of the heart's electrical current flows toward its positive axis. This lead gives the best view of the ECG waves and best reflects the activity of the cardiac conduction system.


T. K. Koley, *Rapid Review of ECG*,
https://doi.org/10.1007/978-981-99-9116-7_28

## 28.1 Indications for Cardiac Monitoring

Cardiac monitoring is not required for all patients coming to the emergency of a hospital or admitted in a hospital. American College of Cardiology Emergency Cardiac Care Committee for cardiac monitoring has developed the following categories for indications of cardiac monitoring.

- Class I: Cardiac monitoring is indicated in most, if not all, patients in this group.
- Class II: Cardiac monitoring may be beneficial to some patients but not considered essential for all patients.
- Class III: Cardiac monitoring is not indicated because a patient's risk of a serious event is so low that monitoring has no therapeutic monitoring benefit.

Cardiac monitoring is indicated in most, if not all, patients in the following patients:

- Patients resuscitated from cardiac arrest
- Patients in the early phase of acute coronary syndrome
- Patients with major trauma, acute respiratory failure, sepsis, shock, pulmonary embolus, major noncardiac surgery, drug overdose or other indications for intensive care
- Patients with acute heart failure, pulmonary oedema
- Patients with any haemodynamically unstable arrhythmia
- Patients after cardiac surgery
- Patients with temporary or transcutaneous pacemaker
- Patients with AV block after myocardial infarction
- Patients with drug-induced long Q-T syndrome

Often patients present with features suggestive of acute coronary syndrome. However, ECG does not reveal any change. In these patients, serial ECG is required every 5–10 min to make the right diagnosis. Continuous S-T segment monitoring is extremely valuable for these patients until they become symptom free for 12–24 h.

For patients suffering from uncomplicated acute myocardial infarction, it is recommended that monitoring begins as soon as the patient presents to the ED and continues uninterrupted for a minimum of 24 h. All patients who receive early reperfusion therapy should undergo uninterrupted ECG monitoring. In patients with a more complicated course, such as those with ongoing or recurrent ischaemia, development of acute heart failure or cardiogenic shock, and arrhythmias requiring an intervention such as temporary pacing, defibrillation or intravenous antiarrhythmics, monitoring should continue for 24 h after complications have resolved.

Cardiac monitoring is indicated for patients with Mobitz type II block, advanced (2:1 or higher) second-degree AV block, complete heart block or new-onset bundle-branch block in the setting of acute (especially anterior wall) myocardial infarction.

Q-T interval monitoring is an extremely important indication of cardiac monitoring. Q-T interval prolongation is associated with Torsade de Pointes which is often associated with sudden cardiac death.

Acute heart failure is a major risk factor for atrial and ventricular arrhythmias. Some therapies for heart failure, especially intravenous positive inotropic drugs including milrinone and dobutamine, have significant proarrhythmic properties.

Therefore, continuous monitoring is recommended for all patients until the signs and symptoms of acute heart failure have resolved and cardiac monitoring reveals no haemodynamically significant arrhythmias for at least 24 h.

Continuous cardiac monitoring is highly recommended in critical patients suffering from major trauma, shock, acute respiratory failure, sepsis, major noncardiac surgery (especially in older adult patients with a history of coronary artery disease or coronary risk factors), renal failure with electrolyte abnormalities (e.g. hyperkalaemia), acute pulmonary embolism, drug overdose (especially from known arrhythmogenics, e.g. digitalis, tricyclic antidepressants, phenothiazines, antiarrhythmics) and other illnesses admitted in intensive care unit. Supraventricular as well as life threatening ventricular arrhythmias are common in critically ill patients. Often these patients are on mechanical ventilators. Monitoring should be continued till these patients are weaned off from ventilator and are stable haemodynamically.

## 28.2 Types of Bedside Cardiac Monitoring

There are two types of bedside cardiac monitoring:

1. Hardwire monitoring (cable monitoring)
2. Telemetry (wireless monitoring)

### *28.2.1 Hardwire Bedside Cardiac Monitoring*

In this type of monitoring, electrodes are applied on the chest wall and these are attached to a bedside cardiac monitor by lead cable system. The cardiac monitor provides a continuous display of ECG and transmits the same to a console at the nurse's station. Both have alarms and can print rhythm strips. It is possible to monitor blood pressure, pulse oximetry in the commonly used cardiac monitors. The main disadvantage of hardwire monitoring is it limits the mobility of the patient. Hardwire monitoring is again of two types:

- Five leadwire system
- Three leadwire system

In five leadwire system, five electrodes and five leadwires are used. In cardiac monitoring, the electrodes from the extremities are shifted to the trunk to avoid artifacts due to movements and the patient can be handled well if the limbs are free. In this system (Fig. 28.1), one electrode is placed at each second intercostal space on right and left midclavicular line, one electrode is placed at each eighth intercostal space on left and right midclavicular line and one electrode is placed at chest lead position (leads V1–V6). In general, V1 is selected because of its value in arrhythmia monitoring. However the limitation of this system is lead V1 that is not very effective in S-T segment monitoring. Cardiac monitors with this lead system often have two

Fig. 28.1 Five leadwire system of hardwire monitoring

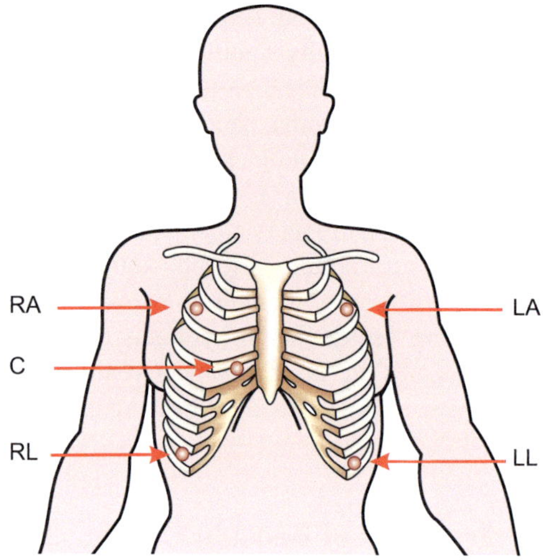


Fig. 28.2 Three leadwire system of hardwire monitoring

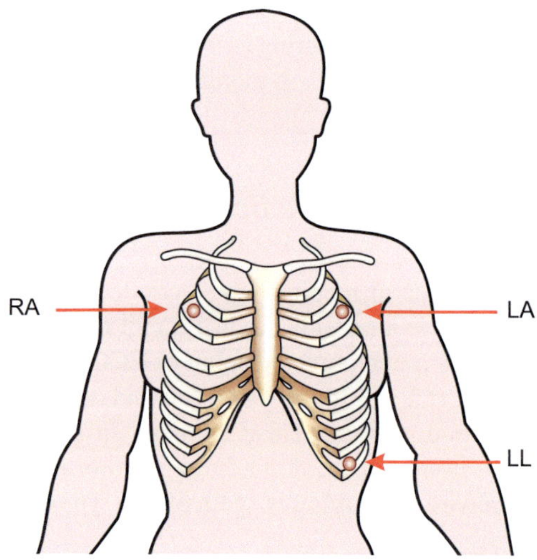


channels generally for ECG display so that one limb lead and one precordial lead can be displayed simultaneously.

In the five leadwire system, all the 12 leads can be monitored, but usually, either lead II or lead V1 is used for cardiac monitoring.

In three leadwire system, three electrodes and three leadwires are used for monitoring (Fig. 28.2). Here, one electrode is placed at right second intercostal space below the right clavicle at midclavicular line, second electrode is placed at left second intercostal space below the left clavicle at midclavicular line and the third electrode is placed at left eighth intercostal space at left midclavicular line.

In three leadwire system, lead I, lead II and lead III can be monitored by adjusting the lead selector on the cardiac monitor. The oldest and simplest of all cardiac

Fig. 28.3 Lead MCL1

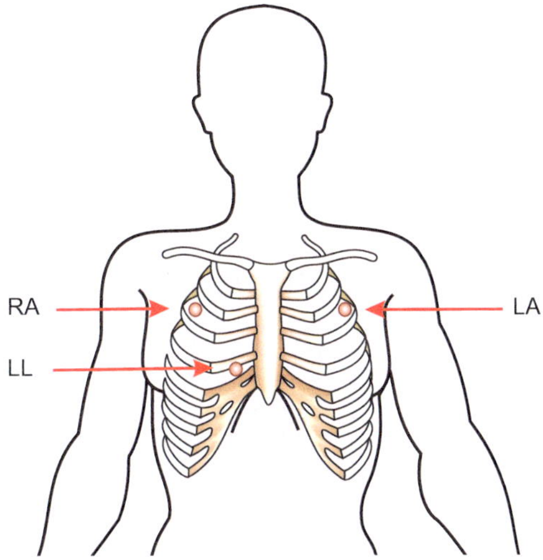


Fig. 28.4 Lead MCL6

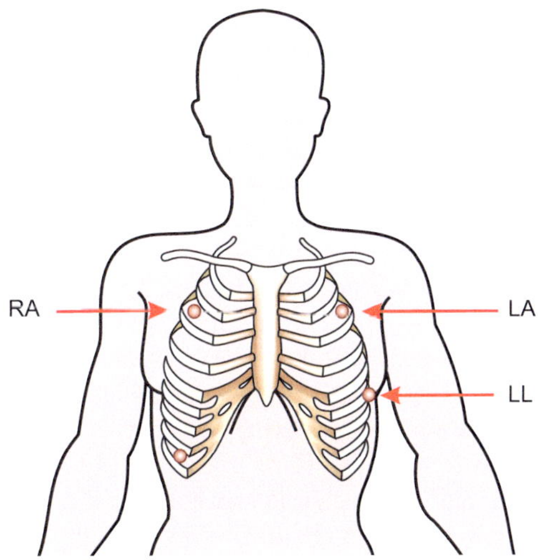


monitoring lead systems are bipolar leads. Usually, lead II is monitored. In this system one can also monitor the chest leads by a modification of the placement of leads which is called modified or Marriot's chest lead system. Bipolar lead system is very useful to track the heart rate, detect R waves for synchronized direct-current shock in electrocardioversion and detect ventricular fibrillation. It is however inadequate for sophisticated arrhythmia monitoring and S-T segment monitoring.

Modified chest lead V1 (MCL1) can be produced by shifting the left leg electrode (which is placed at left eighth intercostal space) to right fourth intercostal space by the side of the sternum (Fig. 28.3), and modified chest lead V6 (MCL6) can be produced by placing this electrode at fifth intercostal space at left midaxillary line (Fig. 28.4).

### 28.2.2 *Telemetry Monitoring*

Telemetry is wireless monitoring. It displays the patient's heart rhythm and electrical activity at a central nurses' station but may not display it at the patient's bed side. Telemetry uses a transmitter connected to the ambulatory patient instead of bedside monitor and sends signal to a remote place for display in a monitor. The transmitter is placed in a telemetry pouch. The patient is free to move around because of absence of cables. Besides this the patient is safely isolated from accidental electric shock occasionally seen in hardwire monitoring. Telemetry was introduced in hospitals during the 1960s to provide continuous cardiac monitoring in cardiac intensive care units. Over the last several decades, the use of telemetry has expanded beyond the ICU setting to non-critical care settings. Both three-wire and five-wire lead system can be used in this system. In telemetry system, many patients can be monitored at a time with the help of central monitor.

Cardiac monitors produce a printed record of cardiac rhythm and sound an alarm if the heart rate falls or exceeds a specified limit.

## 28.3 Setting Up of Cardiac Monitoring

Confirm the identity of the patient before starting the procedure. Check the hospital admission number along with name, age and sex of the patient. Full information about the procedure should be explained to the patient. The patient should be provided with privacy, and the patient is requested to expose his chest wall for attachment of electrodes.

After washing the hands, the chest wall should be cleaned and excess hair should be removed with a razor. Clean the area with alcohol and let it dry completely. It is important to check the lead system before applying the electrodes. After identifying the lead positions, pregelled electrodes should be placed and pressure should be applied for a proper fixing.

Once the ECG starts appearing in the monitor, check its quality carefully. If required use the gain control to adjust the size of the QRS complex. Verify the heart rate displayed in the monitor by carefully counting the radial pulse of the patient. After this the upper and lower limits of the heart rate alarm are set and the alarm is turned on.

For setting up telemetry, all the above mentioned steps need to be followed. However after attaching the electrodes the transmitter is placed in the telemetry pouch and the pouch strings are tied around the neck and waist of the patient.

In both hardwire monitoring and telemetry, take a print out of the rhythm strip, label it carefully and keep them inside the case sheet of the patient. All print outs taken should be carefully preserved with the medical record. Documentation is extremely important in all cases of cardiac monitoring.

## 28.4 Monitor Problems and Their Solution

Various types of problems may be seen during monitoring. Some problems are serious and may threaten life of the patient, whereas others may be simple and not life threatening.

1. Muscle tremor (artifacts)
   (a) Causes
      - Patient uncomfortable, tense or cold
      - 60-cycle interference
   (b) Correction
      - Ensure patient comfort. Provide a cover if room is cold. Encourage the patient to relax.
      - Ensure patient is not holding anything in their hand
      - Ensure feet are not touching the wall or foot board
2. 60-cycle interference (thick, unreadable baseline)
   (a) Causes
      - Ungrounded electrocardiograph
      - Ungrounded electrical outlet
      - Ungrounded equipment that is connected to same electrical outlet
   (b) Correction
      - Change electrical outlets
      - Remove excess electrical appliances from the room
      - Change electrocardiograph machine, if possible
3. Wandering baseline
   (a) Causes
      - Poor electrode contact
      - Cable pulling on electrodes
      - Cable moving with respirations due to respiratory distress
      - Patient restless
   (b) Correction
      - Check electrodes to ensure good contact
      - Check patient cable
      - Move cable off abdomen and guide under patient's arm to stabilize from moving
      - Encourage the patient to relax

4. No waveform

   (a) Causes

   - Disconnection of electrode
   - Dry electrode gel
   - Cable failure

   (b) Correction

   - At first, check the patient, then check and reconnect electrodes
   - Check and reapply electrode gel
   - Replace faulty wires or cable

5. False high rate alarm

   (a) Causes

   - False interpretation of tall T waves as QRS complex
   - Muscle tremor

   (b) Correction

   - Lead repositioning in which T wave is shorter than QRS complex

6. False low rate alarm

   (a) Causes

   - Low amplitude of QRS complex
   - Poor contact between the skin and the electrode

   (b) Correction

   - Increase gain
   - Reapply electrodes

7. Skin excoriation under the electrode

   (a) Causes

   - Prolonged skin contact with electrode
   - Allergy to electrode adhesive

   (b) Correction

   - Clean the site after removing the electrode and reapply new electrodes at a new site
   - Remove the electrodes and use hypoallergenic electrodes

If continuous low waveforms are recorded, then turn up the amplitude (gain) on the monitor or change the lead positions. If intermittent low voltage waveforms are recorded, then change the lead positions. High voltage waveforms are usually recorded due to movement of patient. Seizure may also lead to high voltage waveforms. Telemetry related interference can be corrected by changing the batteries. If there is false high alarm rate, set alarm limits according to the patient's heart rate.

However, it is most important to evaluate the patient before evaluating the monitor. Remember to treat the patient, not the monitor.

**Tips and Tricks**

- One of the most overlooked aspect of cardiac monitoring is loose contact between the skin and the electrodes due to sweating resulting in poor monitoring.
- Premature termination of cardiac monitoring should be avoided at all cost.
- With every alarm, patient should be assessed immediately and record should be maintained.
- If a patient is on permanent pacemaker, check that the pacing spikes are seen in the monitor.
- Patients diagnosed with dextrocardia will need to have the leads swapped to opposite side of the body.
- Do not forget to remove the electrodes once monitoring is over.
- If a patient on telemetry becomes unstable, he should be switched to continuous bedside cardiac monitoring.

**Self-Assessment Questions**

1. Bedside cardiac monitoring means continuous ECG monitoring of a patient's heart rhythm. True or False?
2. ECG electrodes are placed on specific areas of the body surface to capture electrical signals from the heart. True or False?
3. Bedside cardiac monitoring can provide information about the rate and regularity of the patient's cardiac rhythm. True or False?
4. ECG electrodes must be attached directly on the patient's skin for accurate monitoring. True or False?
5. Bedside cardiac monitoring cannot detect the presence of arrhythmias, such as atrial fibrillation, ventricular tachycardia or ventricular fibrillation. True or False?
6. Bedside cardiac monitoring can help identify the efficacy of certain cardiac medicines. True or False?
7. Prolonged Q-T interval on an ECG is associated with an increased risk of ventricular arrhythmias. True or False?
8. **What do you mean by the term telemetry in cardiac monitoring?**

    a. Monitoring the patient's respiratory rate at the patient's bedside
    b. Monitoring the patient's heart rhythm remotely from a central monitoring station
    c. Monitoring the patient's oxygen saturation at the patient's bedside
    d. Monitoring the patient's heart rhythm at the patient's bedside

9. **What is the purpose of ECG telemetry in a healthcare setting?**

    a. To monitor body temperature
    b. To monitor respiratory function
    c. To monitor cardiac rhythm and detect abnormalities
    d. To monitor blood glucose levels

10. **A wandering baseline artifact on an ECG tracing is most likely caused by:**
    a. Electrical interference
    b. Patient movement
    c. Loose electrode connections
    d. Ventricular fibrillation

11. **Which of the following leads is most commonly used for cardiac monitoring?**
    a. Lead V2 b. Lead aVL c. Lead V6 d. Lead II

12. **Which of the following is a potential problem with cardiac monitoring?**
    a. Poor electrode attachment
    b. Electrical interference
    c. No wave form
    d. All of the above

13. **What can be done to address the problem of poor electrode attachment in cardiac monitoring?**
    a. Adjust the gain settings on the monitor
    b. Change the patient's position
    c. Ensure proper skin preparation and reapply the electrodes
    d. None of the above

**Case Study**

Twenty rhythm strips are given below (Figs. 28.5, 28.6, 28.7, 28.8, 28.9, 28.10, 28.11, 28.12, 28.13, 28.14, 28.15, 28.16, 28.17, 28.18, 28.19, 28.20, 28.21, 28.22, 28.23 and 28.24), which were recorded during cardiac monitoring. Identify them and right your diagnosis.

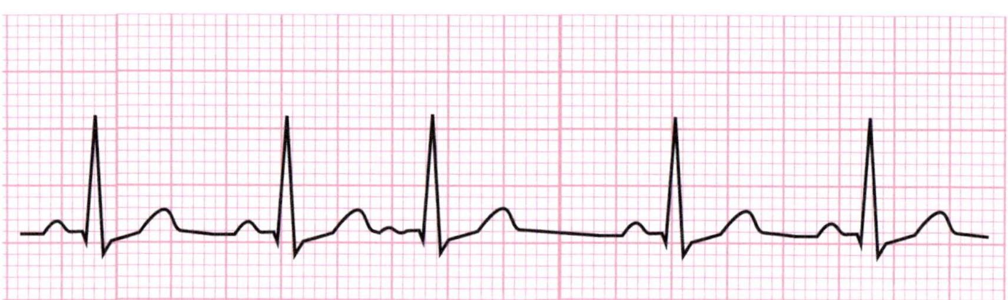

**Fig. 28.5** Identify the rhythm strip

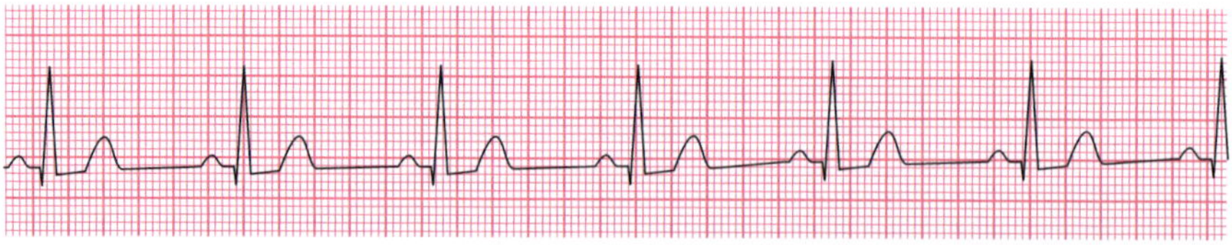

**Fig. 28.6** Identify the rhythm strip

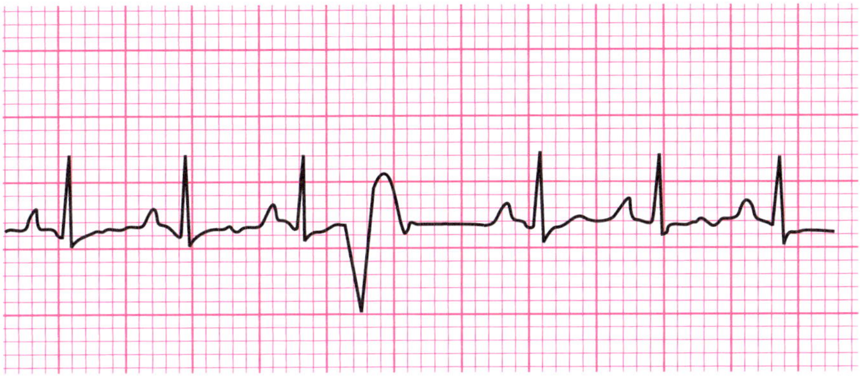

**Fig. 28.7** Identify the rhythm strip

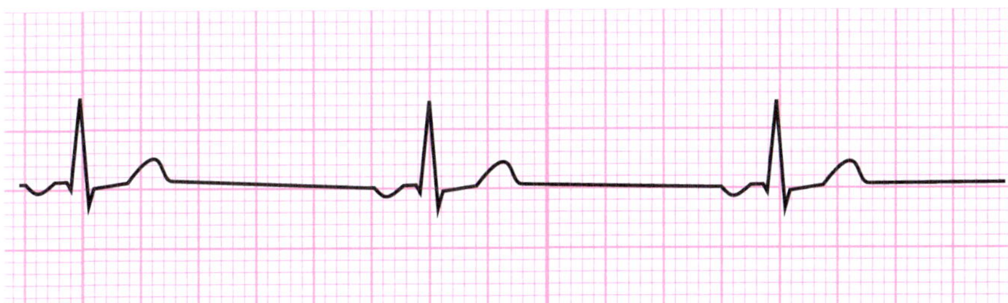

**Fig. 28.8** Identify the rhythm strip

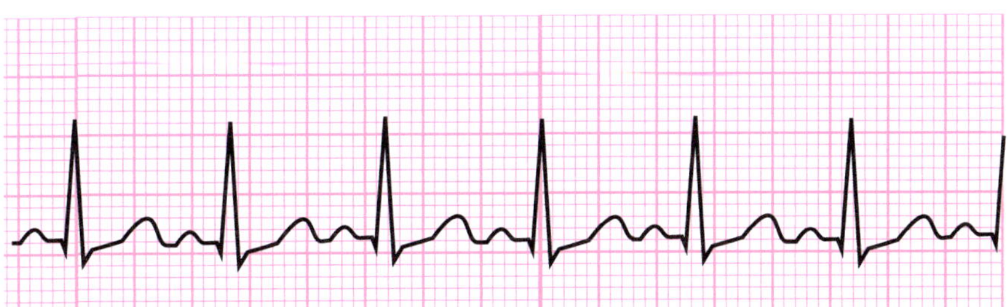

**Fig. 28.9** Identify the rhythm strip

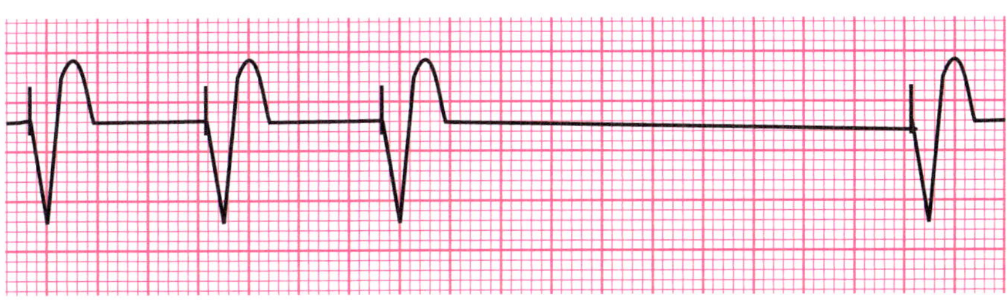

**Fig. 28.10** Identify the rhythm strip

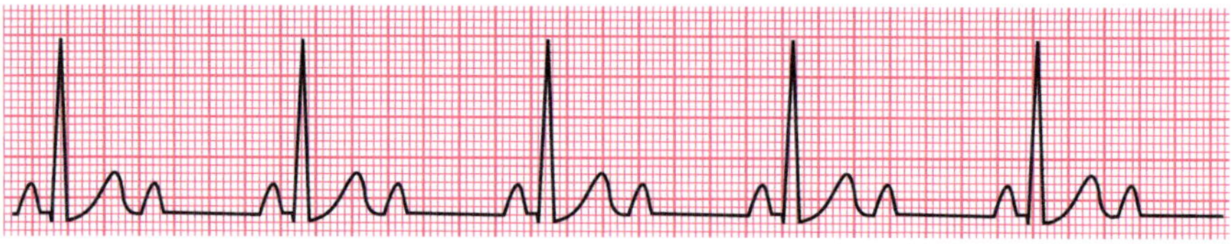

**Fig. 28.11** Identify the rhythm strip

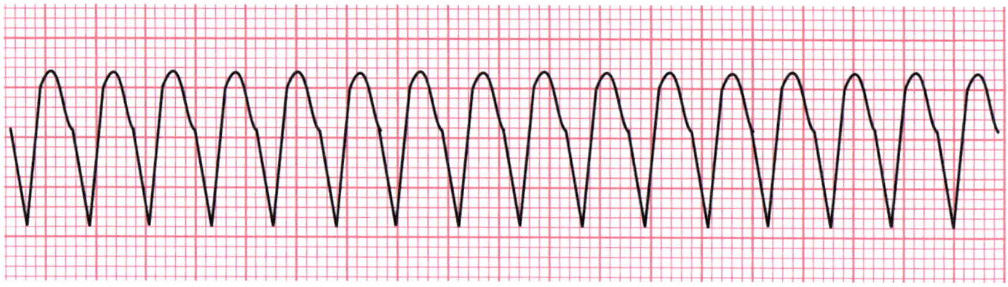

**Fig. 28.12** Identify the rhythm strip

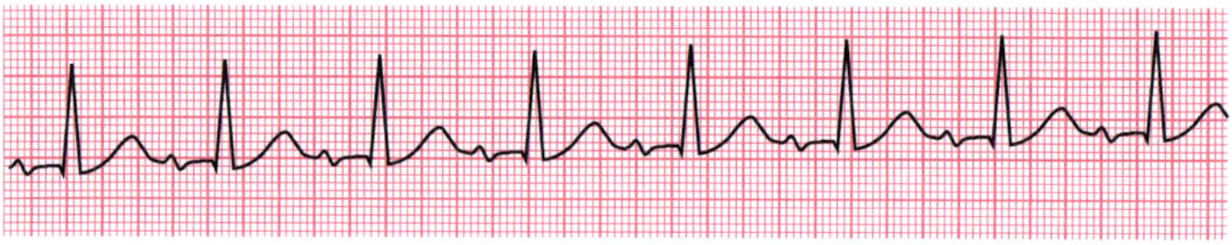

**Fig. 28.13** Identify the rhythm strip

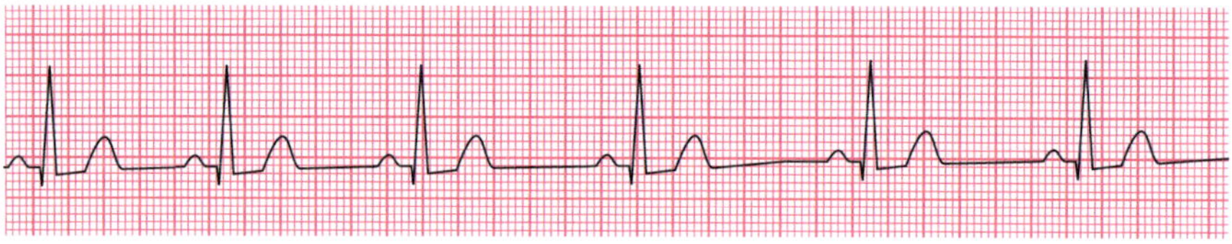

**Fig. 28.14** Identify the rhythm strip

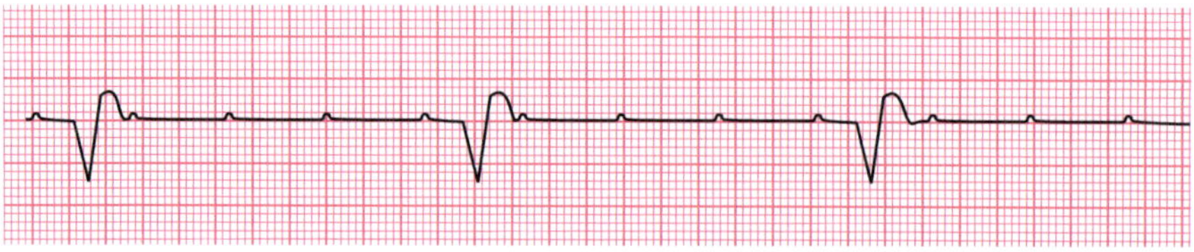

**Fig. 28.15** Identify the rhythm strip

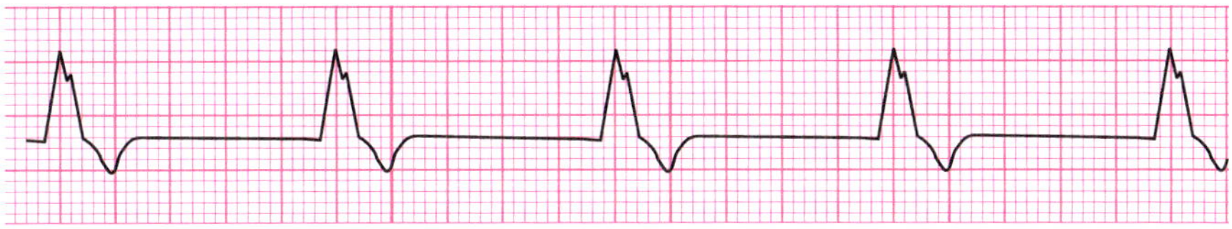

**Fig. 28.16** Identify the rhythm strip

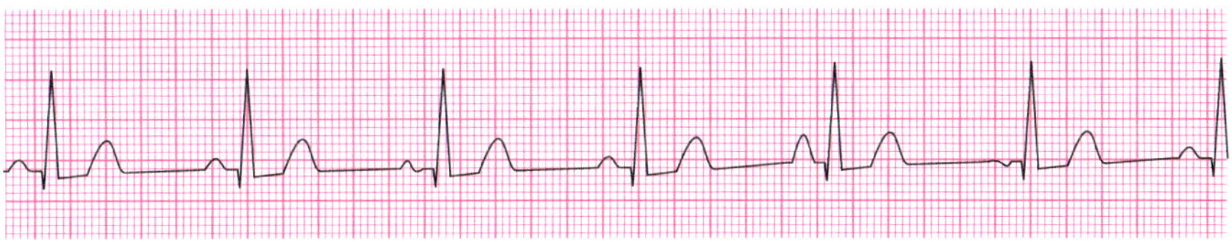

**Fig. 28.17** Identify the rhythm strip

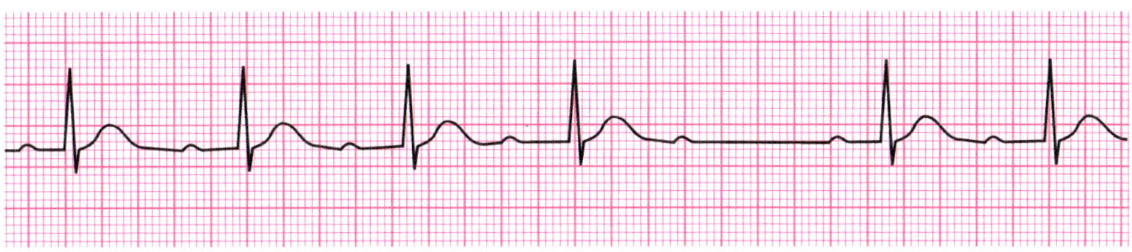

**Fig. 28.18** Identify the rhythm strip

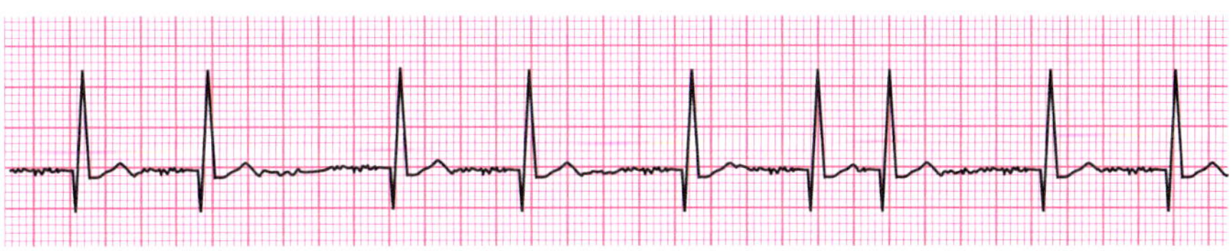

**Fig. 28.19** Identify the rhythm strip

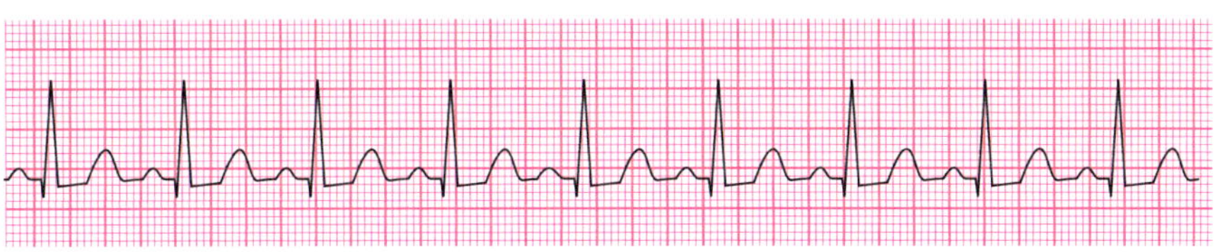

**Fig. 28.20** Identify the rhythm strip

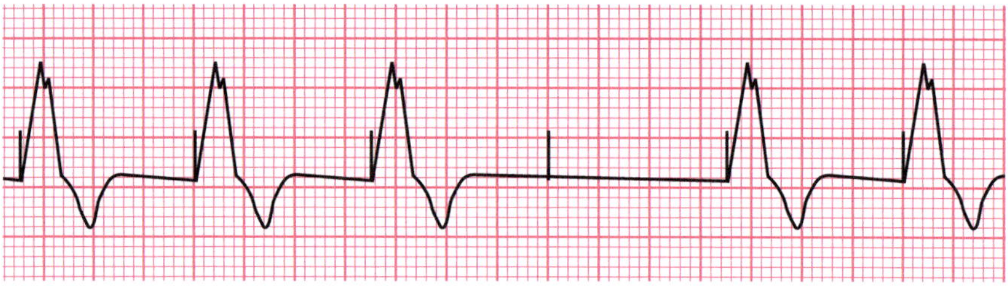

**Fig. 28.21** Identify the rhythm strip

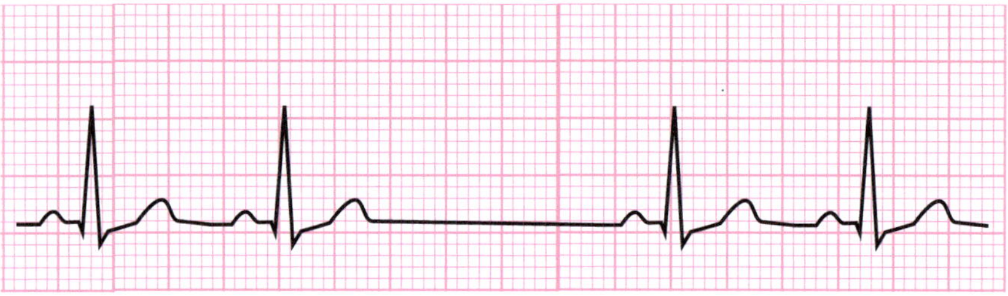

**Fig. 28.22** Identify the rhythm strip

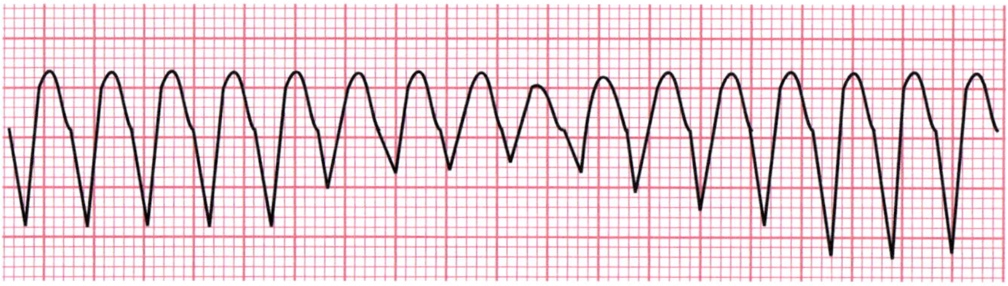

**Fig. 28.23** Identify the rhythm strip

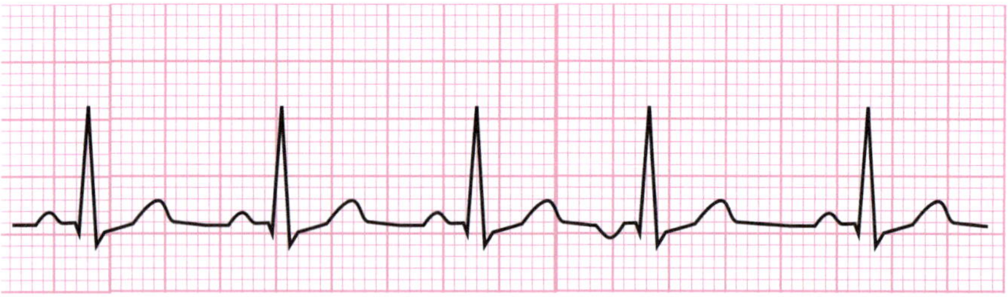

**Fig. 28.24** Identify the rhythm strip

**Answers**

1. True 2. True 3. True 4. True 5. False 6. True 7. True 8. b 9. c 10. c 11. d 12. d 13. c

**Case Studies**

The diagnosis of each rhythm strip is given below.

Figure 28.5: The rhythm strip shows PAC. The third PQRS complex is premature in timing. There is compensatory pause. The QRS complex is normal like the others. It is not wide. The P′ wave is different from the other P waves.

Figure 28.6: The rhythm strip shows sinus bradycardia. All the PQRS complexes are normal and regular. Heart rate is 55 bpm.

Figure 28.7: The rhythm strip shows VPC. The third QRS complex is wide, premature in timing and is followed by compensatory pause.

Figure 28.8: The rhythm strip shows junctional rhythm. The P waves of all the three PQRS complexes are inverted and the heart rate is 50 bpm.

Figure 28.9: The rhythm strip shows sinus tachycardia. All the PQRS complexes are normal and regular and the heart rate is 115 bpm.

Figure 28.10: The rhythm strip shows failure to pace. The pacing spike is visible before the first three and the last QRS complexes. In between there is a pause as the pacing spike as well as the QRS complexes are absent. The QRS complexes are wide.

Figure 28.11: The rhythm strip shows 2:1 AV block. The first P wave is followed by a normal QRS complex. The second P wave is there but the QRS complex is absent. This indicates that the impulse originated at the SA node but fails to pass on to the ventricles and as a result the ventricles are not activated. This sequence continues. For every two P waves, there is one QRS complex.

Figure 28.12: The rhythm strip shows VT. There are wide QRS complexes which are of ventricular origin and occurring at a rate more than 100 bpm. This is a wide complex tachycardia.

Figure 28.13: The rhythm strip shows first degree AV block. The P-R interval is 0.28 s in each complex and each P wave is followed by a normal QRS complex.

Figure 28.14: The rhythm strip shows sinus arrhythmia. The first three QRS complexes are occurring at a faster rate as compared to the last three. All the P waves are normal and every P wave is followed by a normal QRS complex. The R-R intervals are varying.

Figure 28.15: The rhythm strip shows complete heart block. There is complete AV dissociation. The atria are beating at their own pace and none of them is able to pass on to the ventricles. The ventricles are activated by a beat generated in the ventricle at a very slow rate. The P waves are marching through the rhythm strip.

Figure 28.16: The rhythm strip shows AIVR. Wide QRS complexes are occurring at a rate of 60 bpm. There are no P waves. This is also called slow VT.

Figure 28.17: The rhythm strip shows wandering atrial pacemaker. The third, fifth and sixth P waves are of different morphologies. Rest of the ECG is normal.

Figure 28.18: The rhythm strip shows Wenckebach phenomenon. There is progressive prolongation of P-R interval in first four PQRS complexes. This is followed by a P wave but it is not followed by QRS complex.

Figure 28.19: The rhythm strip shows AF. There are irregularly irregular narrow QRS complexes. The P waves are absent and they are replaced by fibrillatory waves.

Figure 28.20: The rhythm strip shows normal sinus rhythm. All the PQRS complexes are of normal morphology. Each P wave is smooth, rounded and upright indicating origin from SA node. Each P wave is followed by QRS complex. The heart rate is 83 bpm.

Figure 28.21: The rhythm strip shows failure to capture. The pacing spikes are followed by wide QRS complex in the first three complexes. After the fourth pacing spike, there is no QRS complex. The pacemaker has fired, but the ventricle is not activated. There is a pause as a result. The last two complexes are again preceded by the pacing spikes.

Figure 28.22: The rhythm strip shows SA block. An entire PQRS complex is missing after the first two PQRS complexes followed by resumption of normal rhythm.

Figure 28.23: The rhythm strip shows Torsades de Pointes. There is wide complex tachycardia with big amplitude complexes at the beginning and end of the rhythm strip and in between lies the small amplitude complexes.

Figure 28.24: The rhythm strip shows premature junctional complex. The P wave in the fourth PQRS complex is inverted. Rest of the P waves are upright, smooth and rounded and each P wave is followed by QRS complexes.

# Chapter 29
# ECG Reminders

In this chapter, short reminders are written which will help in refreshing knowledge of ECG at a glance. This chapter should be read only after going through all the previous chapters. This chapter is also useful at bedside of patient. If you suspect some abnormality in ECG like RBBB or RVH but fail to remember the characteristic ECG finding of RBBB or RVH, this chapter is going to be of immense help. Happy reading.

## 29.1 Cardiac Electrophysiology

- Willem Einthoven is considered the father of electrocardiography.
- The cardiac cell has a resting membrane potential of −90 mV.
- The resting membrane potential is mainly due to concentration gradient of potassium ions across the cell membrane.
- The action potential of cardiac cell starts with rapid inward diffusion of sodium ions.
- Depolarization starts with onset of action potential.
- Depolarization and repolarization propagate from one cell to another, resulting in generation of electric current which is recorded as ECG.
- SA node acts as the pacemaker of heart.
- The electric impulse generated at SA node passes via the conducting system of heart, i.e. internodal tracts, AV node, bundle of His, left and right bundle branch and Purkinje fibres.
- The maximum velocity of conduction of impulse is through the Purkinje fibres.
- The minimum speed of conduction of impulse is through the AV node.


T. K. Koley, *Rapid Review of ECG*,
https://doi.org/10.1007/978-981-99-9116-7_29

## 29.2 ECG Paper and Leads

- ECG paper is in the form of a grid, in which, small squares are 1 mm square and the large squares are 5 mm square.
- Horizontal axis represents time and the vertical axis represents voltage.
- 12 conventional leads (six frontal plane and six horizontal plane leads) are used to record ECG.
- Einthoven's equation → Lead II = Lead I + Lead III.
- Leads V1–V6 are oriented to the anterior wall of heart.
- Leads II, III and aVF are oriented to the inferior surface of the heart.
- Lead aVR is directed to cavity of the heart.
- Right-sided chest leads are used to record the electrical activity of the right ventricle.
- Standardization: 1 mV = 10 mm.

## 29.3 Normal ECG and Its Variants

- P wave is the first wave of the ECG. It is due to depolarization of both the atria.
- Ta or Tp wave is due to atrial repolarization.
- QRS complex is due to depolarization of both the ventricles.
- Q wave is the first negative deflection of the QS complex.
- R wave is the first positive deflection after Q wave.
- S wave is the first negative deflection after the R wave.
- T wave is due to ventricular repolarization.
- P wave is positive in lead II and negative in lead aVR. It indicates that impulse has originated from SA node.
- In lead aVR, all the waves are negative.
- The T wave generally follows the main deflection of the QRS complex in any lead.
- In chest leads, P wave may be positive, negative or biphasic in lead V1.
- In lead V1, rS complex is recorded, and in lead V6, qRs complex is recorded.
- There is progression of R wave amplitude and the transition zone is recorded in lead V3 or lead V4.
- In electrically vertical heart, QRS complexes in lead aVF and lead V6 are similar.
- In electrically horizontal heart, QRS complexes in lead aVL and lead V6 are similar.
- S-T segment is isoelectric.
- The normal P-R interval is 0.12–0.20 s.
- The normal QRS interval is less than 0.12 s.
- The normal range of Q-Tc is 0.35–0.44 s (men) or 0.45 s (women).
- Heart rate = 1500/R-R interval.
- In clockwise rotation, the transition zone is shifted to lead V5 or lead V6.

- In counterclockwise rotation, the transition zone is shifted to lead V1 or lead V2.
- In early repolarization syndrome, there is concave elevation of S-T segment.
- In persistent juvenile pattern, T waves are inverted in leads V1–V4.

## 29.4 Electrical Axis

- Electrical axis refers to the direction of the mean electrical vector. It is defined in frontal plane only.
- The normal QRS axis lies between −30° and +90°.
- In right axis deviation, the axis lies between +90° and +180°.
- In left axis deviation, the axis lies between −30° and −90°.

## 29.5 Chamber Enlargement

- Hypertrophy means thickening of muscular wall of a chamber of heart.
- Pressure and/or volume overload leads to hypertrophy.
- ECG is specific but not very sensitive for diagnosis of hypertrophy.
- Atrial hypertrophy/enlargement is mainly diagnosed by changes in P wave.
- Ventricular hypertrophy is mainly diagnosed by changes in QRS complex.
- *P. pulmonale* is seen in right atrial hypertrophy/enlargement.
- *P. mitrale* is seen in left atrial hypertrophy/enlargement.
- R:S ratio is more than one in lead V1 in RVH.
- SV1 + RV5 or RV6 is more than 35 mm in LVH.

## 29.6 Conduction Disturbance

- Conduction disturbance is an abnormality in the transmission of an electrical impulse through the normal conducting system of the heart.
- In SA block, the sinus impulse is blocked at the junction of SA node and atrial myocardium.
- SA block is characterized by pause due to complete absence of PQRS complexes.
- AV block is the disturbance in conduction of atrial impulse through the AV junction, i.e. the AV node, the bundle of His or His-Purkinje system. There are three degrees of AV block.
- First degree AV block is characterized by prolongation of P-R interval beyond 0.12 s.
- Mobitz type I (Wenckebach) second degree AV block is characterized by gradual prolongation of P-R interval followed by a blocked P wave, i.e. a P wave without the following QRS complex.

- Mobitz type II second degree AV block is characterized by blocked P waves (P waves that are not followed by QRS complexes) without any preceding prolongation of P-R interval.
- Complete AV block is characterized by independent beating of atria and ventricles (AV dissociation). The atrial rate is more than the ventricular rate and there is constant varying of P-R interval. Actually these are not true P-R intervals, but they help in identifying the degree of AV block.
- RBBB is characterized by rsR' pattern (rabbit ear pattern) in lead V1 with QRS duration more than 0.12 s.
- LBBB is characterized by wide and slurred QRS complex in lead V6 with QRS duration more than 0.12 s. There may be notch in QRS complex in lead V6 (M pattern).
- In LAHB, QRS axis lies beyond −45°. The duration of QRS complex is normal.
- In LPHB, the QRS axis is beyond +120°. The duration of QRS complex is normal.
- Bifascicular block is a combination of RBBB with either LAHB or LPHB.
- Trifascicular block is a combination of bifascicular block with first degree AV block.

## 29.7 Myocardial Ischaemia and Infarction

- Myocardial ischaemia occurs when adequate blood supply is not available to the myocardium to meet its requirement.
- The commonest cause of myocardial ischaemia is atherosclerosis.
- S-T segment depression and T wave inversion are the main ECG features of myocardial ischaemia.
- Three types of S-T segment depression: horizontal, upsloping and downsloping.
- Three zones of myocardial infarction: myocardial necrosis, myocardial injury and myocardial ischaemia.
- Myocardial necrosis is represented by pathological Q waves.
- The pathological Q wave is more than 0.04 s in duration and more than 4 mm in depth or more than 25% deep than the height of R wave.
- Myocardial ischaemia is represented by S-T segment depression.
- Myocardial injury is represented by T wave inversion.
- The characteristic ECG changes of anterior wall infarction are located in leads V1 to V6, lead I and lead aVL.
- The characteristic ECG changes of inferior wall infarction are located in leads II, III and aVF.
- The characteristic ECG changes of right ventricular infarction are located in right-sided chest leads.

## 29.8 Drugs and Electrolyte Disturbance

- Reverse check sign is seen in digitalis effect.
- Nonparoxysmal atrial tachycardia with variable AV block is characteristic of digitalis toxicity.
- Hypokalaemia precipitates digitalis toxicity.
- Tall, tented T wave is seen in hyperkalaemia
- Sine wave pattern is seen in severe hyperkalaemia.
- Prominent U waves are seen in hypokalaemia.
- Short Q-T interval is seen in hypercalcaemia.
- Prolongation of Q-T interval is seen in hypocalcaemia.

## 29.9 ECG in Miscellaneous Conditions

- P mitrale is seen in mitral stenosis.
- S-T segment elevation with upward concavity is seen in pericarditis.
- Electrical alternans is seen in pericardial effusion.
- rsR’ complex in lead V1 with right axis deviation is seen in ostium primum ASD.
- Delta wave and short P-R interval are characteristic of WPW syndrome.
- In dextrocardia P, QRS and T waves in aVL resemble that of aVR and vice versa.
- SI, QIII, TIII pattern is classically seen in acute pulmonary embolism.
- P pulmonale is seen in COPD with pulmonary hypertension.
- J wave is seen in hypothermia.

## 29.10 Pacemaker and Cardiac Monitoring

- There are two types of pacing: temporary and permanent.
- Pacemaker fires and produces a pacing spike.
- Wide QRS complex is produced by pacemaker.
- Failure to capture, oversensing and undersensing are important pacemaker problems.
- Hardwire monitoring and telemetry are the two types of cardiac monitoring.
- Lead II and lead V1 are commonly monitored continuously.
- Muscle tremor, wandering baseline, 60 cycle interference are important monitor problems.

MIX
Papier aus verantwortungsvollen Quellen
Paper from responsible sources
FSC® C105338

If you have any concerns about our products,
you can contact us on
**ProductSafety@springernature.com**

In case Publisher is established outside the EU,
the EU authorized representative is:
**Springer Nature Customer Service Center GmbH**
**Europaplatz 3, 69115 Heidelberg, Germany**

Printed by Libri Plureos GmbH
in Hamburg, Germany